Song of Haiti

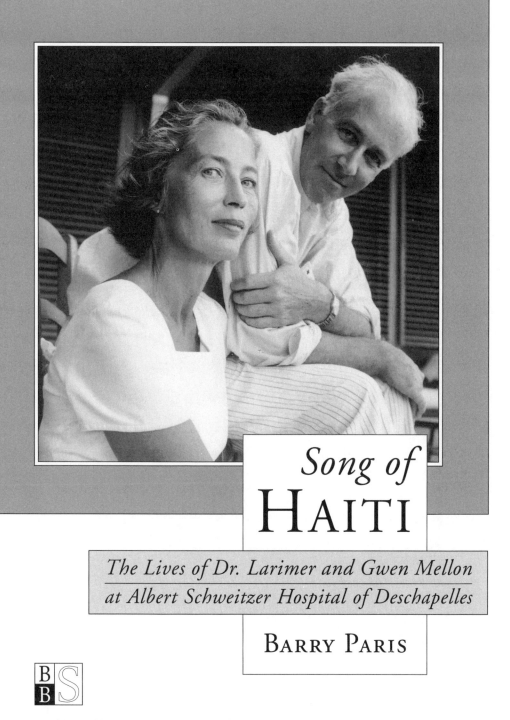

Song of
HAITI

The Lives of Dr. Larimer and Gwen Mellon
at Albert Schweitzer Hospital of Deschapelles

BARRY PARIS

PublicAffairs NEW YORK

Copyright © 2000 by Barry Paris.

Published in the United States by PublicAffairs™, a member of the Perseus Books Group.

All rights reserved.

Printed in the United States of America.

Book design by Jenny Dossin.

LIBRARY OF CONGRESS CATALOGING-IN-PUBLICATION DATA

Paris, Barry.

Song of Haiti: the lives of Dr. Larimer and Gwen Mellon at Albert Schweitzer Hospital of Deschapelles/by Barry Paris.—1st ed.

p. cm.

Includes bibliographical references and index.

ISBN 1-891620-13-4 (hc)

Mellon, William Larimer, 1910–1989.

Mellon, Gwen Grant.

Physicians—Haiti—Biography.

Hôpital Albert Schweitzer.

Medicine—Haiti—History.

I. Title.

R154.M53 P37 2000

610'.92'27294—dc21

99-046266

First Edition

10 9 8 7 6 5 4 3 2 1

Contents

For Wyoming Benjamin Paris III, William Larimer Mellon III, and all other restless mavericks with a burdensome III after their names.

IN POSTWAR PITTSBURGH, there was no way to avoid the name and pervasive presence of the Mellons. Pittsburgh steel had defeated Hitler, and Mellon money had financed the mills. Mellon Bank held the mortgage to our parents' homes. Mellon Institute was doing crucial research for Carnegie Tech (now Carnegie Mellon University) and developing a strange new thing called the computer. Mellon philanthropic funds subsidized a hundred other educational and cultural institutions in town. In history class, we studied Treasury Secretary Andrew Mellon's financial feats. His nephew Richard King Mellon was in our local news every day, spearheading the "Renaissance" to revive Pittsburgh and clean up its famously polluted air.

The one we never read about was William Larimer Mellon Jr.—the odd Mellon out, who had quit Pittsburgh and the banking business decades earlier to become a rancher out West and later devoted his life and his own portion of the family fortune to the poorest people in the hemisphere.

In 1954, while I was putting dimes in my Mellon savings account, Larimer Mellon, at the tender age of 45, was in his fourth year of medical school. As a kid, I vaguely recall, I heard something about "Dr. Mellon's" hospital project in Haiti. But I never thought any more about it until 1990, when I was in Port-au-Prince, doing a magazine piece on the miracle of Haitian art. "You're from Pittsburgh?" someone there asked. "Then you must know the Mellons' l'Hôpital Schweitzer in Deschapelles."

I didn't but soon would.

On my first visit to Deschapelles, when Gwen Grant Mellon and I were discussing a possible collaboration on this book, she asked what other projects I had in the works. I said I was just finishing the autobiography of Tony Curtis, co-written by him and me. I waited for her pro-or-con opinion of Curtis and his films. Silence. "Tony Curtis, the actor—*Some Like It Hot* . . . ," I prompted.

Mrs. Mellon didn't know the name. How could that be? She was quite knowledgeable about Garbo and other actors and films we talked about earlier. Suddenly it dawned on me that she had lived and worked in Haiti since the early 1950s: Her *au courant* film-going had ceased well before Curtis or *Some Like It Hot* hit it big. The ignorance was mine, not hers, but I had embarrassed her a little and hurried to change the subject.

There was no shortage of subjects. Several days later, for instance, recounting her medical training for me, she mentioned that she had dissected mosquitoes for an experimental syphilis-treatment program at Tulane University in New Orleans. I asked her to describe the process.

"Are you really interested?" she asked skeptically, not wanting to waste time if I were just humoring her. "If you are, I'll tell you. If you're not, I won't."

I assured her I really was. In eccentric childhood, I was an avid amateur entomologist, ornithologist, and philatelist, and in eccentric adulthood developed fascinations with irregular Ukrainian verbs, duck-billed platypi, and funeral-home thermometers. I truly wanted to hear about the mosquitoes.

Convinced of my sincerity, Gwen held forth in detail. She had been trained in malaria control and tropical entomology at Charity Hospital, which was then trying out induced-malaria therapy to treat mental illness resulting from syphilis. That new procedure tended to reduce syphilitic spirochetes in the brain, and helped in some cases. Gwen learned how to raise, feed, breed, infect, and anatomize anopheles mosquitoes—removing their heads, salivary glands, stomachs, and eggs under a dissection microscope at the rate of 40 mosquitoes an hour.

Her recap of this important medical experience was riveting. She clearly could have performed the exercise then and there, on the spot. I exclaimed something to the effect of, "What a specialized skill, and you still know how to do it!"

Pause. She looked out at the Cahos Mountains and then, glancing at me from profile position, closed the subject on a sardonic note:

"I may not know Tony Curtis, but I know a *few* things."

A MONG THE THINGS Gwen Mellon knows is how to overcome the obstacles to founding, building, and running, for 45 years, the greatest hospital in the poorest country of our hemisphere. It was her husband's idea, inspired by Albert Schweitzer. But the remarkable Dr. Larimer Mellon could never have accomplished it without her. They did it together, relatively late in life, after first knowing a few things about ranching and raising children and managing a fortune.

I could never have accomplished this book without her, or without the support of the Mellon and long-suffering Paris families, who put up with many demands and disappearances during my five trips to Haiti over six years. The full list of acknowledgments is included later. But special thanks must be given here to the most crucial folks in my literary life-support system.

The extended Mellon family: Michael Rawson, Jenifer Rawson Grant and Ron Noe, Ian and Lucy Rawson, LeGrand Mellon and Herb Sargent, Rachel Mellon Walton, Farley Walton Wetzel, Bill and Kathleen Simpson, Bill and Irene Dunn. Most of all, the late Paul Mellon, his brilliant assistant, Lisa Cox, and the anonymous "angel" who brought us together.

The Hôpital Schweitzer stalwarts in Deschapelles: Tim and Carol Dutton, Dr. Steve and Karen Williams, Dr. Dick Pantalone, Anny

Frédérique, Dr. Harold May, Dr. Michel Jean-Baptiste, Frédérique Pierre-Jules . . . and my beloved Melanj.

The Pittsburgh/New York stalwarts: Bill Bollendorf and Dr. Madeline Simasek, Maria Ciaccia, Daniel Strone, Peter Osnos, Lisa Kaufman, and Myrna, Merica, and Ben Paris.

The important thing is not that these people helped a writer with a book. It's that they opened up a whole country and a profound new experience for me, so that we could collectively open it up for the world. For that, I will always be indebted to them and, above all, to the noble people of Haiti.

BARRY PARIS

Pittsburgh, March 2000

Song of Haiti

IN THE BEGINNING, God created heaven and earth. Something like hell was created later by man, on a Caribbean island which heaven and earth had combined to make a tropical paradise before the Europeans arrived. By the time they withdrew, Haiti's native population was exterminated, its land exhausted, and its brutally imported Africans left to rot in poverty.

Haiti became the world's first black republic in 1804, but over the next 150 years, its economic misery remained unchanged. It was an easy place for North Americans to ignore, and the Mellon banking family of Pittsburgh was no different from any other. Mellons do not have to work, but the best of them always have. They worked at making money, brilliantly. One of them, however, would work for sick people in a remote part of the western hemisphere's poorest country, but its richest in spirit.

The Haitians have a Creole proverb: *Maladi gaté vayan.* "Illness spoils the most valiant."

Albert Schweitzer had a motto: "Help life where you find it."

Larry Mellon had a midlife identity crisis.

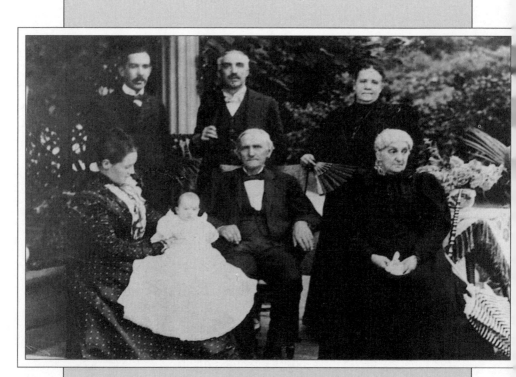

FOUR GENERATIONS OF MELLONS

Standing: William "Big Pa" Larimer Mellon, James Ross Mellon, Rachel H. Larimer; *seated:* Mary "May" Hill Taylor, Matthew "Matt" Taylor Mellon, Judge Thomas Mellon, Sarah Jane Negley.

CHAPTER 1

ANDANTE
Princes and Paupers

ILLIAM LARIMER MELLON JR. was heir to part of a great family fortune that then rivaled, and now dwarfs, that of the Rockefellers. "I was born in opulence," Larry would say. His branch of the clan was not ostentatious—few Mellons were or are—but "There were times when I felt ashamed to be from a family that was known only for wealth."[1]

His great-grandfather, Judge Tom Mellon (1813–1908), founded the family's banking empire, with assets valued at about $56 billion today. His brilliant grand-uncle, Andrew W. Mellon (1855–1937), developed the Aluminum Corporation of America (Alcoa) and served as secretary of the treasury under Presidents Harding, Coolidge, and Hoover. Larry's father, William Larimer "W. L." Mellon Sr., was cofounder and president of Gulf Oil Corporation, where Larry was expected to take his own rightful place one day.

"Idle rich" was an oxymoron in this family's lexicon. W. L. Sr. (1868–1949), unlike other such scions, had not been raised to loll about but to learn about, and actively advance, the whole spectrum of Mellon concerns. At age nine, W. L.'s assignment was to stand by the side of a turnpike in western Pennsylvania's Ligonier Valley to record the number and nature of horse-drawn commercial loads passing by, then relay that information to the Mellons' competitive haulers. Before and during his adolescence, it was also W. L.'s job to peddle the produce from his grandfather's estate—spring rhubarb, summer tomatoes, fall sweet corn. Nothing so delighted old Judge Mellon, the grandson said years later, as "the sight of me, the donkey and the produce-laden wagon, setting off for some market I had found for myself, most likely down on [Pittsburgh's] Penn Avenue."[2]

At fifteen, W. L. spent the first of several hot, buggy summers in Bismarck, N.D., helping plow a thousand acres of winter wheat with no more technical assistance than a team of oxen. Two years later, in 1885, he mastered and installed a tricky new thing called electricity in his grandfather's house, no mean feat for a seventeen-year-old. His additional areas of expertise came to include coal, steel, railroads, lumber, and, above all, oil.

Until the late 1890s, notes one Mellon chronicler, David Koskoff, "oil country" meant western Pennsylvania, "where pure green oil literally oozed from the rocks and stream beds." Long before the riches beneath Texas and Oklahoma were known, America's oil-rush epicenter was the Keystone State, home to such boomtowns as Petrolia, Wellsville, and Oil City, and nobody was more adept than W. L. Mellon at persuading dubious farmers to lease drilling rights on their land. If oil were struck, the farmer got a one-eighth share of the profits; if not, the Mellons took the loss.[3]

W. L.'s wells more often hit than missed. He made a great deal of money for his family from exploration and drilling, but there the profit stopped to his annoyance. The price he and other wildcatters got for their crude oil was dictated by Standard Oil Co., the one (and virtually only) big buyer, in control of most pipelines and refineries. John D. Rockefeller's monopoly would soon come in for a challenge from W. L. Mellon, twenty-three, who steered his family's operation through the creation of its own small but effective pipeline, 200 railroad tank-car force, and refinery. By 1895, the Mellons were sufficiently serious competitors to be disposed of the way shrewd entrepreneurs like best: Standard Oil bought them out.[4]

They didn't stay out for long. New Mellon oil interests, including J. M. Guffey Petroleum, were gradually obtained and, in 1907, reorganized into an expanded corporate entity called the Gulf Oil Company.

A. W. Mellon was president, soon succeeded by W. L., who ran it with fabulous profitability for the next four decades.

His family's enterprises embraced Alcoa, Union Trust and Mellon National Bank, Koppers, Standard Steel Car, Monongahela River Consolidated Coal & Coke Co., Pittsburgh Coal, and Mellon Securities, plus assorted utility companies and huge tracts of real estate—combined resources of enormous industrial power and importance to America. But the single biggest element of the empire was Gulf Oil, and W. L. Mellon was the one who built it.

"It is very hard for me to be patient with incompetents," W. L. once said, yet by all accounts he was kind and generous. A contemporary reporter called him "pleasant personally, but not particularly stimulating and with no distinguishing traits to lift him above the average."[5]

Not so, his wife.

Mary "May" Taylor Mellon was the daughter of a Scottish civil engineer who worked throughout the British Isles surveying railroads and, in America, was a bookkeeper and manual laborer, laying asphalt side-

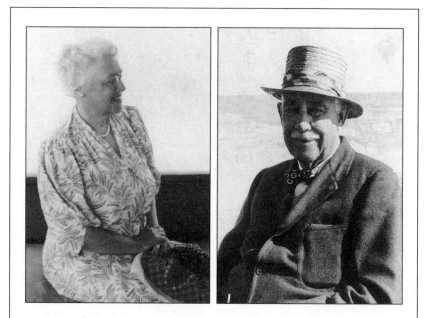

MARY "MAY" TAYLOR MELLON AND WILLIAM L. MELLON SR.

walks in Brooklyn, before his eventual success in a Wall Street brokerage firm. Matthew Taylor shared his eccentric devotions to astronomy, poetry, botany, magic, and especially music with his children. May emerged with the most sensitive refinement. She loathed any display of wealth, declining even to wear jewelry, and evidenced a wit largely lacking in her in-laws.

In 1896, May Taylor and W. L. Mellon were married in Florida, and a trainload of Mellons showed up for the event. As they disembarked, W. L. identified them for his bride by their beloved initials: "There's T. A., that's A. W. . . . " and so on. According to family legend, when ancient Grandma Sarah Jane, Judge Tom's wife, stepped down onto the platform, May could not resist asking W. L., "Who is that—B. C.?"[6]

Once married, May Taylor Mellon ("M. T.," a posthumous trust fund would list her) shunned society and devoted herself to family, Presbyterian church activities, and music. She bore W. L. four children: Matthew in 1897, Rachel in 1899, and Peggy in 1901—the three they had planned—plus William Larimer Jr., "Larry," the surprise, who debuted June 26, 1910, nearly a decade later.

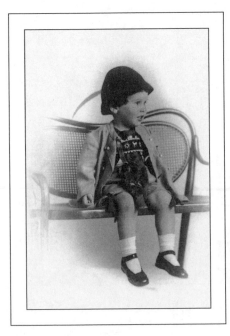

"BABY LARIMER" IN 1913

His mother said that "when she first came to Pittsburgh, it was a great hardship to be among the Mellons," Larry told a family biographer, Burton Hersh. "She meant they weren't very 'couth' people [and] didn't have the kind of manners her mother and father had." He remembered his grandfather, James Ross "J. R." Mellon, once asking him, "Do you ever covet anything?" Larry couldn't come up with anything. "I only covet one thing," said J. R., "whenever I pass a big pile o' manure."

"That's how they were," Larry concluded. "They spoke like farmers." May didn't like it, "but she was loyal, she'd signed up. Father told me once, 'I've been lucky, my wife never interfered in my affairs. I couldn't have taken that.'"[7]

Larry called his mother "the great spiritual force in my life"[8] and identified with her alienation more than any of his siblings did. "To be thrust into a pompous atmosphere was difficult for her," said Larry, who had the same difficulty. "I felt more at home with chambermaids than with my own group. Wealth really can't work for you. Either you get a cockeyed notion of your own importance or you get an inferiority complex. I guess [the latter] is what I had. Once I got the idea that dollars were foolish, the people chasing them seemed foolish."[9]

There was no shortage of chambermaids or dollar-chasers at Ben Elm, the family manse in Pittsburgh's tree-sheltered Squirrel Hill section. That huge homestead bustled with life. The Mellons' more idyllic residence was in Beaumaris, Ontario, where "Big Pa"—as W. L.'s children called him—owned Squirrel Island on beautiful Lake Muskoka, plus the smaller Blueberry Island and a portion of the mainland, all of it perfect for summer fishing and fall hunting. As the family grew, so did its boat fleet for excursions to the upper lake and picnics on Blueberry Island (whence everyone always returned with blue teeth).[10] W. L. and the older children were vacationing in Beaumaris in 1910 while May was delivering in Pittsburgh. It was a jubilant day when she arrived to unveil baby Larimer and join them for the rest of the summer.

Back at Ben Elm, the Mellon children adapted to their nurses and governesses and the rigorous ways their father structured their lives. Most of every Sabbath, for example, was spent in Sunday school. "There was no escape," said Larry's brother, Matthew. "We were locked in closets and spanked with hairbrushes when we offended the code, yet we knew intuitively that our parents loved us and were doing it all for our good, which reminds me of an old hymn we sang down at the Presbyterian Church: 'Trust and obey, there's no other way.'"[11]

W. L. was a busy and important man, imbued with more money-making than parenting skills. Old Judge Tom might have had his grandson in mind when he wrote late in life: "As a general rule parents, especially such as are in easy circumstances or engaged in extensive enterprises, hold their children at too great a distance from them."[12]

Big Pa was an aloof and austere father. But May's warm, caring nature provided the balance. As her father had done with her, she imbued her own children with humanist compassion and a deep feeling for the arts.

"Larry used to tell me about being on the family yacht as a little boy, which he really didn't like much, except when his mother would cradle him in her arms and sing to him," says Bill Dunn, a close friend of later years, "or when he was lulled to sleep by the crew members' singing belowdecks at night. Those were precious times for him, and the source of his love of music."*[13]

May was also the source of Larry's gentleness and sense of responsibility to help others. Larry called her "a pacifist, anything to avoid a row" and remembered her putting in long hours at the Home for Crippled Children and the Women's Exchange.

"Their relationship was very affectionate," says his sister Rachel, ten years older, who celebrated her 100th birthday in 1999. "Mother became ill after she had Larimer, but she just adored him. She would have her breakfast in bed, Larry would get in, and she'd give him little 'birdie bites' of toast. She was just crazy about him."

Rachel remembered their mother as constantly bedridden:

We always traveled with a nurse and never knew exactly what her illness was. She never complained, but she had such awful pain and went to so many different doctors. I went to New York with her to a hospital where they thought it was cancer and operated, but it did no

---

*By contrast, the only music his father ever expressed a fondness for was a banjo record called "Chicken Charlie."

good. Then we went to Philadelphia and they operated again. Finally, another Philadelphia doctor said it was a certain nerve in her back. He practiced on animals for months, examining all the nerves in their spines until he found the right one, cut it a little and found that it deadened the animal's leg.

It was very scary. If there had been one slip, she might never have walked again. But Mother was desperate. We all were. So she had this procedure, and he told her, "Be careful, because you won't have much feeling—don't lean against a radiator." But he found the right nerve. It was the first time that had ever been done, and it worked.[14]

By that time, May's beloved baby was a feisty adolescent. At twelve, Larry loathed the dance classes he was forced to attend, especially the preparations when "Mother would straighten out my jacket and jam the stiff collar into my neck. I wasn't too faithful to dancing school. I used to escape by the fire escape which, at the bottom, had about a ten-foot drop to the street."

At Pittsburgh's Shady Side Academy, he once asked a girl to meet him by a pond. When she said another boy had asked her first, Larry plotted to ruin his rival. On a school typewriter, he and a friend pecked out a note to the girl's parents full of scurrilous reasons why the other boy was not to be trusted with their daughter. Of course the authorship was discovered (the typewriter had a telltale broken key), and Larry and his pal were both expelled for a week.

"I always felt kind of sorry for Larry as a boy," Rachel said, "because Father was in the process of retiring then and didn't seem to have much time for him. He and Mother had a yacht, the *Vagabondia*, in Florida and went down there every year. Sometimes they'd take us, but often Larry would have to stay home for school, and I'd be home too because I was the older one *out* of school and wasn't married yet. We'd be the only two left behind [unless] Mother would call and say, 'Bring Larry down for Easter.' Then we'd come, and on the steamer Larry and Matthew would hide awful things in my stateroom, maybe dangle a crab over my bed. They had fun with me."[15]

For Big Pa, the highlight of nautical life in Florida was deep-sea fish-

ing and harpooning the occasional sting ray. The Mellons also loved
side-trip river cruises to explore the tidelands and to blast alligators at
will. "It was," Matthew wrote, "a wonderful world of unrestricted
slaughter without a thought to disturb our consciences. The oil wells
were gushing over in Texas, and we could keep every penny they made
because nasty things like income taxes had not yet been thought of and
capitalist was a proud name, and not, as now, a dirty word."[16]

Now and then, a moment of excitement leavened the leisure, such as
the time a wave washed the *Vagabondia's* corpulent cook overboard in
shark-infested waters on a 1926 cruise to Venezuela. A lifeboat reached
the cook just ahead of a shark. Otherwise, Larry spent most of his ship-
board time that trip studying Spanish. His gift for languages was remarkable. He learned French from his Swiss governess. At Choate, the
exclusive boarding school in Wallingford, Connecticut, he picked up
Portuguese from a Brazilian friend. In adulthood, he added Russian,
Arabic, Hebrew, Greek, and Creole to his linguistic arsenal—all self-
taught or privately tutored, similar to the way he mastered an amazing
variety of musical instruments. Larry always learned and fared better on
his own than in a formal classroom situation.

"He could play any instrument he picked up," recalled George Lockhardt, a lifelong friend, and later financial handler, who roomed with
him for two years at Choate. "Our room was on the third floor of a
building near the chapel, and Larry liked to sit out on the roof there,
strumming his guitar."[17] Newt Chapin, another good friend from
Choate, says his interests were almost exclusively in music: "He be-
longed to the orchestra, the jazz band, the [concert] band, and the
banjo club. He often strolled around with his ukelele, playing and
singing 'Mon Bleu Heaven.'"

Choate's 1928 yearbook reveals that Larry, at seventeen, was five feet
nine inches tall and weighed 145 pounds. The maxim beneath his graduation picture is: "Beware the fury of a patient man." That seems to have
had its origin in a campus musicale at which Larry was playing bass viol:
a string broke, provoking a major tantrum. "He busted up his bass,
made it into matchwood," says Chapin. "He had a bad temper then."[18]

Evidently, both the fiddle and the fiddler were a little high-strung. As a private person rather than performing *artiste*, Larry was moody, Chapin remembers, but also "charming, with a wonderful mind and great charisma. Everybody liked him. He had the most winning smile and personality when you and he were getting along. But if he took a dislike to someone, he could be very arbitrary."[19]

He could also be unlawful, in nonobservance of Prohibition. The Mellons were not heavy drinkers, but they regularly enjoyed a cocktail or two in the evening and, like millions of other Americans, would not be deprived by the 19th Amendment. At their separate prep schools, both Larry and a cousin Ned Mellon, rigged up stills. According to Ned, Larry's operation was the better of the two—until tragically terminated by an explosion.[20]

With or without moonshine, W. L. Mellon Jr. was not a happy preppie, as another, perhaps symbolic, incident suggests: One day, fooling around outdoors instead of studying, he threw a rope over a high tree branch and almost accidentally hanged himself before managing to pull up and out of the noose. Another time, he impulsively decided to chuck Choate and took off, AWOL, for home. He got to Pittsburgh fine that night, but Big Pa issued a stern reprimand, spun him around and sped him back to Connecticut the next morning.*

All in all, Larimer finished prep school feeling as ambivalent as when he began. He tried to put his finger on it in an introspective little essay, "Farewell to Choate":

Now that there's but a single week of school left, the thought of part-ing does grow a bit harder. Perhaps the old sixth Former who described to me the lump of affection which swelled his throat dur-ing the last week of his school days wasn't just lying after all. I [have] turned out to be one of those persons who either like a thing or dis-

---

*This was rather hypocritical on the part of Mellon *père*. His own father, James Ross ("J. R.") Mellon, had sent W. L. to the Pennsylvania Military Academy in Chester, PA, from which "he had the good sense to run away after a short exposure," his son Matthew observed. Nobody forced W. L. to go back.

like a thing. There's no halfway in anything with me. [But] what is my feeling for Choate? I can't seem to decide. God knows I've had my troubles here . . . I never minded being on "pro" [probation], nor did I mind paying for the windows I smashed. What I did mind was having to row in a shell all afternoon. Athletics—God, how I hate them. . . . In spite of all that, I might have cultivated a real love for this place if it hadn't been for that damned chapel every evening with its clanking bells. Still, the old place [has] been my home for five years and there's something I do love about it anyway. Maybe it's just the fields. I don't know. Perhaps I shall someday.

The course had been charted for Larry Mellon, who had little to say in the matter. He was now accepted into Princeton. It was assumed he would enter the banking business or join one of the companies Mellon Bank owned, the thought of which depressed him. "In those days," he said, "everyone wanted to be a bond salesman and belong to the right clubs. That was the limit of their ambition." His own ambitions were, in fact, nonexistent. Certainly, he exhibited no special interest in medicine or the Caribbean, except as a family playground aboard the *Vagabondia*. The Mellons did not always go ashore on their tropical cruises and seldom mixed with the natives when they did. Least of all were they curious about the natives on western Hispaniola, citizens of the first and poorest black republic in the world.

·   ·   ·

IN THE HAITIAN CAPITAL OF PORT-AU-PRINCE, the most exciting time of year is *Ra-Ra,* a wild pre-Mardi Gras festival when the streets are filled with noisy parades of young celebrants, many dressed as Haiti's aboriginal Arawak Indians in pink feathers and long white hemp braids, brandishing homemade bows and arrows as they sing and dance through the city.*[21]

*In colonial times, just before Lent, plantation owners allowed their slaves to leave—supervised by whip-wielding bosses—for visits to other plantations near and far, with much dancing and music-making along the way. It was the nearest thing to a "vacation" slaves ever

Haiti's friendly, docile Arawaks were mostly slaughtered by the Spanish crews of Christopher Columbus, who "discovered" that unfortunate island on December 6, 1492. The surviving natives had been polished off by disease and brutal servitude when France took possession of western Hispaniola in 1697 and stepped up the importation of slaves from Benin, the Congo, Dahomey, and Guinea in staggering numbers. African forced labor would make the colony fabulously profitable through the eighteenth century.

Such was French greed at its peak that, by 1791, there were 500,000 slaves in Haiti, eleven blacks for every European. The situation was ripe for insurrection and a long, bloody independence struggle led by the great freedom fighter, Toussaint L'Ouverture. Despite concerted international efforts to suppress it, history's first successful slave revolt finally triumphed in 1804 under Jean-Jacques Dessalines and was secured by Henri Christophe. The latter renamed himself King Henri I (his daughters became Princess Athénaire and Princess Améthyste), but royally failed to improve the lot of his subjects.

Certainly, he got no help from the young United States of America, which repaid the favor of French help in its own revolution by joining France's furious effort to quash Haiti's. The American government, moreover, was opposed to the thought—let alone reality—of a nearby black republic. Fearing similar slave revolts, the United States refused to recognize Haiti until 1862, when the island struck Abraham Lincoln as a potential dumping-ground for freed slaves. Liberia was recognized the same year for much the same reason.[22]

Racked by poverty, internal power struggles, black-mulatto racial strife, and disputes with neighboring Santo Domingo nineteenth-century Haiti was bankrupt by the twentieth and had no choice but to accept a U.S. Customs receivership forced upon it in 1905. Direct American rule began in 1915 after Haitian President Vilbrun Sam had his heart torn out by an angry mob—an act that sufficiently appalled

---

got, but its purpose was hardly humane. The masters' motive was to mix and strengthen the gene pool for next year's crop of slave babies. The name *Ra-Ra* comes from a Creole corruption of the legal maxim, *Le roi ha dit,* "The king has said."

Woodrow Wilson to send in American marines to occupy the country and calm its political tumult. Haiti's parliament was disbanded for refusing to accept a new U.S. corporate-designed constitution. U.S. troops organized a plebiscite in which that constitution was ratified by a 99.9 percent majority (of the 5 percent of Haitians who voted).[23]

The marines were commanded, and Haiti ruled, by fierce Gen. Smedley Butler throughout the "Cacos War" of 1918–1922, a long and hopeless guerrilla struggle against Yankee occupation.

However brutal and self-serving, U.S. military domination of Haiti brought relative stability to the hemisphere's most densely populated nation and was regarded by whites as a humanitarian mission. The marines and the few Americans back home who cared were shocked by Haiti's squalor and even more repelled by its superstitious religion, voodoo, mocked and misunderstood in North America and Europe.

Contrary to frightened foreign impressions and Hollywood depictions, Haitian voodoo wasn't and isn't concerned with sticking pins in dolls to destroy enemies, but rather with a lofty set of beliefs in African spirits called *loas*, who can be summoned when needed and who rule daily life as well as death. Among voodoo's phenomena is the belief in zombies—"work-slaves"—raised up from their tombs by *houngauns*, the voodoo priests. Many Haitians live better dead than alive: Relatives often spend a year's income to erect huge, heavy tombstones over their loved ones' graves to prevent them from being dug up and turned into zombies. Sometimes the deceased are seated at tables with cigarettes or food and allowed to decompose a bit before burial so they will be less appealing candidates for zombification.

But voodoo and its magic permeate life more often in light-hearted than in morbid ways, as in Africa, whence Haitian culture springs. Dr. Albert Schweitzer provided a fine illustration from his medical mission in Gabon:

There was a lumberman with a glass eye who had supervision over many local workers. One day he had to leave for a week and when he returned, he discovered his office and compound in utter confusion.

When he had to leave again, he took out his glass eye and put it on his desk. He told his workers, "I shall be watching you while I am gone." Sure enough, when he returned, everything was in perfect order. However, the next time, when he tried that trick, utter confusion. What had happened? Why had the eye failed? One of the workers had taken the lumberman's hat and put it over the glass eye. He had discovered what we already knew, that in Africa, every magic has a countermagic.[24]

Haitian voodoo is "Africa reblended": the spiritual practices of Congo, Dahomey, and Yorubaland merged with Christian beliefs and the social turbulence of the New World. It is less a religion than a pervasive way of life, cleverly grafted onto French Catholicism and Caribbean conditions. Its earthy mysticism is as impenetrable to the outside world today as it was to the French colonials. Voodoo was the only thing that couldn't be beaten or stolen from the slaves over the centuries.

The restlessness of slave and Arawak spirits is palpable in today's Haitians, especially at *Ra-Ra* time, as they revel, with a tinge of anger, in the full-moon shadows of breadfruit trees descended from those brought by Capt. Cook from the South Seas. Ancient yearnings and injustices remain.

Not until Franklin Roosevelt's administration in 1934 was Haiti's government restored to the Haitians, but during and after that decade of Depression, the country slid further downhill. Deeper poverty brought deeper political corruption and deeper cynicism among the peasantry. It was also a time of economic crisis in the United States, of course. There, nobody in or out of Larimer Mellon's family was worried about Haiti.

.   .   .

JUST SHY OF HIS 19TH BIRTHDAY, Larry self-published a thin volume called *Tales, Verses, and Essays* through the Princeton Press. He had no illusions about its literary quality and said so in his foreword: "Herein is to be found the writing of a schoolboy during a period of six long monotonous years—five spent at Choate and one at Princeton. Although the faults in the earlier compositions especially are both obvious and numerous, the work has been left entirely untouched and unsupplemented. [This collection] has been published purely out of vanity, the desire to display in print the fruit of my literary labors."

The tales were humorous parables, precocious juvenilia. Best of them was "Pipa de Arcilla":

Even before I was old enough to be able to enjoy her, still there seemed to be a bond between us, which . . . I can in no wise account for. But am I to blame for not knowing the roots of the matter? For not understanding the lure which she always had for me, for being so jealous at seeing her with another man, for being willing to throw aside my honor and good reputation when she but got near enough to intoxicate me with the aroma of her warm breath? . . .

My father had adopted her immediately upon the death of his best friend . . . I shall never forget the day she came to live with us: I was 9½ years old. How wonderful we all thought it that father should consent to take her into his keeping . . . As we came rushing out to meet her, he lifted her high into the air for us all to admire. Mother was the least enthusiastic over the new arrival . . . I now have reason to believe that she hated her from the very moment when she first saw her. But in spite of this hate, oddly enough, we lived peacefully together for years. It was not until I had reached my fifteenth birthday that the discovery was made . . .

On this festive occasion, what violent passion seized me! . . . My brain suddenly overflowed with lustful and licentious thoughts which centered about this legal addition to our household. I determined to put her to the use for which she was made, and satisfy myself with her once and for all . . . I waited impatiently until I was quite sure no one was stirring, until it seemed as if everyone *must* be asleep.

Then it was that I crept noiselessly toward the room—her room, purposing in my heart to conquer her unsuspecting and defenseless . . . I crept on until I reached the very doorway of her room, then softly I turned the knob and gently pushed the door open wide enough to allow myself a full view of her as she lay there motionless with not so much as a single cover to conceal her smooth curves from the downy moonbeams. . . . In another moment, I had entered, closed and locked the door behind me, and tiptoed over to where she lay. Even as I pressed my feverish lips to hers, she appeared to sleep on, or be impassive to my invasion. . . . But wait!—did not I hear mother step outside the door? . . . Oh, God! What was I to do? She would find out everything.

Then her voice rang out sharply from behind the door, "*Lirro, tu estás fumando addentro?*" [Larry, are you smoking in there?] It was all over. . . . In English, this little clay pipe loses all her feminine charm and becomes nothing more than a cold, neuter *it*. . . . As soon as I had unlocked the door, Mother ran in and seized her. Now her fingers closed tight around her neck. Then, she dashed her to the hearth. As I looked sorrowfully down, I saw there at my feet father's *pipa de arcilla* smashed to a thousand bits.

His poetry included three sonnets, an "Invocation to Venus" (translated from Lucretius' *De Rerum Natura*), and miscellaneous amusing doggerel, such as:

On New Year's Eve in '28—
I never shall forget that date—
Not only 'cause we stayed up late
But after quite a long debate
On why she shouldn't hesitate
My brain has tried to cogitate
On what could make it fluctuate
Much more than when I osculate . . .

Later, the teenaged poet put a more melancholy meditation into a more polished verse titled "Life":

Confucius has ended his lecture;
The heathen were crowding the door
But yet one decrepit old female

Still mirrored the prayer-holey floor.
As soon as the audience vanished
She hastened her steps to his side
To finally reach the conclusion
Her own feeble brain had denied.
Croaked she, "What's this life that we're living?"
Oh genius that gasped not for breath,
Thou answered as true as man's knowledge:
"That predicament preceding death."

Larry's essays contained no more or less wisdom than could be expected of any late adolescent but there were samples of his wry humor. "On Babies" addressed the way grown males approached infants: "If the man be young, he will walk on his hands and knees, growl like a bear, stand on his head, or possibly resort to tossing the child high into the air and catching it just as it is about to strike the ground—any one of which is most alarming to the baby and serves only to terrorize it to the *bawling point*. (Apologies to the reader, young mothers, and pharmaceutical technicians.)"

In "Popular Fallacy," he ruminated on punctuality:

The United States of America would be better off if she had never entered the [first] world war at all, and a gentleman would avoid ever so much embarrassment by simply not going to a banquet in lieu of presenting himself tardy. . . . Likewise, cutting chapel at Choate and [hoping to be] overlooked is far wiser than entering after the service has begun, which is as good as confessing one's sin before the entire congregation. This should be published [nationally] to eradicate the popular fallacy "BETTER LATE THAN NEVER."

His final essay, "On Beauty," was deeply serious:

No sooner are we born upon this earth, where evolution is proclaimed material creator and God proclaimed master of intellects, than we become aware . . . that we are living in an atmosphere of mystery and that we are by no means able to find out the "truth" of even the most familiar matter. . . .

Let us consider the wide range of beauty that we receive through the eye alone. Probably the earliest form is scenic beauty . . . [Other beauty] comes to us through the ear. Since the world was first created, there has been the dismal drum of dreary rain, the roar of angry waves, the echoing voice of thunder and the shrill whistle of midnight wind. Wordsworth speaks of his delight in streams as "beauty born of murmuring sound." And who is there who has not been aware of beauty in a loving voice? . . . Next to the human voice in expressing sentiment comes the violin. . . .

Beauty is inherent in nature; realized through man, and explained through God.

Larry was reunited at Princeton with his Choate friend Newt Chapin, who remembers Larry describing his brief time there as "a fi-

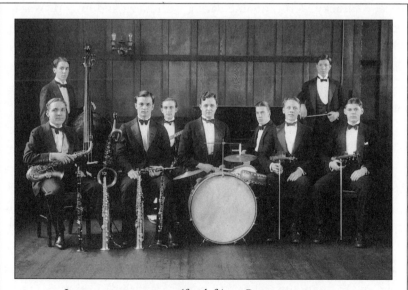

LARRY ON THE BASS *(far left)* IN PRINCETON BAND

asco." Seventy years later, Chapin disagreed: "A year that produced this little book should not be called a fiasco."[25]

Larimer Mellon was a reflective renegade, a sensitive misfit, no better suited to college than prep school. One year in the Ivy League was enough. "I didn't know what I wanted," he said years later, "but I knew I wouldn't get it at Princeton."

.   .   .

RETREATING TO PITTSBURGH, he spent much of his time courting a girl named Grace Rowley. "She seemed very inappropriate to my family," he said, not least because her father was a maker of artificial limbs. Her relatives lived beneath the smoke of the steel mills. Her whole milieu was the diametric, and romantic, opposite of his own: "To me it was an attraction. I used to help the old man make rubber feet down in the cellar. I could have seen myself doing that a lot sooner than working for Gulf. . . . Wealth, social position—to me, it was just one more snare."[26]

The stock market had just crashed, but so what? The Mellons and their fiscally sound empire were not severely affected. Larry took Grace to the Kentucky Derby, double-dating with Newt and his girl. Was it a crime to have some fun? To savor the conjugal joys? In late 1929, they slipped away to Wellsburg, West Virginia, and without telling anyone, got married. The groom was nineteen, the bride a bit younger. They rented a bungalow and lived together clandestinely for nearly a year before Larry finally persuaded his parents to approve their "engagement."

There was, and still is, no bigger social news in Pittsburgh than a Mellon marriage. A grand society wedding was announced for November 1930 and much publicized in Pittsburgh's half dozen daily papers. Arrangements had progressed to the eve of the rehearsal dinner, seventy-two hours before the event, when word reached a certain Wellsburg magistrate who had previously married the currently betrothed.

"That was terrible," recalls Larry's sister Rachel. "All the plans were made. People were sending presents. But then the man who married them saw the announcement and said, 'If you don't give me so much money, I'm going to tell the papers.' Blackmail from a justice of the peace! Father would never fall for that, of course."[27]

Indeed, Big Pa was not intimidated, just *furious*—at the son more than the blackmailer. Larry felt he had done nothing wrong but, to everyone's embarrassment, W. L. abruptly canceled the wedding, uninvited all guests, including Secretary of the Treasury Andrew Mellon, who was en route, and ordered every gift to be returned. It didn't bode well for the non-newlyweds. The marriage continued but did not flourish, even after the birth of their son Billy—William Larimer Mellon III—in 1932.

"It seemed to me that what Grace really wanted was things for her home," Larry told author Burton Hersh. "She engaged an interior decorator to do over a small house Father had bought for us in Sewickley. He designed a table with a very thick top which had to be especially cast at Pittsburgh Plate Glass and cost a good many thousand dollars. Highly stylized kinds of pictures kept arriving, big bills. I got less and less enthusiastic—the very thing I was trying to escape was just what Grace was trying to cling to."[28] His sister Rachel recalls how mortified Larry was by his wife's extravagance and the need "to go to stores and tell them not to accept her credit."

Grace liked the social circuit as much as Larry didn't. "How I hated those parties," he said. "I came to despise that jaded group of remit-

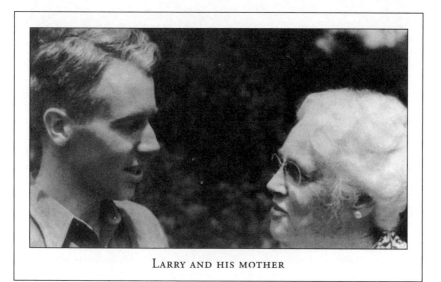

LARRY AND HIS MOTHER

tance people who lived on trust accounts. I felt a man should try to do something on his own, be a professional baseball player or a carpenter, it didn't matter what. Nobody has much respect for a kept woman and neither should they for a kept man."[29]

Larimer had reluctantly joined the family enterprises, first trying out the banking side and then apprenticing with his father at Gulf. Under W. L.'s brilliant direction, Gulf rebounded from a $23 million deficit in 1931 to a $10.5 million profit in 1935. It became and remained the Mellons' single biggest asset for the next half century, thanks to their cofinancing and exploitation of vast new crude oil discoveries in the Indian Territory, the later state of Oklahoma—"Pennsylvania quality in Texas quantities," said W. L.—and to the rights retained by Gulf in 1927 on the fabulous deposits beneath Kuwait.

Larry began at the bottom rung of that gilded corporate ladder, as a glorified errand boy for his father. "I rather liked that," he said. "I got to carry a lunch."[30] After six months, Big Pa promoted him to the sales department, where he worked for two or three gloomy years. ("I'm any-

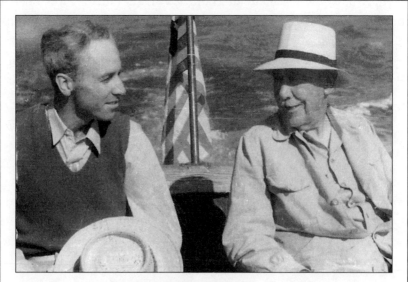

LARIMER MELLON JR. AND SR.

thing but a salesman," he reflected.[31]) It was a time when Pittsburgh was itself gloomy. Nearly a third of its children died before age five, and the death rate of miners from tuberculosis and black lung was alarming. So thick was the mill smoke that city streetlights came on at noon. Larry found it deeply depressing. His one enduring legacy at the Mellons' oil company was to design with Thomas "Buddy" Evans the famous orange Gulf sign. But his only really happy times then were spent in his pickup truck or on his horse, Goldy, getting as far away as he could from Pittsburgh, and from Grace.

An overpowering need to escape confinement—of his job, his white collar, his marriage, Pittsburgh—prompted Larry to take his horse and himself to Arizona, not for a vacation but for permanent relocation. It was the outdoors he loved and longed for. Lots of American boys dream of becoming cowboys. He was one of the few in a financial position to fulfill the fantasy, and he did so, says friend Bill Dunn, "in keeping with the pattern of a man who was out of step with his contemporaries but who was a purist in doing things by the book, whether the book was tax law or his own principles."

When Larry announced his decision to move West and become a rancher, Big Pa said he should have his head examined. "Father was disappointed because Matthew had flaked out, too," Larry recalled.* Even so, W. L. Sr. would rise above his disapproval and give W. L. Jr. a pragmatic suggestion: Go talk to the head of Gulf's geophysical department, one Dr. Foot.

"Dr. Foot pulled down a big map of Pecos County, Texas," Larry recalled, "and told me, 'If I were a young man, this is [where] I would start out.' . . . He was trying to tell me there was so much oil in that section that if I bought three acres there I'd soon be rich enough to buy up the state of Arizona, if I still wanted it."[32]

The young man thanked him politely and ignored the advice. There were no gushers in Larry Mellon's cards, just the firm intention to load

---

*Matthew Mellon (1897–1983), Larimer's older brother, likewise abandoned his father's corporate world to become a kind of freelance intellectual and writer, living much of his life in Germany. His early public enthusiasm for the Nazi regime would much embarrass the family.

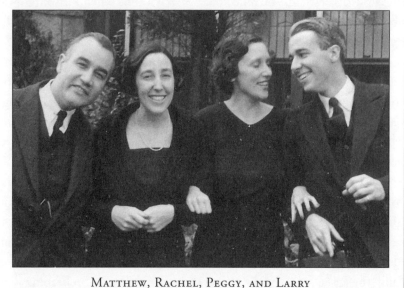

MATTHEW, RACHEL, PEGGY, AND LARRY

up Goldy into a trailer hitch, set out for the Southwest, and do things HIS way.

The first vistas were less than alluring.

"All I could see was baking clay and derricks and a few skinny old longhorns just standin' there, lookin' at the sludge comin' up," he said. "So I kept going."[33] Big Pa had offered to send an agent ahead to buy cattle in Mexico, but Larry declined that assistance, too. He found a proper cattle ranch that suited him, in Arizona, on his own.

There, the Mellon-heir loner now became a dawn-to-dusk working cowboy. He built fences, rode herd, did his own branding, and learned to wield a blacksmith's hammer. He lived simply in what his horrified sister Peggy called a "one-peg shack." Soon, in partnership with his father, he bought another thousand head of cattle and a 110,000-acre ranch at Fort Rock. That venture turned a $25,000 profit by 1938, prompting Big Pa's facetious complaint about losing a tax deduction he'd counted on.

Larry Mellon's marriage was over before he left Pittsburgh. Grace never joined him out West, and he supported her from afar. Eventually, she filed for divorce on the grounds of desertion. When Big Pa learned of it, he summoned Grace and gave her a check and a warning: "I don't want you ever to bother my son again." By all accounts, she never did.

.   .   .

LARIMER MELLON'S FIRST RESIDENCE in Arizona was little more than a chuck wagon. Soon enough, it would graduate to a bunk house and later to comfortable ranch homes in Oak Creek Canyon and Rimrock. But from the start, he loved the new life he was forging. Although he knew nothing about the theory let alone the practice of cattle ranching at first, he learned fast. His ability to pick up new skills quickly and to enjoy long hours of hard work aided him then and for the rest of his life. One day as he and a hired hand, Bill Jones, were riding into a sand-storm, Jones shook his head and asked, "How did we ever get into this goddamn business?" "I don't know," Larry replied, "but look at the fun were having!"[34]

Oddly but typically enough, he was serious.

To augment income, Larry took on the job of fattening and dehorn-ing a large herd owned by a rancher in Mexico, where grazing range was meager. "We dehorned the entire thousand head, blood all over the place," Larry remembered. "It rained that summer, and pretty soon the animals were covered with blowflies, and after that, we spent most of our time chasing them around so we could doctor them."[35]

It was a rugged, gritty life, but it was the one he had been seeking and the one that brought him a measure of satisfaction and tranquility for the first time.

World politics, on the other hand, were far from tranquil and fast de-teriorating as the decade drew to its close. In 1940, the Nazis overran Holland, Belgium, and France. In early 1941, Larry received word of his mother's decline and went east immediately, spending an emotional week with her in Florida. It was their last reunion. On March 18, 1941, soon after his visit, May Mellon's long battle with cancer ended. She died aboard the family yacht in Miami Bay.

Though America was not yet a belligerent in the European war, Larry had been seriously contemplating enlistment for undercover work, holding off only because he knew it would upset his mother—who thought espionage was contemptible. ("Son," she told him more than once, "I know you would never stoop to becoming a spy."[36]) Saddened but released by her death, he now signed up for duty with the Office of Strategic Services (OSS), forerunner of the Central Intelligence Agency. His proficiency with languages in general, and Portuguese in particular, was a valuable counterintelligence tool possessed by few Americans at the time. He was ordered to report immediately to spy school outside of Washington, D.C.

There was more comedy than secrecy in his first assignment, which involved a cryptic set of instructions for getting to the school itself: He was to appear at the corner of Eighth and L Streets, where a car would pull up and the driver would say, "Are you waiting for Mr. X?" Larry was to say yes, get in, and not reveal his real identity under any circumstances. He found the corner all right. The car pulled up according to plan. But instead of inquiring about Mr. X, the man at the wheel exclaimed, "Mr. Larimer! What are you doing here?" This particular OSS driver had been the W. L. Mellon family's beloved chauffeur in Pittsburgh for years.

Thereafter, his training began in earnest. One frequent exercise was escaping from a certain place or situation without detection. Another was building a lean-to with nothing more than a small pile of wood, some nails and a saw to work with. His carpentry skills were fine and the task no great challenge except for the fact that, as he was assembling his shed, a "helper" kept hitting him in the back of the head with lumber. Larry retained his usual calm and got battered around a lot before catching on that the guy was there specifically to annoy him. The object was to weed out the hotheads. Larry Mellon was decidedly cool.

More significant was Mellon's instruction in the political and economic skullduggery inside Portugal, whose neutrality made it a haven for international spies and a staging ground for all manner of "Casablanca"-style intrigues throughout the war. For fascists and democrats alike, few things were more important than oil. The Allies were disturbed by reports that Venezuelan ships were stopping in the course of trans-Atlantic oil transports and refueling Nazi submarines at sea—in which case, they would arrive in Europe with less than a full load. Larry's job was to observe oil tankers in Lisbon harbor, estimate how much fuel they were carrying, then find out and inform the Allied command where they were headed next.

He carried out those and other undercover tasks for the next two and a half years, working with such colleagues as Allen Dulles and William Casey* in Spain, Portugal, and France, spying on enemy ships and escorting important refugees and informants in and out of belligerent territory. Mellon's fluent French, Portuguese, and Spanish were highly useful in hustling Underground agents or rescued Allied fliers across the French-Basque border at night.

It was "nothing spectacular," he said. "You expected to get killed if you were caught behind the lines, but you understood that."[37] He never told war stories and was "really irritated" years later, his sister Rachel said, "about that book by the girl who was some kind of spy and said he made love to her."

The offending tome was *The Spy Wore Red* and "the girl" author was Aline Griffith Romanelli, who claimed to have been recruited for cloak-and-dagger work by Mellon. Her hinted romance with Larry is unlikely, but her book suggests a real knowledge of OSS operations in Portugal. The following breathless passage, to be taken with many grains of salt, paints a man of James Bond-like proportions:

> Larry Mellon warmly shook my hand [and I] followed him to an upper deck [of their airplane]. Larry and the general sat across from a fellow who was introduced as Bill Casey . . . The general explained [our circuitous flight]: "The route is changed for extra precaution. The Germans attack everything crossing the Atlantic. Not long ago, they downed a plane from Lisbon with [actor] Leslie Howard aboard. . . .
>
> Lisbon lay below. It was as if we were arriving at a gigantic party in

---

*Both Allen Dulles, the brother of John Foster Dulles, Dwight Eisenhower's secretary of state, and Casey were future directors of the CIA.

full swing. [On the ground,] jabbering Portuguese in long red-tailed woolen caps transported us to the dock.

"Look!" Larry Mellon pointed to some rowboats nearby. "The Japanese. Their intelligence center operates out of Lisbon and Madrid.

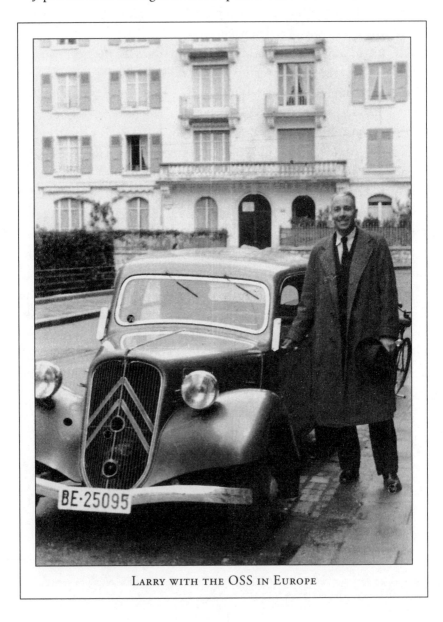

LARRY WITH THE OSS IN EUROPE

When a Pan Am Clipper crashed a month ago, the Japs were cruising the wreckage before anyone could get to the scene, picking up pouches destined for Allied embassies, leaving wounded passengers to drown while salvaging top-secret documents. Beware. Under Lisbon's frivolity lurks a city of deadly intrigue. . . . Can you change into evening clothes in 20 minutes? I must go to the casino, and you should see it too."[38]

It didn't sound like anything that could ever come out of Larry Mellon's mouth, but Griffith presses on:

Inside, the scene was breathtaking, because of the sheer scale of its opulence. . . . Larry pointed to the Japanese milling about. . . . "They're contacting agents here in the casino, picking up messages transmitted by the numbers played at the roulette table—right under our noses." . . .

We wandered through the game rooms for a while, Mellon scanning the faces. Then he guided me down a wide corridor to the WonderBar [nightclub]. At midnight the crowd was at its peak and every table was taken; the floor was filled with couples moving to the music of a rumba band. . . .

Suddenly the piercing shriek of a woman resounded through the wide corridor. In an instant the scene before us became a bedlam of people running. Larry sprinted ahead, and I followed. . . . A crowd was gathering around something on the red-carpeted floor. I stared down at the crumpled body of a man lying facedown. . . . A knife protruded from the center of the man's black dinner jacket! . . .

Kneeling down, Larry felt the man's pulse while the crowd pushed and shoved to get a better look. [I saw] that Larry recognized [him]. Straightening, Mellon braced his hands on my shoulders and pivoted me around, propelling me . . . through the crowded hall toward the entrance.

"Is he dead?"

"Very much so."

"Do you know him?"

"Of course not. Come on, we can't get involved."

"How can we not get involved? Won't we be questioned?"

"Aline, where do you think we are? Wake up—this is Lisbon. The only thing anybody in there cares about is getting rid of the body so they can get back to the tables."[39]

The next day, according to Griffith, Mellon led her into a Lisbon cellar where ten men sat in a circle, engulfed in cigarette smoke. She claims that Casey was one of them and that Larry went to the center of the circle to address them:

> "The news stinks," Mellon announced in his slow drawl. "The head of one of our [saboteur units] was captured and our transmitter reports the Krauts began the torture by pulling out his fingernails one by one." . . . .
>
> "How about our agent bumped off last night in the casino?" asked a skinny young American seated next to me.
>
> "Forget that incident," Mellon advised sharply.[40]

Griffith's melodramatic reportage is hardly reliable, but the bold use of Mellon's and other OSS agents' actual names when they were still alive, plus such details as Larry's "slow drawl," indicate she indeed knew him. Larry acknowledged as much to his friend Art Bergner, long after, describing Griffith as "a knockout" with such a creative imagination that her book should be classified as fiction.*

A less colorful but more certifiable OSS mission of Larry's at the end of the war was the assignment to unearth Benito Mussolini's diary. After much searching, he located the Duce's daughter, but she had sold it. Eventually, he tracked down the new owner and bought back the dicta-

---

*Griffith subsequently married a European aristocrat and became "Countess Romanelli," an international jet-setter. She and Larry Mellon had a final encounter decades later at a fund-raising dinner where they were seated together on the dais, laughing and having a good time, while Larry's wife sat below with her dull dinner companion in pique. "Do you think she's jealous?" Aline asked cattily at one point. "I hope so," was Larry's reply.

tor's journal for $10,000. It turned out to contain nothing more signifi-
cant or fascinating than his dentist and barber appointments.

Upon discharge in 1945, Larry returned to Arizona. It was time to get
back to ranch life—and to the woman who would be his match in every
way.

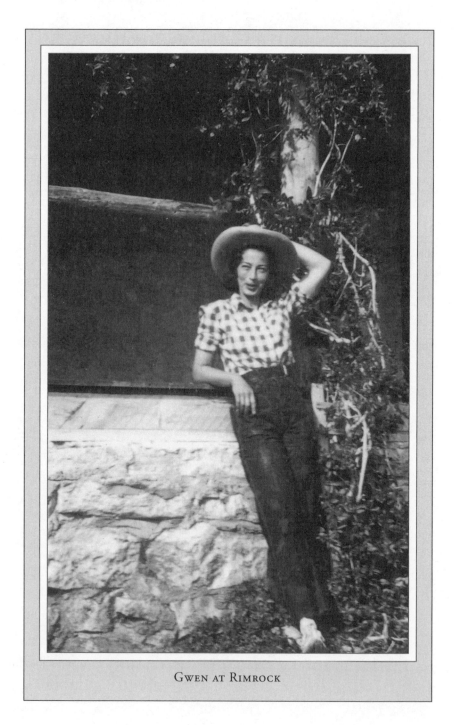

Gwen at Rimrock

CHAPTER 2

ALLEGRO VIVACE
Homes on the Range

GWENDOLYN GRANT WAS a Shipley- and Smith-educated maverick not unlike Larimer Mellon. Her family divided its time between urban residence in New York City and idyllic summers upstate on the Hudson River in Geneva. There, mother Katherine Hall Grant maintained the genteel lifestyle in which she had been raised as a debutante, while father William Wright Grant, a prosperous construction engineer, took Gwen and her sisters and brother for fine long walks and ornithology lessons in the woods. His devotion to nature was matched by an equally keen interest in civic affairs and in equipping his children with practical skills for useful lives.

"My mother didn't know how to do a thing," said Gwen, with characteristic offhand honesty, "so my father was determined that all four of us—my brother, too—would learn typing, shorthand, sewing, cooking, carpentry, and farming."[1]

She grew into a fair, willowy, regal young woman with distinctively high cheekbones and straight, un-"done" hair that, at the end of the century, looked much as it did when she and the century were in their twenties. Gwen was an excellent horsewoman, an adventurous lover of the outdoors and, by 1942, when she met Larry, the mother of three young children, whom she supported by working on an Arizona dude ranch. But much life was lived, and tough wisdom gained, before the eastern equestrienne became a western divorcee.

She speaks with a twinkle in her eye and its equivalent in her voice, the words punctuated by energetic bursts of laughter that seem to take her by surprise. But the voice grows soft and serious when she recalls life before Larry:

> I met John Rawson when I was going to Smith. He was very attractive, and I was pretty deeply in love with him. So he became my husband and the father of my children. But I had other interests, too.
>
> I heard Walter White talk at Smith—a black man. He later became very radical, but he was inspiring then. He was the NAACP secretary when it was at its inception, and I was very excited about it. I spoke to him after his lecture and he said, "We have a WPA [Works Progress Administration] project coming up in the Virgin Islands to educate black children, and there's a job opening for two years. Would you be interested?" I said yes, and he said, "Then have lunch with me next week at the Algonquin and we'll discuss it."
>
> So John drove me there and said, "When do I pick you up?" I said, "In two hours." Well, it was almost four hours, and he was furious! I said, "I've signed up." He said, "If you think I'm going to wait two years for you, forget it." I thought about it a couple of days and decided not to go, even though I'd agreed to and was gung-ho for it. It was a terrible disappointment.

It was a watershed moment. Women weren't supposed to think about careers. But at twenty-three, this woman was predisposed to the kind of idea that only took hold of Larry Mellon at thirty-eight.

"I had no hesitation about it," she muses. "I didn't mention it to Larry until years later, and it wasn't a big factor in what we decided to do in Haiti—but he knew I'd thought of going, all right. Anyway, at the time, I was married to John and I didn't regret it because I got my wonderful kids."

Three kids in four years, to be exact—Michael, Jenifer, and Ian. While Rawson went to law school in Albany, New York, Gwen took care of the children and kept the home show running, on meager income, in a house her family built for them. Yet even as the knot of domesticity tightened, she couldn't forget her lost project or abandon what it signified: "I knew I was treading water. I felt I was wasting my life. I wasn't doing anything for anybody except my kids. I wanted to do something worthwhile."

For openers, she took a night-school class in carpentry, where she was the only woman. "I had the best time there," she says, brightening at the memory. "They were lighthearted guys my age. They'd say, 'The girls sweep up!' and watch and clap—'More under there!' But I was obtaining skills that would be useful later on."

After Pearl Harbor, John Rawson, a dabbler in law and real estate, was offered a job in New York City with the U.S. Office of War Information and snapped it up, moving the family to a high-rise in the Jackson Heights area. For Gwen, that small, dark apartment became a cage: no grass, trees, or hint of the outdoors she loved. She did not love alcohol and the fact that her husband drank heavily. Adding to her misery was a serious back operation, followed by weeks of lying immobile at home. She was just getting back on her feet, literally, when Rawson informed her he'd be making a career move to Europe. Without her.

That was it for the marriage. There would be more of a separation than he bargained for: She'd be moving, too.

"I told him, 'I'm going to make myself a new life—I'm leaving,'" she recalls. "He said, 'You wouldn't dare.' I said, 'Yes, I would dare.' I don't know how I had the nerve, with three kids and no job. But I went out West."

She never liked big-city life. Now, in 1942, with money enough to keep them afloat for about six months, she took herself and her children to Arizona. She found a dude ranch in Rimrock where they could stay, a job as a riding instructor—and William Larimer Mellon Jr. Actually, her daughter found him first.

"I met the most wonderful man, Mr. Maloon," Jenny told her mother on their first day at the ranch. "You're going to see him at supper."

After their introduction, the first thing Larry said to Gwen was, "I hear you have two other kids. Where are they? I'd like to see them."

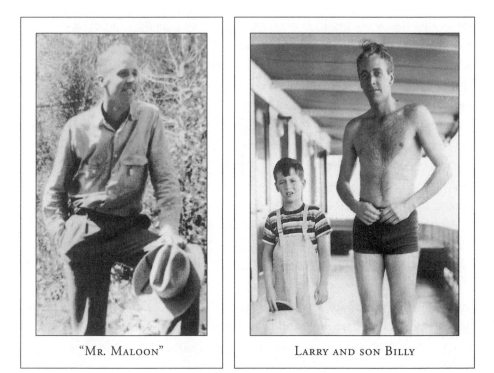

"MR. MALOON"   LARRY AND SON BILLY

Michael and Ian were presented. Larry surveyed the full quartet of Raw-
sons and remarked wistfully that he wished his own son, Billy, then at
school in California, could join them. He couldn't make that happen,
but he could take Gwen and her youngsters for a long, pleasant ride
that evening and many subsequent evenings. Then came a crisis, as
Gwen relates:

> We rode very late one evening and later, in the middle of the night, I
> had terrible pain. I knocked on Larry's door and said, "I'm in trouble."
> He woke up the manager of the ranch, and they took me to the hospi-
> tal in Jerome, an old copper-mining town. The head nurse said later,
> "I thought you were dead when they brought you in."[2]

Gwen had double pneumonia and spent days in an oxygen tent.
Straightaway, Larry assumed responsibility for her kids and took them

to visit her at the hospital. "They came up the stairs and looked in—Jenny's pigtails sticking way out on the sides," Gwen remembers. "Larry had braided them and put on blue ribbons. They saw me in this terrible shape. Then they left, and Larry came back up. He said, 'I want you to get better. It makes a difference to me.' From that moment on, I began to care whether I lived or died. Before that, I didn't."

They had known each other all of three weeks.

Through the end of her hospital stay, Larry tended to the welfare of the kids. He liked them more and more, and they liked him. But if a romance was budding, it would have to wait to bloom. As John Rawson had gone overseas for the OWI, so now did Larry for the OSS. "If you want to do something for me while I'm away," he told her, "learn to be a good cowgirl."[3]

Gwen did exactly that, as much to please herself as Larry. She got a job gathering wild horses at Mormon Lake and taught riding at a Squaw Peak dude ranch in Phoenix. When the war ended, both John Rawson and Larry Mellon returned to the States around the same time,

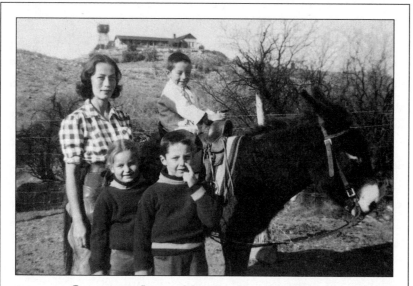

GWEN WITH JENNY, MICHAEL, AND IAN RAWSON

and both of them went straight to Gwen. Her mind was firmly made up by then: She told Rawson she was divorcing him. "You'll never do it," he replied.

In a confrontation with *this* lady, that was invariably the wrong thing to say.

.   .   .

WHEN GWEN ASKED LARRY why he wanted a thirty-seven-year-old woman with three children, Larry's answer was, "Probably just for that reason." "I wouldn't take you without them," he said.

He loved her kids from the start. Jenifer recalls that when she first met this unusual man, "He took me for a ride in his pickup truck, and as we bounced over the Arizona countryside, he grinned at me and said, 'See, out here we don't need roads.' His words were more prophetic than they were probably meant to be, because all through his life he seemed to chart courses where no roads previously existed. It was my privilege to be a peripheral part of his journey and to witness his joy in pursuing these uncharted paths. Every day, I thank my lucky stars that I was lucky enough to be part of the package Larry signed on for when he asked my mom to marry him."[4]

So they joined forces and families, and from then on would negotiate the ups and downs of Arizona ranch life together. "I think I was one of the many people that Larry picked up that needed help," Gwen reflects, with tough honesty about herself as about others. "There were a lot of them."

Shortly after Larry's marriage to Grace, for instance, he took on and took in a Latin American psychiatric patient he knew, much to the bride's chagrin. He later did the same for Hub Hruby, a Czechoslovak exile, who lived with the Mellons at length, while Larry managed his rehabilitation from wartime tribulations. But none of Larry's needy cases was more colorful or enduring than Jack Beau.

When they met out west, Beau said he'd been in the French cavalry, knew horses, and needed a job. With more charity than wisdom, Larry made him manager of his ranch, Breezy Bench. Beau's "management" largely consisted of counting the sheets, towels, and dishes, totally trivial in Larry's view, but central to Jack's idea of how to run the ranch. He could never quite connect with the mindset and larger view of his boss.

One day, Beau came in bubbling with excitement: "Larry! The telephone line is coming right across the front gate of Breezy Bench. What room do you want it in?" Larry said to put it in the saddle shed—as far away from the house as possible. Beau couldn't believe it. Why there? "Because I can use it if I need to," said Larry, "but I don't have to hear it." Jack was crestfallen. But the saddle shed was where the phone was put, and stayed.

Dishes and telephones bored Larry. The rancher's hardest outdoor work was what he loved. One spring when the cattle were brought down from the winter range and the calves gathered for inoculation against "black leg," the roping and throwing turned to chaos as the calves were separated from their mothers for the first time. Gwen was wielding the needle and syringe, but in the dust and confusion, "somehow I gave Larry a full shot of black-leg vaccine through his blue jeans," she recalls. "I was frantic, but he just said, 'It doesn't kill the calves, does it?'"

Far more life-threatening were the chaps Larry made from a kangaroo

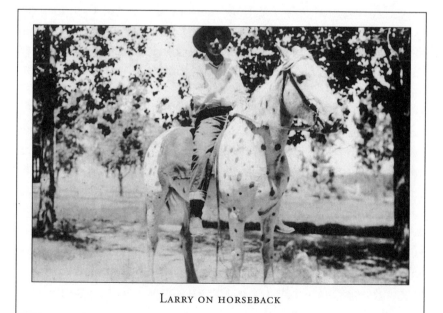

LARRY ON HORSEBACK

hide given him by a friend who had visited Australia. The process was time-honored: You cut two pieces to size, strapped them on, stepped into a water trough to soak them, and then struggled hard—wet leather being extremely heavy—to mount your horse. You rode all day and by the time you got off in the afternoon, they'd be dry and they'd be *yours*—shaped like you, and only you, forever. Nobody else could wear them.

Larry followed procedure, soaked his chaps in the trough, and scrambled aboard a colt named Cowboy—"a pretty calm, sensible horse," Gwen remembers. "We left together early in the morning and rode way down to a place called Grandpa Wash, thirteen miles from the ranch. But coming back late in the afternoon, Cowboy stepped on a tin can and threw Larry up out of the saddle. He had big heavy metal taps on his stirrups, and there he was, on the neck of the horse, with his feet caught by those taps."

Gwen jumped off her own horse and tried to grab hold and control Cowboy, but he only bucked worse. Larry was holding on for dear life, too far forward to get back in the saddle and too tangled up in his stirrups to get free. "Stand away!" he shouted, "I'm going to try to jump clear." He managed only to get one foot out of the taps. The other was stuck, snapping him to the ground full-force on his shoulder. Gwen took one look, remounted, and raced to the ranch house, then sped back in the pickup for an emergency run to the hospital in nearby Cottonwood.

The shoulder was badly broken, and the timing could not have been worse: Shortly before Cowboy and the kangaroo chaps laid Larry low, he and Gwen had decided to be married, traveling East to meet each other's families first. The trip had been elaborately planned, plane tickets purchased, children arranged for. Now here he was in Cottonwood Lawrence Hospital, encased in a body cast with his left arm stuck ridiculously high in the air.

On New Year's Day, 1946, Gwen finished packing for herself and for Larry, who could only sit and watch and nurse his broken wing. The next morning, they left Breezy Bench in a station wagon, depositing the

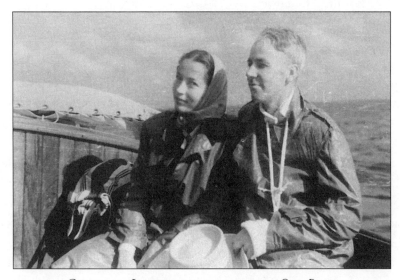

GWEN AND LARRY WITH CAST ON THE *OLD RIVER*

kids at Orme Ranch School on their way to the Phoenix airport. Commercial flying in 1946 was a risky, unpredictable business. They got as far as Texarkana, Arkansas, where the plane was grounded by bad weather. The passengers stampeded down to the local train station. Gwen ran with them and got the last berth, as luck would have it, an upper. "I don't know how we got him up there in that full body cast," she says, but somehow they did. Once in place, Larry remained shelved there for two days. Grand Central Station looked pretty good by the time the train crept in and the duo staggered out. Back in the bosom of her family, Gwen breathed a sigh of relief, happily announced her wedding plans—and got hit with a surprise in return:

> When I told my mother and sister Kathleen in New York, they said, "Do you know who you're marrying?" I said, "Sure, Larry Mellon." "But do you know who he is?" I said, "He has a ranch out West. In fact, he has three ranches." Kathleen said, "No, I mean his *family*." When she told me, I was paralyzed with fear. My God, I was a wreck. I'd been brought up very nicely, but this was completely unexpected.

The fact that I'd known Larry all that time and he never revealed it. I must have been dumb.

Or Larry must have been deliberately concealing the fact. In either case, the Grants sized up and gave high marks to their prospective in-law. Despite the absurdly oversized cast that encased him, he and Gwen took their blood tests for the marriage license and then headed down to Florida to meet Larry's family.

Rachel Walton, the only one of the Mellons who'd met Gwen earlier out West, liked her very much and remembers how nervous she was about meeting the Mellon patriarch. Gwen had been told he was "on the boat, fishing," says Rachel, "and she was expecting one of those little things with a motor in the back."

Not exactly. He was on the grand family houseboat, *Old River*. The *Vagabondia* had been even grander, but when America entered the war, Big Pa did his patriotic duty and turned over the seaworthy *Vag* to the Navy for military use.* Most pleasure boats had been ordered off the waters, but in exchange for his considerable gift, William Mellon was granted permission to continue his beloved fishing pastime—more or less uninterrupted by World War II—on his smaller, flat-bottomed craft, which was moored in the Miami River.

So it was on board the *Old River* where Gwen met Larry's father, brother Matthew, and sister Peggy for the first time and where she spent the next two weeks cruising around Cape Florida. Larry couldn't participate in the fishing and was not allowed near the rail because if he had fallen in with his enormously heavy cast, he'd have drowned for sure. But Big Pa made sure his Gwen was initiated and fully included in the family obsession. They snagged barracuda, grouper, sharks, and red snapper by day. By night, Larry joined them at the card table for gin rummy or lollapalooza; cumulative scores were kept for the whole trip.

Gwen won over Big Pa in many ways, not least of which was by

---

*Years later in the Haitian port of St. Marc, a friend of the Mellons noticed an unusual vessel in the harbor and, upon examining it more closely, made out the very faint word "Vagabondia." Big Pa's once proud craft was a stripped-down cargo boat.

catching on fast to the challenge of bonefishing. Considered one of the finest of angling arts, it is also one of the trickiest, requiring just the right equipment, bait, casting—and silence:

> We went down in very shallow water, maybe a foot and a half, no deeper. You had to be careful not to let the pole bump the side of the boat and make noise. No talking. You just sat there and waited for the tide to come in, until you saw the bonefish's tail—it puts its tail up in the air and feeds on seaweed—and then you cast right in front of them.
>
> If they take the bait, which has to be shrimp, you let them swallow it hard for a long time, because the inside of the mouth is solid bone and you can't hook it in there. Then you strike hard, and the bonefish makes a run. You slowly reel it in, but when it sees the boat it makes another huge run. You can do this five or six times before you land them. It takes a lot of patience and it's nerve-racking.

She was not only a good fisherman on that trip but a good hunter, too, according to Larry's diary: "Gwen shot two little snipe on the beach."

She denies it.

"I'd never fired a gun before. I'd shoot—the bird would jump up. I'm not sure I killed it. I just made it a nervous wreck. I did the same thing with quail out on the ranch. Larry wasn't much of a hunter, either, and after a while, he gave it up. He felt badly about it. We both did. The killing. It was exciting to know how to do it, but then it would be upsetting to see the animal dead."

More important than the field-and-stream activities to Gwen was the opportunity to observe first-hand the relationship, and enormous differences, between William Larimer Mellon Sr. and William Larimer Mellon Jr.:

> Big Pa wasn't affectionate. He was a man of few words, even when we first arrived. "Hello, son, how are you, haven't see you in a long while. We'll be sailing as soon as things get under way." Then the captain

came up and said, "We're delayed. The port terlet is under water." I ask Mr. Mellon, "What's a terlet?" It sounded so nautical. Larry never let me forget it. Oh God, they laughed. They had a maid, a chef, a butler who took care of Mr. Mellon's clothes—and of course the best fishing equipment for the Keys and Bahamas chain. They always decided the night before where they were going and what time we'd leave. Like clockwork. Wonderful picnics would be packed for you. . . .

Big Pa loved it when it got tough going. We went into Bimini in rough weather once. The waves were crashing, you could see the rocks. We couldn't get back in to shore, and I was scared to death, but Big Pa just thought it was great. Other times, Peggy was the one who had a special way and could make him a little more fun. Normally, Big Pa wasn't "fun."

William Mellon always wore a captain's hat on the yacht and dressed for dinner every night. Wardrobe represented one of many great contrasts between the father and the son: Once, on the ranch, Larry got a telegram from Big Pa asking him to join the family in Los Angeles for a cruise to Peru. He did so, more dutifully than enthusiastically, and the voyage was pleasant enough. Toward the end of it, as they were approaching the Lima harbor, Big Pa casually told Larry, "We'll stop in town before dinner and get your suit pressed first." Larry said he had no suit. Big Pa was stunned but resourceful, as only a Mellon could be. First he got Larry's measurements. Next, he ordered his bilingual radio man to put out an open shortwave inquiry: *Who is the fastest tailor in Lima?* Some helpful yachtsman nearby soon radioed back with the name and address of a sartorial speed demon, and the rush order was immediately dispatched by wire.

Larry's suit was ready for him when he got to the tailor shop, just in time for dinner.

The postscript and fillip took place ten years later in Washington. Larry was there visiting his friends Averell and Helen Clark, who had been among the Mellon family's guests on that South American cruise. "I remember so well when your father wired ahead to Lima to get you that suit," Helen laughed. Larry jumped up and said, "I've got it on right now!" He then turned the pocket inside out, proudly revealing the Peruvian label.

"That's how *a la mode* he was about his clothes," says Gwen.

.   .   .

IN THE GRIM PITTSBURGH PAST, Big Pa had brusquely aborted Larry's first public wedding for its violation of propriety. But in a sunnier present, the premarital cohabitation of Gwen and Larry didn't disturb him or mar his opinion of her a bit.

"He might not have known," she says with typical candor. "He had no reason to, actually, unless somebody wrote and told him, which I doubt. But he did investigate me. Someone came around and asked my mother, 'What kind of person is Gwen?' She said, 'She's one of the most determined people I've ever known.' My mother didn't know what the hell this man was doing."

The private eyes pronounced her "clean," she was a good fishing companion, and it was plain that Larry loved her. That was enough for Big Pa to give his blessing, and later to give Gwen a beautiful diamond ring he'd given his much-adored wife, May. Its symbolic importance to him was deep, and the gift of it symbolized his burgeoning fondness for Gwen.*

At the end of the month and the cruise, Larry finally had his cast removed in Miami. As Gwen vividly recalls: "I stood there watching while the doctor took this big, heavy thing off, and as soon as he was done, Larry fainted dead away. People often do. The cast gets to be like a part of your body. It's like having your arm cut off."

Revived and liberated from his cocoon, Larry with Gwen made the return trip north for their wedding. In New York, they stayed at the Savoy Plaza and one night had dinner at 21 with Larry's sister Peggy and

---

*He also gave her a fur coat, which was not terribly practical for life in Arizona or the Caribbean: "I didn't know what to do with it. I mean, if I lived in Alaska, maybe, but . . . I kept thinking, 'I've got to give it to somebody who's *cold*.'" Better late than never, in the 1990s, after half a century in storage, the coat was delivered to a cold person—a relative of a friend in Poland.

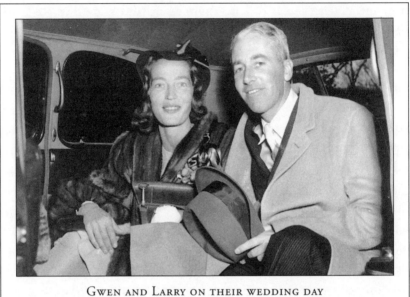

GWEN AND LARRY ON THEIR WEDDING DAY

Serge Oblenski, a war hero whose parachuting exploits behind enemy lines were famous. "We had drinks and I was nervous," says Gwen, "and I knocked mine over on Serge and on myself. All the waiters rushed up to brush off his suit—from Dunhill's, undoubtedly. Nobody paid any attention to me."

Larry thought it was hilarious. Gwen was not so amused. But she forgot about it an hour later when Larry escorted her down Shubert Alley and into the St. James Theater to see *Oklahoma!*, the Broadway musical phenomenon of that decade. The next night, wedding eve, they were the stars of an intimate reception for Gwen's family and Larry's New York friends, hosted by Peggy in her elegant Gracie Square apartment.*

They were married the following day, February 2, 1946, in the Con-

---

*Peggy Mellon originally married steel-family heir Alec Laughlin of Pittsburgh. After his death, on one of many medical trips with her mother to New York, she met a businessman Tommy Hitchcock. They married and settled into the social life and philanthropic prominence of Manhattan. Peggy was a dynamic part of the opera, fashion, and horseracing worlds of California and South America, as well as New York. The Hitchcocks had five children. They also had their own amphibian plane, enabling them to fly *beneath* bridges for convenient landings in the East River.

gregational Church of Wilton, Connecticut, where Gwen's sister Kathleen Van Wyck lived, and then returned to New York City for supper. They got up the next morning and visited the Central Park Zoo. It was a charming if eccentric thing for a bride and groom to do after the wedding night.

"Well, we didn't want to go see anybody, so we decided we'd rather go see the monkeys," Gwen explains. "We'd been living together for years, after all. The marriage was primarily for the family. It wasn't necessary for us."

Three days later, after catching a matinee of *Showboat*, they left for Pittsburgh on the PRR *Golden Arrow*. Larry Mellon would visit Pittsburgh a total of three times during the rest of his life. This was the first of those occasions, with the purpose of formally presenting his bride at Ben Elm. The comic complications were supplied by an extremely short Brazilian named Tony Lage, Larry's best man, and Tony's wife, Zetti, who was even shorter.

"They stuck right with us the whole time in New York," says Gwen. "We didn't mind too much, although we thought maybe we'd have a little time alone. Anyway, when Larry went to say 'Good-bye, we're going to Pittsburgh,' Tony and Zetti said, 'Oh, we want to go, too!' He didn't have the heart to refuse them, I think because they were so *small*. So we all took the night train to Pittsburgh together. And then a few hours after we got there, Larry went down to the bank, and Dick Mellon told him, 'I saw you getting off the train this morning with your wife and two new children.' That's how short Tony and Zetti were."

Thus did Gwen and the Brazilians make their Pittsburgh debut jointly. "Larry would leave me alone and go off to introduce 'my friend from Rio de Janeiro and his wife,'" she recalls. "It amused me. The Mellons had no idea who Larry was marrying, but from the word go, they were wonderful to me."

The evening's entertainment was home movies. Big Pa had many tins of film from family voyages on the *Vagabondia* to the South Seas, the Straits of Magellan and the Mediterranean, often in the company of a privately engaged scientist for educational cachet. In a lower room of the mansion, beneath larger-than-life portraits of William Mellon's wife and daughters, Gwen and the assembled guests watched. Larry discreetly yawned.

Ben Elm was a huge, three-story, dark red stone house. "It was a stiff place," as Gwen remembers it. "No levity. It was what Larry grew up with: dark, like so many houses in Pittsburgh. Depressing. It was the first house I was ever in that had air-conditioning. Not because it was so hot, but to help clear out the coal and steel smoke." The nearby mansion of Uncle Andrew Mellon, which she later visited, had an even more extravagant innovation: a full-size swimming pool in its basement, said to be the first private indoor pool in the United States Gwen recalls: "It was ghastly and dank down there. A pool is supposed to be out in the fresh air. But it was an amazing thing for the time."

Pittsburgh, of course, was a hotbed of wealth. In addition to the Mellons, it was home to the Carnegie, Frick, Heinz, Thaw, and Jones and Laughlin families. They and the city's other millionaire-industrialists rivaled each other not just in business, but also in philanthropy. The Mellons won, hands down.

William Mellon prided himself on keeping up with technology, and his favorite of many personal philanthropies was a "futuristic" project his Mellon Institute was then subsidizing for Carnegie Institute of Technology, now Carnegie Mellon University. "Go over to Carnegie Tech," Big Pa told Larry and Gwen during their visit. "In the cellar, there's a wild Russian who's doing something very interesting—something new that's going to be very valuable."

He was very excited about it, and so they went to inspect. "Sure enough," says Gwen, "we found this tiny little blond man there—hair flying out to his shoulders—with the first-ever computer. It was so huge, it took up the whole cellar of the business school. We said, 'What can you do with it?' He said, 'Play tic-tac-toe.' And he did. The wheels turned. We didn't think too much about it at the time."

Larimer never went back to Pittsburgh if he could avoid it. He wasn't comfortable there and didn't pretend to be. The Mellons' need to uphold their image as leading family in the city—if not the state, if not the

nation—went against his grain. But life amidst the Mellons was no culture shock for Gwen.

"My family was stiff, too," she muses. "Like Larry, I had to dress for
dinner, sit with proper manners, use the silver correctly. Mother was
warm and friendly, but the household was stiff. Anyone who came to
see me had to be formally introduced to my mother and father. No one
ever 'dropped in.' In that sense, I was prepared for the Mellons."

It was home movies the first night, the Pittsburgh Symphony under
the baton of Fritz Reiner the second, the Rolling Rock races next, and
much discussion of the raging steel strike in between. At the end of the
week, Larry and Gwen filed their passport applications at the Pittsburgh Post Office building in preparation for a south-of-the-border so-
journ. His family viewed that plan skeptically: It was unusual for
well-to-do Americans in general, Mellons in particular, to focus on
Latin America in their travels.

But first, Larry and Gwen felt a pressing need to get back to Arizona,
the children, and the ranch. Jack Beau met their train in Flagstaff during
a snowstorm and drove them to Breezy Bench, where there was a lot of
work to be done. Larry and Jack drove a truck to Phoenix the next morning to pick up five tons of cottonseed cake and to prepare for more wedding celebration, Western-style: A few days later, sixty people crowded
into the Mellons' living room for a big shivaree, the traditional noisy hoe-
down for newlyweds. Next came a few days of business: Larry rode to
Fort Rock to look over a new ranch site and land-exchange deal for 240
prime valley acres. There was a meeting of the Yavapai Cattle Growers
Association to attend in Prescott, after which he and his cowboys
branded six new Thompson bulls.

Finally, on March 6, he and Gwen were able to leave for their delayed
honeymoon trip, by romantic pickup truck, to Mexico. As always,
Larry meticulously recorded their progress:

March 8: Drive from Tucson to El Paso, put up at a Mexican tourist
camp—all hotels full. March 10: Gwen and I spend pleasant day in
Chihuahua, seeing a bullfight (Ameliano Vega) and a lovely circus. . . .

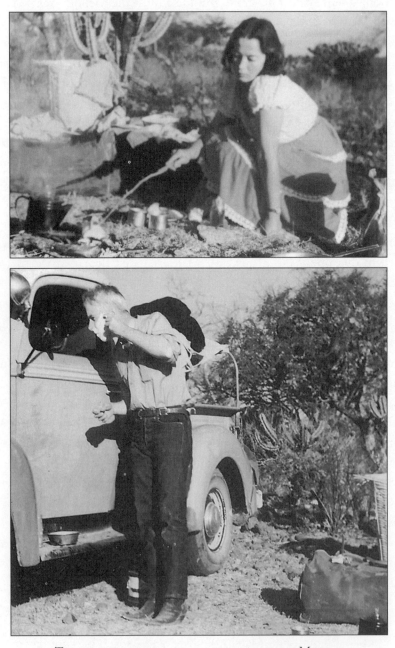

The newlyweds on their honeymoon in Mexico

March 12: Jimenez to Torreon in 12 hours. Dust, dust, DUST. March 14: Torreon to Saltillo. Buy *azulejos* [tiles] for bathrooms and kitchen floor in new Ft. Rock house. March 16: Saltillo to Monterey. Stop and camp for night along roadside. March 17: Drive to San Luis Potosi, a filthy town with very little charm.

They took thirteen leisurely days getting to Mexico City, and celebrated there by hitting the clubs and dancing more than one night away. Then it was on to Cuernavaca, Tepoztlan, and a 1567 Franciscan monastery. Near Mitla, Gwen bought an Aztec stone idol from a *campesino* who had dug it out of his own garden. In Taxco, they ordered hand-painted curtains and then drove on to Acapulco—"a lovely restful place," wrote Larry, "excluding the town itself, which is filthy and ill provisioned." Swinging back to Mexico City, they shopped for Victrola records and sheet music before visiting the archeological ruins at Oaxaca. They found a rare movie theater in Guadalajara and took in the relatively new *Picture of Dorian Gray* with Spanish subtitles before moving on to Guaymas and a day of fishing for mackerel and barracuda, "the latter regarded as highly edible by the local population," Larry observed.

His terse, often unintentionally humorous diary entries recorded the day's activities with precious few slivers of emotion or elaboration, to wit: "April 19: No music due to Good Friday. April 20: Swim in pool and work at Russian verbs all day. . . . April 22: Marlin fishing in the [Baja]. Gwen lands a 130-pounder after a three-hour tussle. It's grand here but we miss our kids and wish our car would hurry and arrive."

Deep in southern Mexico and afflicted by homesickness, they shipped the pickup ahead by rail to Nogales, flush on the Arizona border, then flew there to collect it for the short drive home. "Even a honeymoon isn't successful if you're not glad to get home again," said Larry's ebullient journal entry that night.

Ebullience declined the next day. Before putting their truck on the train, Larry had been required to drain the gas and oil for fire-safety reasons. Upon replacing both, they hit the road but had driven only a short while when the truck suddenly overheated, its engine fatally fried: He had forgotten to close the crankcase's stopcock and thus poured all the new oil straight through into the ground from whence it came. They now needed a rebuilt motor (at a cost of $207.67, Larry noted with shocked disapproval) before they could head back to Arizona.

Once home, their first callers were Barry and Peggy Goldwater, who drove down from Rainbow Bridge to spend the night. "Barry was a good cowboy friend," says Gwen, who had known him from the time she worked on the dude ranch near Phoenix and from the famous Goldwater Department Store. "Larry bought all our saddles there—beautiful saddles—and Peggy was adorable." She can recall no political conversations or foreshadowings with the controversial GOP presidential candidate-to-be of 1964.

The newlyweds quickly settled back into ranch life at Breezy Bench, their winter headquarters, which included a working barn and everything else needed to hold horses and cattle. It was where Larry first lived when he moved to Arizona, in a kind of shed, until his mother and sister Peggy came to visit, viewed his residence with restrained horror, and stepped in to build him a proper two-bedroom place. That was fine for a few men, but after Gwen and her children moved in, followed by a tutor and Mr. and Mrs. Jack Beau, the house was cramped to say the least. Hence the move to Fort Rock where, during the long time it took to finish the new house, the Mellons lived in a bunkhouse without electricity.

Between the Apache Maid summer range and Breezy Bench, the elevation sloped up to a 7,000-foot peak. As the weather grew colder, the cattle instinctively began the downward trek by themselves and hardly needed to be driven. "The north range had snow in winter, the south practically none," says Gwen. "That gives you an idea of the size. It went practically from snow to banana country."

The Fort Rock spread was likewise vast: 110,000 acres, moist and beautiful, with a subirrigated meadow that was rare in northwest Arizona. Larry said the land around there reminded him of *The Grapes of Wrath,* which he loved. "Every time we left the ranch and were on

Highway 1 to Seligman, he relived the Joad family's long trip," wrote Gwen in *My Road to Deschapelles*, her 1997 memoir. "His heart always ached for Rose of Sharon. . . . In Arizona, the backbone of the country was broken-boned cowboys who were used to heavy daily work. Two I know had lost their thumbs roping cattle. Many had pains and aches from past riding injuries, but none stopped working. Larry was one of them."[5]

The Mellons fared better than the Joads. Fort Rock was soon turned into a fine profitable ranch, where it was not uncommon for Larry, Michael, Ian, and two other cowboys to brand 250 cattle in a day. How many head did they have altogether? "You don't ever ask that," replies Gwen in an instructional tone. "It's like saying, 'How much money do you have?' We had white-faced Herefords." Pause. "A lot of them."

At Fort Rock, as everywhere the Mellons lived, time was carved out and set aside for entertainment. Though Easterners might think it the middle of nowhere, Southwest rancher society had its moments and Gwen and Larry enjoyed them. All work and no play would have made Jack Beau, for one, a dull boy.

"Gwen and I go to Cottonwood to hunt music for a dance at Breezy Bench in honor of Jack and Anne next Saturday," Larry recorded in his journal. No fewer than 135 guests showed up for that event, which "came off May 11 as scheduled and was generally proclaimed a success," he noted.

Gwen remembers wonderful parties to which almost everyone in the valley would be invited. They were the kind of people who often made their start by driving cattle up from Mexico, getting them on a train to Chicago, holding them there for some time, and then selling them. The more successful ones then came down to Arizona, bought a piece of land and built a good house on it. Gwen describes one such person, Livy Burrill, fondly:

> Livy came from a very good family in Long Island, but he drank and made a mess of himself, and then came out to start a new life. When Larry went to Europe and made Livy ranch manager, Livy never took

another drink. Straightened up. There were many men like that who came out to get away from Chicago or wherever and start over. A lot of girls came out for the same reason.

It was a funny life. Everybody you knew from around the general store would come to a dance, the cowboys would bring their wives and kids. It was a mixed bag. The music was a banjo, nothing too great—and believe me, it was the two-step. But it was a lot of fun. Larry played the guitar and accordion. We both liked to dance, but Larry was not a good dancer. He was always looking at the instruments and kind of beating time. Heavy going. We never got off the dime. But some of the square dancing was great.

A wealthy rancher named Charlie Ward came down periodically in the winter with a great planeload of his Chicago friends, with saddles and belts and hats heavily adorned with silver. "Really doggy," says Gwen. They would be installed on horses to have their pictures taken, and at the end of the visit Charlie would always throw a fine party for them, to which all the local ranchers were invited as well.

The social scene was more active in winter but, in any season, "pretty rare," says Gwen. "Real ranchers got up early, went to bed early, and had to drive a long way to see people. Your life was where you worked and slept and lived. You were terribly isolated, and so you drew pretty close to the people in your little community orbit and relied on each other. The big deal for the kids was going to the Green Frog Restaurant in Prescott and then up to the Hacienda Hotel to call Pittsburgh. That was our big excitement." The bulk of her time was devoted to the ranchwoman's traditional duties of raising the kids, keeping house, and, most of all, cooking:

Quite a few people ate at our house—the cowboys, hired hands, Sam the tutor, all different kinds of people. The quality of the conversation was pretty low. You'd sit down to breakfast Sunday morning and Lyman, one of the cowboys, would say, 'Lemme tell you 'bout this movie I saw last night. This here fella, he knocked on the door and turned the knob and walked in and closed the door, not quite all the way, you could see through a little crack, and then this other fella comes in and turns to the right and'—Step by step, every detail, the whole Saturday evening movie! They'd laugh and somebody would say, 'No, no, he turned to the *left*, not the right!' It took the whole breakfast, almost to lunch, to get the full story, blow by blow. Then another cowboy might tell us in great detail about a cow that was someplace it shouldn't have been—nothing about politics, nothing about the world. They had their own world.

Often, especially during roundups, Gwen made breakfast for fifteen men, prepared a fully-stocked chuckwagon for their lunch on the range, and saw to it that they were all fed, saddled up, and off by dawn. Appetites called for coffee, biscuits, hot cereal, grits, pancakes, fried eggs, "and of course cowboys always have to have meat for breakfast, usually fried steak, which I'd cut from a hanging quarter of beef in the storeroom." When the meat supply ran low, a steer would be slaughtered, hung up, and quartered just before nightfall, to reduce the hazard of flies.

Once during a torrential rain and electrical storm, they saw lightning strike a big tree near the place where four beautiful young bulls were pastured. "We all ran out, because we were pretty sure they would push up under the tree in a storm," she recalls, "and all four of them were lying dead. It was tragic. We tried to butcher them quickly, but the meat was no good at all—the lightning exploded every red cell in their bodies."

The Fort Rock ranch was thirty miles from the nearest school, so the children were tutored in the mornings at home and otherwise lived the normal life of ranch kids with their own horses and growing pains. Once during family dinner with the cowboys, Michael announced he had a joke to tell. Everyone said, "Good, go ahead," and he delivered an off-color yarn that left them all gasping. A little investigation in his room produced a copy of that ever so slightly racy magazine *Captain Billy's Whiz Bang*, which he had salvaged from some cowboy's trash. "Michael's first significant reading material," said his mother.

Larry and Gwen made many trips to California to visit Larry's son,

Billy, at Cate School in Carpinteria. One of those trips had a business purpose, as well: to deliver a horse. After doing so, they decided to treat themselves to a fancy Hollywood restaurant, and Gwen climbed in the back of the horse van to change her clothes while Larry drove down Sunset Boulevard. The restaurant had a canopy under which they had to drive, very carefully, to the consternation of the valets. Their tall horse trailer cleared it by about an inch and they pulled up in front of the entrance behind some Lincolns and expensive sports cars. The doorman and parking attendant were still gaping when Larry handed over the keys with a nonchalant, "Park it, please."

More typically, they went to California exclusively to see or pick up Billy, watch him play baseball, and take in a Western movie or two. After one such visit, they were bringing him back to Arizona for summer vacation when they stopped at a gas station and encountered a man with an albino raccoon. He said he had to sell it. Billy said he had to have it.

"So Charlie Coon rode in the back of the car with Billy," says Gwen. "I had a lot of material that I'd just bought for curtains and, while we were sleeping, Charlie pulled it out and shredded every single yard."

Back home at the ranch, Larry made a special harness and a house for Charlie, duly recording in his diary: "Coon house is completed. Ranch pets now include one albino coon, one possum, three horn toads, one gopher snake, one dog, two chipmunks." A few days later, the children's prospective French tutor arrived from Paris and Larry chose to interview her while taking Charlie for his daily bath and swim.

"Raccoons can't eat without water," says Gwen, "so they took Charlie down to the water tank, and there was Larry talking exquisite French to the tutor and holding the leash, long after Charlie slipped out of his harness and disappeared. That was the last of Charlie Coon—such a white, unpleasant-looking thing. Even with the right suit on, they're not too charming."

The year 1946 marked the beginning of the McCarthy era, but Larry Mellon wasn't buying it: "Met John P. McHale of the National Republic publication," he noted, "a definite phony with an anti-Communist cover." The greater disturbance that summer was John Rawson's arrival to pick up the three younger children and take them back East through August.

"They didn't want to go," says Gwen. "They were very happy in Arizona, and this was very difficult for them, for me, and for Larry. His involvement with those kids was deep, every single day. Wherever we traveled, the first thing he did after we arrived was rent a suitable schoolroom for them. Larry sent them to college, Europe, did absolutely everything for them—more with my three than with Billy, sadly. He felt he couldn't get very close to Billy."

Larry's son had been raised largely in California by his mother, whose numerous remarriages brought new stepfathers and disputes in which Billy was often the focal point. At first, not surprisingly, he wasn't fond of Gwen and her kids. Their arrival on the Arizona scene was hard on him because he was used to being the center of his father's life whenever they were with one another, especially during their summers together. "But he came around," says Gwen. "He became my most devoted child. It didn't take him long to develop an affectionate relationship with the three younger kids. Then he went to St. Paul's School in Concord, New Hampshire. He was a perfect St. Paul's boy. He and Michael were there at the same time for a while. But he was a lot more sophisticated than my kids were. His life and his ambitions were very different."

Larry worried about him in his diary: "Billy has a tendency to keep changing his mind, to say he'll do something and not do so." Larry was also worried about his father, then in declining health. In August 1946, he and Gwen took a train from Arizona to Toronto, where they were met by Big Pa's chauffeur, who drove them on to Beaumaris for a late supper. William Mellon's place there was still the centerpiece of the family vacation compound—a beautiful basswood-paneled house with a fine fireplace and equally fine cold-water fishing. Sisters Peg and Rachel had separate homes on the island, tennis courts had been added, and some of the old boathouses had been converted into dormitories for the numerous new grandchildren.

One Sunday there, Larry, Gwen, and Big Pa were on their way to church on the mainland when, as Larry leaned over to untie the boat, his cherished Parker pen, a gift from his mother, fell out of his pocket into the dark water. Most men would have said farewell and given up on it. Not Larry. Hurriedly stripping, he said it might not sink because of the air pocket in its rubber ink bladder—if he could just catch a glimpse of it. While his father sat in the boat watching with fascination, Larry jumped in, dove down, and came up with it. He put on his pants and shirt, tied his tie, started up the motor, and zoomed off to church, the prodigal Parker safely returned.[6]

Gwen's other strong memory of Beaumaris was the big annual sailing race, a highly competitive affair:

> Someone in the family had a little sailboat that was beautifully tuned up, and Larry said, "Come on, we'll enter it just for fun." And damned if we didn't win! Larry and I were the hicks from the sticks, and we couldn't have told you why we won. We just got off to a good start. It was a fluke. And it was awful! Other people who were dying to get the cup were mad.

That event and its odd outcome seemed to bolster Larry's general aversion to Beaumaris. From then on, "Whenever we could get away from Arizona, we wouldn't normally choose a place like that," says Gwen. "It was 'vacationland,' and ranchers can never really vacation anyway."

New York City was more their idea of a good time, and after the obligatory week in Ontario they made a beeline for the Savoy Plaza. Larry's journal entry the day they arrived in Manhattan was, "Buy Russian books," followed in succeeding days by, "Get first Arabic grammar. . . . Start Arabic lessons at Berlitz. . . . Gwen and I see *Carousel*. . . . Great reunion of the Grant clan in our room at Savoy with Gran Kitty [Gwen's mother] and 14 of her chicks. . . . Arabic lesson. . . ."

Such was his new obsession with Arabic that he set up a meeting with an Arab from Brooklyn, Habeeb Massabney, and, once satisfied with his credentials, arranged to bring Habeeb, his wife and two children out to Arizona to give him Arabic lessons. The family actually went, after overcoming the terror of the wife, who had never been West but had heard that the deer out there liked to attack and kill human beings.

Why, exactly, did Larry want to learn Arabic?

"He didn't want to waste his time, especially in the winter," Gwen explains. "So he had a lesson every day, and it kept him busy in the off-season. He just wanted to master it because it was a puzzle to him. Most of the languages he learned after the war were more for literary purposes than conversation, though he ended up speaking Arabic very well."*

Before leaving New York, they saw *Harvey* (starring "my old Princeton classmate James Stewart") and *Annie Get Your Gun* and had dinner at Sardi's. "We were starving for entertainment," says Gwen, "and we didn't know what else to do in New York. You couldn't saddle a horse or do any of the things we were used to. We'd go to bed early, get up early and couldn't get breakfast till 8 o'clock." For ranchers, that was shamefully late.

.   .   .

THE MELLONS' RANCH LIFE—dominated by the gathering, branding, and shipping of cattle—is well illustrated by excerpts from Larry's diary entries of a single month:

Sept. 24: Drive small herd from Paso Robles and put them through the drift fence near Devil's Hump. Catch and tie up several yearlings at Basin Tank. Sept. 26: Move camp from Paso Robles to Fort Rock. Boys spend day shoeing horses. Oct. 5: Spent day at Breezy Bench doing carpentry chores, then we all go to see *The Virginian* after supper in Cottonwood. Oct. 9: Tally 320 head of cattle at Badger Flat by run-

---

*He used it for biblical study, too, as he told Albert Schweitzer in 1948: "[You] inspired me to [read] St. Mark in Arabic, which is for me a hard job since my knowledge of this language is incomplete. Nevertheless, this exercise furnishes several advantages. First, it requires that I pay strict attention to detail and that my work not be hurried. Secondly, it obliges me to compare the Arabic text with my own language to be certain of its meaning. Thirdly, having never studied Hebrew or Aramaic, I feel closer to Jesus's words by their proximity to Arabic than I do when I read them in English. . . . Presbyterians, more than other Christians, carry painful [financial] duties and responsibilities. Not necessarily, alas, bringing more spiritual satisfaction."

ning them through the chute and bobbing tails. Oct. 11: 20 degrees
and blowing hard when we get up at 5 a.m., saddle up and gather at
Badger Flat pasture, drive herd of about 1,000 to middle pasture.
Only seven miles, but they won't go any farther. Oct. 19: Finish shipping first bunch of calves from Flagstaff, 355 head. This morning ship
656 head to Calif. Oct. 25: We bob about 500 tails and brand 27
calves. . . . Put 200 head through the Fort Rock chute.

Around Thanksgiving, a hospital in need called for help, a harbinger,
perhaps, of a future hospital and a future call from within. Cottonwood's medical facility had a severe shortage of nurses and of space.
Could Gwen and Larry help out? A few weeks later, Lawrence Hospital
announced a $15,000 fund drive to which the Mellons not only con-
tributed but agreed to "beg money," as Larry put it, from other members of the regional gentry. He hated asking anyone for money and
couldn't remember ever having to do so before. But he and Gwen
worked hard for Cottonwood's Lawrence Hospital, a vital facility with a
good staff, and he later took a place on its board.

Meanwhile, life, languages, and leavings continued, all faithfully
recorded in his journal:

Jan. 6, 1947: Go to Cottonwood in the morning to sell lead out of
used wet cell batteries from FRL power plant. See Bill Gray to get $115
he owes me for horses. All I get is a promise. Jan. 8: I transcribe Mark,
Chapter I, in Arabic. Jan. 9: Leonard Cameron stops in to sell me
70% interest in a gold mine near Yuma! Jan. 14–21: Leave Breezy
Bench for Mexico City, Merida, then Chichén Itzá to inspect ruins.
Feb. 9: Bullfights . . . Feb. 25: Spend a delightful sunny afternoon in
the Maya ball court playing guitar and singing. I work at Arabic com-
position all morning . . . Start Jules Verne's *La Vuelta del Mundo en 80
Dias* [his Spanish translation of *Around the World in 80 Days*]. Children have school all along the way.

A big part of Larry and Gwen's baggage consisted of maps and school books, and the tutor, Brown, always traveled with them, not just for the enlightenment of the kids. Back in Arizona at the end of June, Larry asked Brown to teach him trigonometry. That month, too, they finally settled in at Fort Rock, a move "we hope is our last," Larry wrote. "Since 1929 I have moved at least once every year and more often, twice." The ranch house at Fort Rock was their grandest—six bedrooms, each with its own bath and fireplace, plus lots of space to accommodate transients and a sizeable swimming pool.

Despite a drought that year, Larry's calves averaged around 200 pounds, the yearling steers about 700, the cows about 950, and the prices they fetched were good. In October, it took three trips by five large trucks to get them all to Seligman: 22 bulls, 241 calves, 181 cows, 222 steers, 67 yearling heifers. He could relax with the Goldwaters again and devote time to Gwen and the kids. "More snow today," he wrote one wintry day. "I wound a coyote but lose him. Jenny and I follow the bloody track for a mile."

Once upon a Caribbean island, many years later, Larry surprised Gwen by saying, "I don't think we were ever as good people as when we lived in Arizona." When she asked him why, he replied, "Because we lived so basically." But at the time, he still seemed restless to her. Long after his return from the war and their marriage, his never-unpacked duffel bag was still leaning against their bedstead. "You had better get rid of that," she finally said one day. "It makes me nervous."[7]

Ranch life was good, and satisfying in an honest, elemental way. But not wholly fulfilling. Larimer Mellon didn't quite realize that himself until a magazine article changed the course of his and Gwen's life.

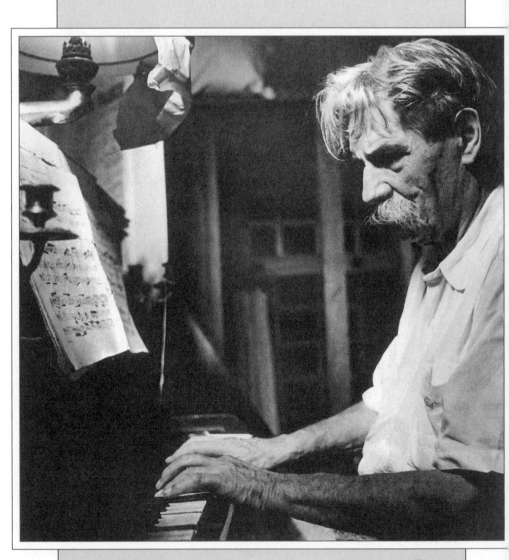

ALBERT SCHWEITZER: BACH ON A JUNGLE-PROOFED ORGAN IN GABON

CHAPTER 3

LARGO
Road to Damascus

L ONG BEFORE THE PEACE CORPS was a gleam in John F. Kennedy's eye, Larimer Mellon came across a *Life* magazine article of October 6, 1947, titled, "The Greatest Man in the World." It was essentially just a photograph layout with brief text of about 750 words, many of them erroneous, to lionize "Albert Schweitzer, Ph.D., Th.D., Mus.D., M.D., a seventy-two-year-old medical missionary who lives among the wild cannibals at Lambaréné, deep in the jungles of French Equatorial Africa."

Dr. Schweitzer (1875–1965) was threatened by many things in Gabon, but cannibalism was not one of them. On the other hand, it was true, as the writer continued, that "natives spread the word up Ogowe River that the white medicine man could kill a patient, cut his belly open, and then bring him back to life painlessly. Carefully catering to native superstitions, he pretends to take some object from sores or incisions and throw it away, thus removing the evil spirit which caused the sickness."

It was not the sensationalism of the piece that so struck Larry Mellon, but the philosophy, even in snippet form, it contained and a reference to the book on which Schweitzer was then working, *Reverence for Life*. "The picture of an old gentleman musing on a log in the jungle," said Larry, "was a novel concept of greatness. It set me thinking."[1] During the last half-century of his life, Schweitzer would provide medically and nutritionally for more than 500 people a day. Even more compelling to Mellon, once he sought and learned more about the doctor's work, were Schweitzer's words behind the deeds:

"It struck me as incomprehensible that I should be allowed to lead such a happy life, while I saw so many people around me wrestling with care and suffering . . . The Fellowship of those who bear the mark of pain: They belong together all the world over. They are united by a secret bond. One and all, they know the horrors of suffering to which man can be exposed, and one and all, they know the longing to be free from pain."

Schweitzer's insight into the way pain diminished humanity struck Mellon to the core. Paul on the road to Damascus experienced no greater conversion.

.   .   .

ONE DAY WHEN Albert Schweitzer was out bicycling with Helene Bresslau, his wife-to-be, he told her a secret: He had promised himself in early youth that he would live for himself and enjoy his own and his family's good fortune until he reached thirty; after that, he would devote himself to the service of humanity. The catalyst, curiously, was virtually identical to Mellon's inspiration four decades later: an article Schweitzer read on the desperate need for medical help in equatorial Africa. Almost immediately, he gave up his principal's position at a Protestant theological seminary, his university teaching and his financial security to become, at the age of thirty-one, a humble medical student.

Due to Schweitzer's prominence as both a theologian and musician, there was considerable excitement at the announcement that he would go to Africa as a doctor, to heal rather than convert the "heathens." Friends and family alike thought he might be mad—that perhaps *he* was the one who needed treatment. But through seven years of study and internship, he never wavered from his goal, often sleeping just four hours a night or sitting at his desk with his feet immersed in a bucket of cold water to stay awake. Meanwhile, he gave organ concerts all over Europe to raise money for the project, always with the support of Helene, who was deeply involved in all his plans and work.

In 1913, they left for Africa to establish their hospital, with seventy-five crates of medical equipment and supplies and a piano. At the remote outpost of Lambaréné (the name meant "let us try" in the local dialect), word of their arrival was sent up and down the Ogowe River by the beating of drums. Even before they unpacked, sick people began to arrive from all directions. The need was far greater than they ever imagined. Some time later, upon returning to Lambaréné from a trip upriver, he told his wife he had discovered "the secret of all secrets" and handed her a piece of paper covered with his agitated scribbling:

Lost in thought, I sat on the deck of a barge, struggling to find the elementary and universal concept of the ethical idea which I had not discovered in any philosophy. Sheet after sheet I covered with disconnected sentences . . . On the third day at sunset, as we were making our way through a herd of hippopotamuses, there flashed upon my mind, unforseen and unsought, the words REVERENCE FOR LIFE . . . Since my life is full of meaning to me, I want others to respect my life. Then I, too, must respect the other life, however strange it may be to me.[2]

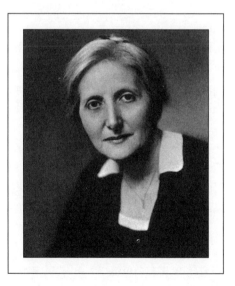

HELENE SCHWEITZER

But the outbreak of World War I soon shattered the Schweitzers' world. They were Alsatians, German subjects, in Gabon, a French colony, and the authorities considered them enemies. The Africans could not understand why French soldiers suddenly imprisoned the doctor and his wife in their own hospital. Schweitzer pleaded to be allowed to continue his work, but in 1917, after four and one-half years there, he and Helene were forced to leave.

They endured a long voyage in the overcrowded hold of a ship with hundreds of other prisoners of war, allowed to walk on deck for one hour a day. In France, they were sent to an internment camp, where Albert was made to do hard labor, when not taking care of the many, including his wife, who fell sick. Upon their release at the end of war, both ill and without money, they returned to the chaos and confusion of Strasbourg. After 48 years of German rule, Alsace was once again part of France. It was painfully ironic: By *not* being French, they had lost their hospital, their years of hard work, and their good health; now, they were French citizens. Helene had in fact contracted tuberculosis, from which she never recovered, and she was pregnant. Their daughter was born on January 14, 1919, Albert's forty-fourth birthday. He had picked out a boy's name—Rhenus, Latin for his beloved River Rhine—and they feminized it to Rhena.

Schweitzer now gave lectures and organ concerts to earn some money to build their house in the Black Forest, where he finished the first two volumes of his *Philosophy of Civilization*. But he was restless, his thoughts still of Africa and the people there. He knew he had to return to Lambaréné, and he knew his wife was too ill to go with him. In February 1924, with her blessing, he left for Africa alone.

Nine years later, after Hitler came to power, Helene fled to Lucerne, Switzerland, because German law considered her Jewish and classified Rhena as "50 percent non-Aryan." It was Helene, not her husband, who led the family's opposition to the Nazis. For now, it was not politics that occupied him:

The morality we have lived by was fragmentary only. We must abandon it in favor of the complete, all-embracing love expressed in "reverence for all life." Concern for human life alone is like a single tone floating in the air, incomplete because the bass tone to produce the harmony is missing. Reverence for life gives us the full chord, the harmony. . . . From the time they start school, young people must be imbued with the idea of reverence for all living things.

·   ·   ·

LIKE ALBERT SCHWEITZER, Larimer Mellon's need to do something extraordinary was born of a restless spirit that, if not manifested before, was dramatically galvanized now. Soon after reading the *Life* piece, he wrote Schweitzer to tell him it had inspired him to establish a medical mission of his own, "perhaps in South America." Schweitzer's response came in the form of two letters written within four days of each other in early 1948:

> You can well imagine how pained I am by the stupid superlatives which the author of the *Life* article abused in describing me. . . . I was very much moved upon reading your letter and felt a certain responsibility towards you, since the knowledge of my life influenced your decision to devote yourself to a similar undertaking. . . . Therefore, I consider you a dear brother, and I speak to you as such.[3]

In those first letters, Schweitzer's utmost seriousness alternated with lighthearted cordiality and a keen awareness of his correspondent's pedigree:

> Perhaps it would interest you to know that your uncle, the Secretary of State Mr. Andrew Mellon, and I both received a Doctorate Honoris Causa at the same time from the University of Edinburgh. At the dinner which followed, Mr. Mellon and I were seated at the same table. He was the one designated to speak for the newly elected doctors and to respond to the Vice Chancellor of the University. When he had finished his speech, a voice rose saying, "So, Mr. Mellon, now that we have made you Doctor of Edinburgh, it is, of course, no

longer a question that Great Britain will repay its debts to the USA. You will take care of all that." . . . Thus, having met the uncle, I also hope to meet the nephew and I am delighted to be in contact with him.

A bond between two mavericks already existed and grew quickly. They would correspond the rest of their lives.

Mellon wasn't even a college graduate, much less a doctor. But he had made up his mind, even though, at 38, his handicap would be considerable, as Schweitzer warned him:

> Do not delude yourself about how difficult it will be. . . . Your age imposes one of the first and most serious difficulties. I myself have had the experience that after a certain age one has more difficulty in assimilating new knowledge than in youth. One's memory is no longer sharp enough to master the required concepts. You will notice it even more than I, since you are studying at a more advanced age. On the other hand, you have the great advantage over me to be able to concentrate entirely on your studies. I had to earn a living on the side, have pastoral duties, and finish writing books. How much I suffered from the state of things I could not change!
>
> The fact that you can concentrate on medicine alone guarantees you will succeed, despite the difficulties that your age imposes. You can rest assured of that.[4]

When that fateful *Life* article appeared, the Mellons were just getting settled in to their new Fort Rock house. Gwen's furniture had finally arrived, as had the material she'd ordered in Mexico on their honeymoon. She was in the act of hanging some new curtains when Larry informed her of a momentous new mission that would radically alter their lives.

His announcement did not shock her.

"I knew he wasn't satisfied with life on the ranch," she says a half century later, "and the idea came at the right moment. He blurted it out—'I think I'll become a doctor and practice in the undeveloped world'—and

I said, 'So that's what's been on your mind lately. You're right, we don't want to sit around looking at the damn cows all our lives.' So really, we both decided."

Gwen's unflappability never ceased to amaze and delight him. She would not only go along for this ride but serve as co-pilot and actively participate by studying medicine herself.

In December 1947, just four days after composing his first letter to Dr. Schweitzer, Larry wrote to inform his father of his medical plans and to request a letter of recommendation from Dr. Edward J. MacCaigue, the prominent Pittsburgh physician who had attended his mother. Big Pa's reply was stiff. "The idea was alien to him," says Gwen, "but he didn't criticize and he wasn't mad or upset. His letter was businesslike, as always: 'Don't keep the ranch if you're not going to be there working. Absentee ownership doesn't work.'"

Dr. MacCaigue, for his part, duly wrote friends at Tulane University in New Orleans on Larry's and Gwen's behalf. The speed of it all was amazing. Larry's letter hadn't even been delivered to Dr. Schweitzer yet. What if Schweitzer had never answered?

"I think he would have become a doctor anyway," thinks Gwen. "The calling was that strong. His mother once told him 'the best thing a man can be is a medical missionary.' Then his brother Matthew, coincidentally around this time, happened to write and mention how important Schweitzer was in the philosophy world.* But the real driving force was the passage in the article that said Schweitzer went to the place with the greatest need. Let me tell you, when Larry read that, he was excited. He was very influenced by the biblical verse that for a rich man to enter the kingdom of heaven was harder than for a camel to go through the eye of a needle. He often used that passage for his translations into different languages."

---

*Matthew Mellon, once a teacher of philosophy at Freiburg University, was interested in Schweitzer the theological thinker, not the medical missionary, as revealed in Schweitzer's brilliant *Quest for the Historical Jesus*. Matthew's own writings dealt with related topics, such as the essay "An Inquiry Into the Ethics of Christianity" in his provocatively titled book, *How God Became Moral*. A director of the International Bach Society, he had contributed organs and met Schweitzer at meetings of the group.

His sister Rachel, asked if she ever had any hint of Larry's interest in becoming a doctor, replies, "No, and he had a terrible time getting into medical school."

Mellon was still far from admission when, on January 5, 1948, he dispatched Jack Beau to Africa for the purpose of delivering to Dr. Schweitzer a crucial letter further explaining his goals and asking for advice. As Larry's scout, Beau was instructed to have an in-depth talk with the doctor and report back in detail. But he insisted on taking along his wife Anne, and they were not quite prepared for what they found. "He hated it," said Larry, "the mosquitoes especially."[5] Hardier souls than the Beaus had experienced trouble with Gabon, the hospital, and its founder.

"It was a very primitive place," says Dr. Arthur Maimon, a later colleague of Mellon's, who met Dr. Schweitzer in Lambaréné in 1946. "Schweitzer could be very gruff. I remember saying to Mrs. Schweitzer through an interpreter that it must be great being married to this world-renowned Nobel prizewinner, and she replied in broken English, 'If you knew Albert like I know Albert. . . .' He was moody and recurrently depressed. But then, aren't we all?

"Dr. Schweitzer never learned the Gabonese language. He talked to his patients through interpreters and referred to them as *mes sauvages* [my savages], which speaks to why he went there in the first place. Those were still colonial days.

"While I was there, a young man showed up from France, bright-eyed and bushy-tailed, and asked Dr. Schweitzer the meaning of life. Schweitzer pointed to a large pile of wood that was to be moved across the compound: Cord it, stack it, and come back and see him in a week. It must have been 105 degrees there and mosquitos were plentiful, but this kid did it and came back, and I overheard some of his conversation: 'Could you now tell me what the meaning of life is, Dr. Schweitzer?' And Schweitzer said, 'Don't you know by now?' Meaning, just get off your butt and get to work—stack the wood and quit thinking about it."[6]

In any case, the Beaus were boggled by Lambaréné and intimidated by Schweitzer, who had a habit of not paying much attention to guests for the first few days. He had set aside time for the end of their visit, but the cancellation of a scheduled boat required Schweitzer to spend the

Beaus' last day in Lambaréné arranging new transportation for them. He sat up most of that night writing Larry the longest, most soul-searching letter of their decades-long correspondence:

> I arranged to be free (as much as I can be in my circumstances) in order to have some quiet time with Mr. Beau on Saturday, February 28th before his departure. [But] I had to spend the entire day looking for a boat that would take him to Port Gentil. [So] the only day that I could have spared to speak to him of matters close to the heart was sacrificed. . . .
>
> [Thank you for all the gifts.] The medicine Mr. Beau "lugged" with him throughout his trip was very precious. . . . I was greatly touched by your kindness. The pen is a marvel. It is extremely useful as it suits my poor hands tortured by writer's cramp. I use it especially when I need to write more neatly than usual. It is always on my desk. The handsome pipe is, unfortunately, an anachronism! I used to be a heavy smoker and smoked pipes as a student. But on January 1st, 1899, while a student in Paris, I made a vow to quit smoking and I have kept it! But, with your permission, I will nevertheless keep this precious pipe in order to give it one day to a smoker who has done me a favor. . . .

A superb illustration of how Schweitzer's pragmatism cohabited with his idealism came in the form of his shrewd advice to Larry for med school:

> At the beginning of your studies, concentrate on the essentials: Anatomy and physiology. As for zoology and botany, only learn what you need in order to pass your exams. I, myself, made the mistake of getting too deeply involved in these two subjects . . . As for chemistry, pay attention above all to what is pertinent to medicine.
>
> The study of medicine before the study of chemistry is a hard test of patience. One finds oneself before an open door without being allowed to enter the building. But you must be patient and not get frustrated. . . .
>
> Be sure from the very beginning that you have a sound base in

practical things: physical examinations and the laboratory procedures for blood and urine. . . . Major surgery, with operations that demand someone highly skilled, is not of interest to you. You should have a theoretical knowledge of it, but you should not aspire to perform it . . .

There is one thing that will astound you coming from me: avoid specialized studies in tropical illnesses! If one day you are in a tropical setting, you can become familiar with the illnesses and treatments on the spot by referring to books. You must have these cases in front of you in order to know them. . . . If you know the standard laboratory and microscopy procedures, you are fully equipped to study on location.

Above all, do not try to pass your exams brilliantly. Be content with getting through them somewhat honorably.

And do not write a pretentious doctoral thesis! Take a limited subject that won't require vast amounts of research . . . just enough to get your degree. For you, what matters most is to have knowledge that is both basic and practical, solid and far-reaching. Keep that well in mind. . . .

If I am still alive, come spend your vacations here once or twice during your studies (June to October) during the dry season. You will be able to acquire practical knowledge from the great amount of human material at your disposition here. It would be a good opportunity to learn how to diagnose and to treat. As you can see, I am already beginning to weave dreams.[7]

Larry was ecstatic—tremendously moved by the warmth and depth of Schweitzer's concern. His reply included a lament that he lacked fifty-eight credits (Gwen, with her B.A., needed only half that many) and a "symposium"-type Glaucon-to-Plato recapitulation of the master's advice:

Your interest and your encouragement came at just the right moment for my wife and me, because the enthusiasm shown by the heads of American medical schools for our getting medical degrees was not encouraging, to say the least . . . Alas, they were suspicious of my grey hair, and I did not even try to tell them the truth, that the first signs appeared at age 12. . . .

So that you are able to see that the time spent in recounting your experiences is not lost, here's a little summary that my wife and I have tried to fix in our minds.

"Avoid humiliating situations.

Stay independent.

Concentrate on the essential . . ."[8]

He would be guided by those points in med school, Mellon pledged to Schweitzer—if and when he ever got *into* med school.

"They all said, 'No, you're too old,'" recalls Rachel. "Gwen's the one who really got him in. She told them at Tulane, 'You'll regret it if you don't take him.' Not as a threat. She meant they'd be sorry they missed their chance to have him. She's wonderfully assertive, you know."

Larry had sent his application and a fervent plea to Tulane, but the initial response was that his lack of any chemistry, biology, or a bachelor's degree made it impossible to accept him.

"We went in person to see the dean, Max Lapham, and said we both wanted to go to medical school," Gwen recalls. "Larry left the room at one point and Max said, 'You, maybe—but Larry, with just one year at Princeton?' I just said, 'If you don't see your way clear to take him, you'll be making a big mistake.'"

Two weeks later, his letter of acceptance arrived.

·   ·   ·

THERE WERE A HUNDRED THINGS to be done before the move to New Orleans: homes to be bought and sold, schools to be lined up for Michael, Jenifer, and Ian. But, as always with Larry, prior commitments were to be kept. The one at hand was a long-planned family trip to Peru "to study the conditions in underdeveloped countries as well as the geography on the west coast of South America," he wrote Schweitzer, with a not-so-hidden agenda of scouting locations for his own future medical mission.[9]

"Packing for Peru," he noted in his diary on January 21, the same day that "Gwen and I tell Michael about our plans to begin studying medicine. Gwen told Jenny yesterday, and the children seem much interested!"

That entry, and the trip to Peru, in fact took place *before* Larry's acceptance by Tulane. Despite that uncertainty, as their ship sailed slowly down the Pacific coasts of Nicaragua, Panama, and Colombia, he and Gwen studied biology together in the mornings. They were soon walking around Lima and he was studying Quechuan, the Andean Indian language, in the afternoons. "I feel my first earthquake," he recorded on February 26.

From Lima, they hired a man to drive them to the mountain town of Arequipa. Hardly had they arrived at a little hotel there, when in rushed an American missionary couple with a very sick little boy.

"They didn't speak any Spanish, and they were absolutely unbalanced by the illness of this child," Gwen remembers. "Larry was no doctor, but his Spanish was excellent and so he took them to a clinic doctor. The boy had appendicitis and had to be operated on, and Larry had to stand by and do all the translating outside the operating room. They'd open the door and say, 'More gauze!' He'd run to the pharmacy. This went on for hours. Larry spent all his waking moments working down there and tended to everything. He was trapped and couldn't extricate himself. The child came out looking white as a sheet, but he made it. I think the parents assumed Larry was part of the hospital staff, and they weren't a bit grateful."

Their next stop was to check out a possible hospital location in the tiny town of Tingo Maria at the headwaters of the Amazon. They took a taxi equipped with oxygen masks for the altitude.* Everyone there seemed to be drinking hot chocolate, they noticed. What the Mellons naively mistook for "cocoa" turned out to be "coco," coffee heavily laced

---

*By coincidence, the exact day, month, and year the Mellons were inspecting Tingo Maria as a possible site for their hospital, Dr. Theodore Binder was in the nearby Peruvian town of Pucallpa doing the same thing. Binder's inspiration was the same as Mellon's, and the name he chose, quite independently, for his own medical center was "Hospital Albert Schweitzer de los Amazones." Some years later, Billy Mellon and his wife, LeGrand, would make an excellent documentary film about it.

with cocaine. "Without it, these people could not survive," said Gwen. "Our driver would stop for a drink, drive wildly, and then after gradually slowing down, he would stop and drink again. We didn't understand this sequence until the trip was over."[10]

On the way back to Arequipa, they marveled at the "prehistoric astronomical trails going towards certain stars and certain seasons." Gwen and Larry took oranges and cigarettes to the 170 prisoners of the Arequipa Jail, breaking the cigarettes in half to stretch out the supply. "Conditions fairly good," Larry noted. "Since someone has stolen the antenna from the roof of the jail, I buy another one and help install it so that the prisoners can listen to the radio."

The Mellons did jail duty repeatedly that week, among other unpredictable things. One day was devoted to inspecting llamas and vicunas and methods of cross-breeding them. Another was spent with a Russian woman who offered to give Larry Russian lessons, which he happily accepted. On Easter, they asked to be taken to the local orphanage, where Michael, Jenny, and Ian passed out bamboo whistles and dolls they had made. The mother superior there showed them the kitchen and mentioned a shortage of plates; the children were eating on leaves.

Gwen and Larry, for their part, were trying to eat some of the local delicacy, *cui* (guinea pig), before packing up their *twenty* pieces of baggage for the return. A separate truck for the luggage was needed to get everything to the embarkation point in Mollendo.

"There were five of us, after all," says Gwen in self-defense. "But the bags were the easy part. Our ship was a freighter, and it was offshore. They warned us, 'It's open seas,' but I didn't know what that entailed: no dock, just a roadstead leading to a bluff at the edge of the sea. The boat's way down, and you're way up on the cliff, with big waves in between. They put you in a basket and swing it across and drop it down to the boat. The guy up above has to tie you just right. That's the only way you can get on. It was terrifying."

On the voyage home, they analyzed the possibilities of practicing medicine in Peru. They had seen a need, but perhaps not the greatest need. There would be no Peruvian future for them, but there would also be no forgetting the country. A few days after their return to Arizona, Larry noted in his diary: "Ordered 400 sets of aluminum dishes for Arequipa orphanage."

.   .   .

THE BIG EXCITEMENT upon their arrival home at Fort Rock was the long-awaited debriefing session with Jack and Anne Beau about their mission in Lambaréné. It had taken them several leisurely months to get back to Arizona, by way of France, and belatedly deliver Dr. Schweitzer's letter and exotic presents. Larry wrote in May 1948 to thank Schweitzer and to relate the fate of his most extraordinary gift:

> The carved stone figures and the mask worked in soft wood are marvels of primitive art which will honor our new home. The little black pen holder with a snake and crocodile sits on my desk and stares at me with an evil eye. The fine grass cloth, as well as the elephant tusk and the hippo wisdom tooth, lend interest to our mantelpiece. On delivering the latter, Jack repeated your warnings that the dry climate would explode the big tooth, and I must tell you that before the night was over there was a great bang which woke my wife and sent her looking for the cause, which was none other than the wisdom tooth which had cracked along its entire length![11]

"It was a huge, terrible-looking thing," Gwen recalls, "and exploded all over the room. Lucky nobody was there. So that was the sad end of the hippopotamus tooth from Dr. Schweitzer."

There was no time to lament it. Within days of their return to the ranch, Tulane informed them that Larry would need to attend summer school plus two full additional years just to make up his premed requirements. It was decided that he should begin immediately. Within a week, he was in New Orleans, leaving Gwen behind with the little task of closing down their ranch.

Only a Mellon, or only *Larry* Mellon, could have made the following diary entries on his first days at Tulane as a student: "May 5: Pick up books for my summer classes, Chemistry 105 and Math 151, algebra and plane trig. May 6: Buy a home in New Orleans, 301 Northline Street. Swimming pool installed."

Then a brief return to Arizona—"May 28: Supper with Bill Jones and crew. Looks like I've seen my last roundup! They've just put 500 cows through. May 29: My last day at Fort Rock."

Next morning, on his father's eightieth birthday, he left again for Tulane and was soon happily enjoying "my first classes for 20 years. It's really fun to be playing schoolboy again. In fact, much more fun than it used to be. Math and simple chemistry are all I have to worry about this summer . . . Confidence in myself regarding schoolwork is returning. These young kids could beat me hollow, but few of them are trying."

He was even happier after Gwen and the children arrived at the end of June: "The novelty of attending class again has not worn off yet, and

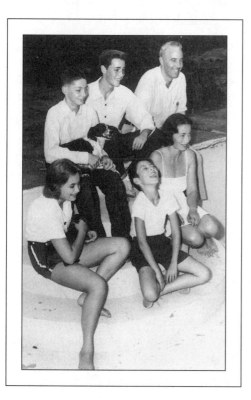

THE MELLONS POOLSIDE
IN NEW ORLEANS

I'm enjoying it 200 percent. Having reached the age of 38, my world has suddenly changed from one of debonair, cowboy joviality to one of compelling effort, and the cares and sacrifices which attend city-dwelling humanity. It would seem a poor exchange if one were not a Christian!"

By July, however, the novelty had worn off.

"I need at least four hours for homework every day. I find oxidation reduction equations difficult to understand . . . Midsemester exams. I take a two-hour math exam this morning. Big chemistry exam—I think I passed, although I confused boiling point with molal freezing-point depression. There's a couple of points shot!"

When the mid-semester marks were posted, he was delighted to find he had made A's in chemistry and math. But in the second term of summer school, things got considerably tougher, thanks to plane trigonometry and qualitative analysis. The marathon four-hour trig final in August "almost finished me off," he noted, but he got the requisite C in the course.

In off hours, he read Dr. Schweitzer's *Indian Thought and Its Development*. Mahatma Gandhi's philosophy of nonviolence appealed deeply to Schweitzer and Mellon alike, even as it threatened and terrified the colonial worlds they cared about, especially following Gandhi's shocking assassination earlier that year. Post-war instability was growing worldwide. "For months," wrote Mellon in September, "the newspapers and radio have been telling us that war with Russia is inevitable."

These days held more of the paradoxical juxtapositions that distinguished Larry Mellon from the average undergraduate. On September 16, he stood in line with everyone else to enroll in courses for the 1948–49 Tulane school year (physics, sociology, biology, and Portuguese), and soon after had his first physics lab "in which we chose partners, two to a desk." The next day, he was summoned to Pittsburgh as a voting member of the W. L. and May T. Mellon Foundation to approve his family's gift of $6 million to create the nation's first Graduate School of Industrial Administration at Pittsburgh's Carnegie Institute of Technology.

On Oct. 1, he dutifully flew to Pittsburgh. His father's chauffeur met him and took him straight to Ben Elm, where his father, siblings, aunt, and uncle were waiting. Mellons do not waste time: The business meeting was conducted swiftly, the gigantic gift approved, and red-eyed Larry was whisked back to the airport for New Orleans at seven the next morning. "He had to get back to school," says Gwen with a sanguine shrug. "You lose a day or two in school and you're lost."

Larry's conscientious involvement in the family foundation activities would have a direct bearing and utility in his own plans. When informed that Gulf Oil was issuing new stock at 4 to 1, Larry asked his attorney about transferring his own considerable shares to the May T. and W. L. Mellon Foundation, in order to avoid paying capital-gains taxes. The lawyers concluded that could not be done but set about exploring other ways to maximize the philanthropic potential of his assets. On October 28, 1948, he and Gwen launched their Yavapai Charitable Foundation with an initial founders' gift of 400 Gulf shares worth $29,450.*

A few months later, in March 1949, Larry allowed his name to be placed on the board of solicitation of the Sara Mayo Hospital in New Orleans, a clinic begun in 1905 by women doctors for needy families. "Gwen has already raised $300,000 to provide more bed space," he noted in his diary.

Unlike the journals of Albert Schweitzer, those of Larry Mellon rarely fail to include his wife's activities as well as his own. She was doing a lot more than just fund-raising:

> Gwen attends Council for Christians and Jews meeting, also tea at the Protestant Home for Babies. . . . Gwen spends day doing chauffeur duty for 280 displaced persons just arrived from central Europe. Their welcome to America consisted of standing for two hours in the

---

*An example of the Mellons' tax burden came in the form of Larry's fourth-quarter IRS bill for 1948: Taxes on his $44,000 Gulf dividends were $39,000. ("Rough!" was the one-word comment in his diary.) The Yavapai Foundation, named for the Arizona county where they had lived and ranched, was forerunner of the Grant Foundation that later served as a conduit by which Larry's and other money could flow to support his hospital in Haiti. The name Grant was chosen to honor his wife, and to avoid the name Mellon, in view of his constant sensitivity to the family's notoriety.

rain listening to six senators they can't understand. . . . Gwen is working very hard at Veterans Hospital in the lab, learning to make blood
counts and studying bacteriology. With Gwen's help, I finish my sociology paper, "An Original Study of Group Conflict," about the forest
service and cattlemen. . . . Gwen assists at her first autopsy at Veterans Hospital. She is pleased to find she could "take it."

Soon enough, for reasons of time and family, Gwen abandoned her
original plan to go through med school and decided on the shorter
course (by two years) of medical technician. Asked if she ever regretted
not becoming a doctor, she replies, "Never. I was terribly busy as it
was." She was even busier after taking on a three-day-a-week job at Veterans Hospital on Lake Pontchartrain, where she worked in the pathology lab and acquired such delicate skills as how to assist at a sternal
marrow tap.

Christmas of 1948 was celebrated in Florida with Big Pa on his
yacht—a full-course turkey dinner and champagne. Brother Matthew's
Melmar was anchored alongside, and each boat had its own beautifully
decorated tree on the stern deck.

At eighty, W. L. had recently retired after forty-six years as chairman
of the board at Gulf, which by then had 42,000 employees and $839
million in assets and was the world's fourth-largest oil producer. Before
leaving, he had designated several blacks to be station operators and
promoted a Jew to head one of Gulf's refineries. The latter appointment
prompted a delegation of stockholder-advisers to come in and say, "You
ought to get him out and put a Presbyterian in there." W. L.'s reply was
relished by the family that holiday: "Go out and find me a better-quali-
fied Presbyterian."[12]

The New Year found Larry reading Sir Edwin Arnold's translation of
the *Bhagavad Gita* ("I find it extremely inspiring in its discipline"), but
not for long. Most of January was devoted to hard studying for his semester finals. On January 28 he was "delighted to find out my [physics
exam] grade of 78 out of 100 was the highest in the class." A week later
he registered for the second semester. He had received special permis-

sion to take seven courses, twenty-four credit hours, even though "fitting them into the daily schedule is better than a chess game." Doing so was a testament to his stellar organizational abilities. "He was just doing it all as fast as possible to get into medical school," says Gwen. He also was cramming for the all-day medical college admissions test that month.

Nevertheless, for balance and sanity, there was a musical and cultural life to live, as well: "Locate a Pincel-Muller used clarinet, in good shape," he noted, "and have fun learning the fingering and trying to get some tone." A few days later he and Jenny spent an evening playing accordion-piano duets, after which the whole family enjoyed seeing James Stewart in the spooky new Hitchcock film, *Rope*.

Their social life was a little more problematic.

"Gwen and I received many invitations to attend this or that Mardi Gras ball," Larry recorded in February 1949. "Fortunately, we have good reason to refuse all or most of them." A week later, Gwen, without Larry, attended a ball given by the elite Mystic Society. She was unimpressed, said Larry, "and termed the whole procedure childish, expensive and boring." Nor did they enjoy the annual Cadaver Ball, a drunken spring ritual beloved by the younger med students. "Good band, though," Gwen recollects.

More their style was dinner at the Beverly Country Club, followed by "the hillbilly songs of Dorothy Shay," and the New Orleans appearance of Carmen Miranda and her five-piece Brazilian orchestra. Dixieland jazz and the periodic local exhibitions of "Mexican jitterbug" were also favorites of Larry's. But all such jottings in his diaries were superseded by the one and only entry in red capital letters, dated March 16, 1949:

WORD ARRIVES FROM TULANE SCHOOL OF MEDICINE SAYING I AM ENROLLED IN NEXT FALL'S FRESHMAN CLASS.

The work that lay ahead was sobering. But his dream was now closer to reality, inspired as always by Schweitzer. That inspiration was heightened by the exciting announcement of Schweitzer's first American visit, to deliver the main address at the Goethe Bicentennial celebration in Aspen, Colorado. Larry was determined to finally meet him face to face.

Schweitzer's ocean liner arrived in the United States in June 1949, and, since he refused to fly, he boarded the Santa Fe Chief for the long trek to Denver. His fellow passengers on the train included two women who kept staring at him and whispering together. Finally, one worked up her nerve to approach and said, "Dr. Einstein, could we have your autograph?" Schweitzer politely took the book and signed "Dr. Albert Einstein, courtesy of Albert Schweitzer."

A week after Schweitzer—not Einstein—appeared on the cover of *Time*, Larry spoke with him by phone and happily accepted an invitation to Sunday lunch at the Gramercy Park apartment of Dr. Emory Ross, where the Schweitzers were staying in New York City.

"Spent from 11:30 until 3:30 with the doctor talking about Africa and the requisites of a medical missionary," Larry recorded after their first meeting, July 17: "Mrs. Schweitzer is extremely charming and bright."

Larry translated for Schweitzer and some pharmaceutical company salesmen who were also present that day. "What can we give you, Dr. Schweitzer?" they kept asking. "I could use three vials of such-and-such," he would reply. "You mean three dozen?" they'd inquire. "No, *three*," he would answer. And so it went.

"Everything he asked for, they wanted to give him ten times the amount," Gwen recalls. "Dr. Schweitzer couldn't get over it, and they couldn't understand that he had no place to put it. It was a matter of storage, and not having it spoil and be wasted."

Finally, Schweitzer said to Larry, "Let's take a walk," and they escaped the crowded apartment for a private stroll around Gramercy Park that produced even greater bonding. "He was so absorbed," Mellon remembered, "that I had to guide him. He did not seem to see traffic lights or traffic. He wanted me to know and to understand everything he had done."[13] At one point during their walk, Schweitzer saw something shiny on the sidewalk and picked it up to examine. A discussion ensued between the two as to whether it was a diamond or just a piece of glass.

Schweitzer finally concluded that it wouldn't be worth much either way, and whimsically tossed it away.

.   .   .

TULANE WASTED no time. On Larry's first day of med school, "We get our cadavers and begin dissecting," he recorded. "A most interesting and inspiring day." He was also excited about his introduction to psychiatry class, offered to freshmen med students that year for the first time. He was less excited, a few days later, when his first anatomy quiz was returned with a large "F." Meanwhile, Gwen was enrolled in her medical technician's course across town at Loyola: "We waved to each other once in a while, in passing."

On October 8, 1949, at age eighty-one, William L. Mellon Sr. died "a relative pauper," said family chronicler David Koskoff. Of his $22 million estate, $15 million worth of Big Pa's Gulf stock had to be sold just to pay the inheritance tax. Of the remainder, his Canadian property went to daughter Peggy, $100,000 to son-in-law John F. Walton Jr., $50,000 to William S. Moorhead (his lawyer and golf buddy), and equal trusts of $1,461,203 apiece to Peggy and his other three children.[14]

Larry flew to Pittsburgh to attend his father's funeral and returned to New Orleans that same night at 1 a.m. The tyrannical demands of med school took precedence over mourning and all else, as his diary entries of the next few weeks suggest:

Oct. 14: Buy my first stethoscope for $7.50 . . . Oct. 21: Practical exam in gross anatomy. 50 structures to identify with 1½ minutes allowed for each. Had the distinct feeling I did not do very well. Oct. 26: Practical exam in histology, identifying 15 tissue structures in 45 minutes. I miss 6 of them, which earns me a failing grade.

Gwen's own unique medical education, meanwhile, continued apace. She was taken under the wing of Dr. R. J. Walker, Tulane's prominent malariologist, who employed her in his lab and trained her in malaria control and tropical entomology.

"Dr. Walker said, 'I want you to come and work for me. I can teach you in one week what you're going to learn in this school.' For my first lesson, he pointed to a big microscope and said, 'All right, Mrs. Lemmon'—there was a famous family in New Orleans named Lemmon and he could never get us straight—'now, take that apart.' You can bet he made sure I learned how to take off every piece and put it back together again—a very valuable lesson. But the main business was to learn about the feeding and breeding of anopheles mosquitoes, and the psychotic ward where a malarial treatment for syphilis was being tried out."

She had to raise, feed, infect, and then dissect these mosquitoes, taking off the heads and the salivary glands and the stomachs with the eggs in them. All this was done under a dissection microscope at a rate of forty an hour.

Charity Hospital was then conducting induced-malaria therapy and insulin and electric-shock treatments for mental illness resulting from syphilis. Those new procedures tended to reduce spirochetes in the brain and help in some cases, and a new ward for such patients had just opened. "The nurses were all locked up in glass booths," Gwen remembers, "and I would walk through carrying my mosquitoes in a cage."

Far from feeling competitive, Larry took huge pride in her achievements, which, academically, were better than his own. "Gwen takes a practical exam in medical technology and makes 100 percent," he noted one night in his diary. Studying came easier to her than to him. "Took final exam in histology, 4 hours," he writes on November 10, 1949. "It put as high a degree of nervous pressure on me as any scholastic experience I've met so far. . . . Study again until midnight."

Larry's prematurely gray hair was getting whiter these days. He looked older than his years and, in fact, was developing an ulcer. "I remember one time I was sitting in a medical movie," he told biographer Burton Hersh, "and next to me was the youngest boy in the class. There was a character on the screen, and I said, 'Hey, that guy looks like Wendell Willkie, doesn't he?' And the fellow said, 'I don't know, Grandpa, he died before I was born.' Another fellow made a very comforting remark to me—he said, 'You know, it's harder to stay the last in your class than the first.' I thought that was a very kind thing to say."[15]

Gwen smiles at the memory: "Larry was very slow. He'd get lost and involved in details. Young kids can read a page and pick it right up, but when you're older, your mind is not quite as agile. Another reason he had so much trouble is that he wanted to get it *all*."

Larry also had more on his mind than the average student. One of his and Gwen's many overlapping interests was the National Leprosarium in Carrville, Louisiana, which they often visited. Gwen once took Schweitzer's own beloved nurse, Emma Hausknecht, to Carrville. She was terrified: "The patients were doctors, ministers and lawyers, but Emma couldn't get over the fact that they all shook hands with me and knew me. She'd never seen anybody with leprosy. People think it's highly contagious, but it's not. It takes close proximity for years."

In late 1949, the Mellons and their friends Edgar and Edith Sterns set up scholarships for African medical students who, it was hoped, would serve with Schweitzer in Lambaréné. Larry and Gwen personally contributed $20,000 to subsidize the education of the first three doctors from Gabon, with the understanding that they would never know the names of their patrons.

"They indeed became the first Gabonese doctors, but none of them went to Dr. Schweitzer's hospital," Gwen says. "It was disgraceful. The obvious reason was financial—to go into more lucrative practice. The sad thing was that Larry did it for Dr. Schweitzer, and no Gabonese doctor to this day has ever worked at the Schweitzer hospital."

The Mellons were way ahead of their time. In February 1950, Larry was exploring "ways we could help financially in African-American relations. Gwen and I decide to help with program to educate American Negroes about Africa and make them proud of their origins." Afro-American studies departments are now *de rigueur* at virtually every university, but the idea was radically new then. The Mellons wanted to establish such a program at Tulane, but the idea was dismissed. Segregation in New Orleans was a deeply entrenched way of life, not conducive to concepts of black awareness in education. No Negro had yet been admitted to Tulane.

Charity Hospital, where Gwen first served as a nurse's aide, was a racial mirror image, one side white patients, the other black. Black nurses and aides were permitted to work on the white side, but no whites on the black side. "It was my first real exposure to hospital work," she says. "Since I was the only married woman in the group, they gave me all the men. I learned how to feed people, bedpan duty— all the basics. It was good, disciplined training. Those Catholic Sisters of Charity were wonderful."

Not so wonderful was the prevailing racism. "A young man around 19 climbs into our living room window," Larry recorded that September. "Police arrest him later in the day and say he has a jail record. Gwen and I are greatly concerned at the shabby and shameful way Negro suspects are treated."

·   ·   ·

THE TURN OF THE NEW DECADE brought no great improvement in Larry's academic fortunes. "Take quiz in neuroanatomy and fail miserably, even after studying it hard last night," he wrote on January 12. "Medical school at times is very discouraging . . . Jan. 31: Final exams in gross anatomy this morning. What a relief to have that course behind me, even if I need to do some additional work this coming summer to work off a 'condition.'"

A "condition" was something like probation, the result of his grades in anatomy and embryology being "LP"—low passing.

"He didn't do famously," says Gwen. "The subject he really had trouble with was anatomy. Head and neck. He had to repeat it, and the whole family to this day can recite every muscle and bone from the shoulders up."

Larry and his fellow students spent February learning how to draw venous blood from one another. ("Al got 10 ccs out of me before coagulation set in and the syringe froze.") A typical day in March was devoted to "getting whirled in a chair in physiology lab, which proved that it's not hard to overstimulate the semicircular canals. I'm still dizzy!" April's highlight was a three-day starvation experiment to produce ketone bodies in his urine and measure chloride loss. In May, he was vaccinated for smallpox, by Gwen, and endured more physiology experiments, "knocking ourselves out with hyperventilation and asphyxia." His biochemistry final left him "plenty worried that I may not have passed. Freshman year lived up to its reputation for being discouraging." On May 28: "I walk the streets from 1 to 4 a.m. trying to get tired enough to sleep. I haven't recovered yet from the effects of that last exam." When the grades came in, there was more to recover from: "Shocked to learn my class standing for first year of med school—117th in a class of 123!"

But that month, his relationship with Albert Schweitzer graduated from mentor-pupil to something more like collegial equality. Schweitzer was now seeking *Mellon's* counsel. "Return from chemistry lab to find a letter waiting for me from Dr. Schweitzer, who says he has two young doctors who have come to stay 'not just for a year or two,'" Larry recorded. One was a European refugee with no passport, a married man involved with a lawyer's wife. The other had personal problems, too. It was a delicate situation, and Schweitzer was anxious about it, even as he was grateful for Larry's ongoing gifts:

The last several months have been extremely difficult. I have often wondered if I would be able to hold up under the strain of all the worries and the work. Since mid-February I have two capable young doctors at my side [and] an excellent surgeon has just arrived [who] will instruct the former in surgery. . . .

At this very moment the three of them are performing an operation on a complicated gynecological tumor by the electric light supplied by your generator! How many times have we blessed you for that. . . . It is working very well and we keep it up as best we can. Upon my return I was able to appreciate the value of all you sent us. Everything is extremely useful to us. You couldn't have chosen better. . . .

I cannot yet rest. From morning till night I am on call down at the hospital in order to initiate the two new doctors in medical and paramedical work. If things are to work smoothly, the doctors must know how to cope with many things besides medicine. I would like to get the hospital functioning so that it can continue when I am no longer here. That is why I am training these two doctors.[16]

Larry eventually helped find new positions for the two troublesome doctors. At the moment, his reply expressed the hope that they might spare Schweitzer some duties, "among them the task of repairing the water pump each time it becomes stubborn and capricious. Maybe what you now need is a mechanic who could maintain the pipes, the famous pump and other annoying machinery? But be careful, Doctor Schweitzer, for you will discover a trap. It is I, the mechanic-cowboy, who would come to your aid!"[17]

Mellon was keeping an eye on Europe, as well as Africa. After the Communist takeover of Czechoslovakia, John Foster Dulles had put him on the mailing list of the National Committee for Free Europe. Dulles' brother Allen, Larry's wartime OSS colleague, now contacted him to report on their mutual friend "Hub," a Czech spy for the West who had barely escaped with his life and for whom they both felt some responsibility. Dulles asked Mellon to help find him a job, and he did so.

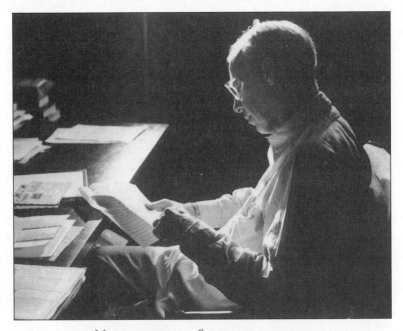

Mellon reading Schweitzer letter

Things were even worse in Asia: On June 25, 1950, the day before Larry's fortieth birthday, Communist North Korea declared war on the South. "Korea is the focus of everyone's attention in these nervous days," Mellon wrote. It was the subject of many more diary entries throughout that year.

His home front, by contrast, was the source of tranquility he much needed and valued. "My good fortune in having such a fine, healthy family and such a good wife overwhelm me at times," he wrote. "I reproach myself for not thanking God oftener." But he had no need to reproach himself for the attentions he paid them. "We have steaks and stop at Chez Wen's Voo Doo Room, where they let tarantulas down from the ceiling," he recorded after an exotic French Quarter outing with Gwen. Soon after, they had a close encounter of the pop-cultural kind: "Attend the drive-in movie. You sit in your car and an amplifier is furnished with a wire. Between shows there's a 10-minute intermission & everyone runs to the concession stand for cokes and popcorn and flirting."

Another night, no fewer than forty-seven teenagers attended a dance given by daughter Jenny at home. Larry and Gwen worked hard "to break the ice and get the dancing started, but it seemed hopeless until a penciled note was delivered to me by one of the boys. It read, 'We the people hereby request that the lights be lowered.'" That done, success was assured.

Dancing was always important to the Mellons; the whole family once trooped down to a local Arthur Murray studio for samba and rhumba lessons, which came in handy for a European cruise in July, where the nightly dancing went on until 3 A.M. In Paris, they walked the Champs Élysées, explored Toulouse-Lautrec's haunts in Montmartre, and met several of Larry's old friends from the French Resistance. From there, it was on to visit Omaha Beach, then Spain and Switzerland in August. By the time they boarded ship in England for the trip home, they had driven 5,000 kilometers in thirty-one days.

.   .   .

LARRY MELLON'S SOPHOMORE YEAR in med school began in September 1950 with the purchase of an intimidating set of pathology, bacteriology, and pharmacology textbooks. He had his medical work cut out for him in school. Outside the classroom, he expanded the WASPish horizons of his upbringing in a whole new academic-social circle of friends. One was Tulane philosophy professor Jim Feibelman, who regaled them with witty talk of a new science he had just invented, "psychosynthesis." It was the opposite of psychoanalysis: The doctor recited his troubles to the patient.

"Jim was a strange, charming man," says Gwen. "He had six Rodin sculptures, one of which was of himself, and we had wonderful dinners there. We later took him to the Yucatan—his first time out of the country—and he was scared to death and wouldn't go out of his room. He was one of many interesting Jewish people in New Orleans. The Sterns were our very close friends, great philanthropists, but they would always leave New Orleans during carnival because they weren't invited to the balls and affairs, due to their religion. When the Israel war started, they were among all the Jewish people called to a meeting in a movie theater. A man sat up on the stage with a roster and called out, 'So-and-so, you have such-and-such business?' Yes. 'Fine. You're signed up for $10,000.' And they all produced it."

In October, UN forces reached the 38th parallel in Korea and Gen. Douglas MacArthur made his surrender ultimatum, subsequently pushing into North Korea. By December, a million Chinese were massed on the border and President Truman declared a national emergency. But life and med school in Louisiana went on.

"Gwen's first day of practical nursing hard and very depressing at the Colored Home for Incurables," Larry noted. The name of the institution spoke volumes—and the volumes could have been written by Tennessee Williams. "That's what it was," remembers Gwen. "People were well kept and comfortable there, but New Orleans was a weird place. So many people had aunts or uncles up in the attic who were alcoholics or drug addicts."

Larry was now studying the pathology of tropical diseases and was very excited about it: "Too busy to eat today. Use every spare moment in bacteriology lab. Gwen & I work at parasitology and look at slides of Ascaris, hookworm, cyclops, etc . . . Gwen teaches me how to make red cell counts." It was not the first or last time she would impart a newly acquired, useful skill to him, an example of how their separate medical training dovetailed. She summed up their lives wryly in a February 14, 1951, poem to Larry:

My valentine,
He has no time . . .
But I have no peeve
I wait the eve
And the evening is mine
From 6:30 to 6:39
When in between bites
He often recites
The PH for something very alkaline . . .
He looks into my eyes at night
But with a machine and a little light . . .

In March, Larry concluded his elaborate x-ray examination with a gall bladder visualization and was "glad Dr. Teitelbaum is finished with me after a week of laxatives, enemas and barium meals!" He was issued a box of 100 blood and bone marrow slides to master and then sent to examine hearts in the wards of Charity Hospital, where the presiding doctor was "interested in my ability to outline the heart by oscillatory percussion." Soon after, he bought an odd Columbia recording of heart murmurs and arrhythmias: "You listen to it with stethoscope on and eyes closed and learn to diagnose the various signs."

In April, as he was attending lectures in neurology, ophthalmology, and psychiatry, Gwen began work in the operating room of Charity Hospital. One night she came home with two living slide specimens, on loan from Dr. Walker's lab, of blood containing microfilaria*: "We're much excited to observe the little fellows pushing their way among the

*Microfilaria are the embryonic or prelarval forms of the filarial worms, found in the bloodstream and tissues, that cause sleeping sickness (encephalitis lethargica).

red blood cells," Larry wrote. "They have survived two days under a cover slip."

Schweitzer wrote to say he would be in Europe that summer, suggesting the Mellons postpone their trip to Lambaréné but visit him in Günsbach. "You will only benefit fully from [Lambaréné] if I am here," he cautioned. But they decided to go both places and duly got vaccinations for yellow fever, smallpox, typhoid, and tetanus. "We shivered all night with chills," Larry recorded, yet they still managed to pack all their instruments and books for the journey.

His classic, unironic diary entry before leaving: "Spend a pleasant day reading Warshaw's *Malaria: The Biography of a Killer*."

.   .   .

FIRST STOP WAS the Savoy Plaza, their favorite New York City hotel. It was there, a few years earlier in their ranch years, that Larry had decided to throw away all his fancy clothes. Gwen did much the same but had stored a few things in the basement, and now, when some relatives invited her to a formal dinner, she went down to retrieve them: "I grabbed a hat and dress and put them on, and we were sitting at dinner, all fancily dressed, polite conversation, music playing. Just as the waiter came to take our orders, there was a big *plunk* in front of me, and everyone turned to watch this big mothball that dropped out of my hat, rolling around and around on the empty plate. It was terrible."

The twinkle in her eye, however, suggests otherwise.

Originally, when the Mellons were about to cancel their African trip because Schweitzer wouldn't be there, Gwen's friend Dr. Walker argued they should go anyway. When Larry countered that he did not like making a trip without a purpose, Dr. Walker secured them positions on a medical team headed for Liberia to do a malaria survey on the Firestone Rubber Co. plantations there.

Before leaving for Africa, Larry and Gwen met Erica Anderson, the great photographer who had achieved international recognition shooting Schweitzer at work in Lambaréné. She and Schweitzer developed a close friendship: When the doctor had a lecture tour, she would ship her car to Europe or Africa for his convenience—and her own.

"It was an open roadster," said Gwen. "The top could go on or off, and they would go place to place giving concerts. He'd pick up people on the road, and Erica had a tape recorder in the car so you could hear the conversation. They had a deep friendship and also a father-daughter kind of relationship. He was very, very fond of her."

Anderson and the Mellons likewise became close when she visited Deschapelles, where she took beautifully lit, soulful pictures of Dr. Mellon as a practicing physician.* But aside from her brilliant photography, Anderson was a colorful character with a colorful background herself. Gwen's favorite example:

Erica had a nice apartment on Central Park West, where she'd brought her mother from Europe after the war. Her mother used to go down and sit in the park, and one day she looked up and saw her beloved childhood friend, Rudy—hadn't seen each other in 20 years. So they fell on each other and had a tearful reunion and agreed to meet for dinner that night, and then went their own way. But they forgot to say where they lived or where they'd meet. So the next day they had to go back to the park and sit and wait again for each other. Isn't that wonderful?

The Mellons set foot on African soil for the first time on June 27, 1951, and, typically, went to work immediately, taking and diagnosing blood samples in Monrovia. That night at a Firestone party, they met the plantation crowd and danced until 2:30 A.M., then paid a courtesy call the next morning to the Liberian minister of health. But they had no interest in being just guests or social members of the team. From then on, for four solid weeks, they did nothing but work, as Larry recorded:

6/30: At hospital by 8 to work on slides. Take 60 more blood tests, over 30 percent positive for malaria. 7/1: Visit nearby villages and hy-

---

*When Schweitzer died in 1965, he left Erica Anderson a sum of money with which, a year later, she founded the Albert Schweitzer Center in Great Barrington, Massachusetts. Erica would later develop Hodgkin's disease and summon Gwen from Haiti to help her in New York in the 1970s. "She lost heart after Dr. Schweitzer died," says Gwen. Anderson passed away in 1976.

droelectric plant. 7/2: Take 50 bloods. Malaria incidence high. 7/4: Tour mosquito breeding places. 7/5: Take smears from 2-month-old baby with sleeping sickness. 7/6: To date, taken blood from 476 children for survey. 7/9: Sleeping sickness conference at Leopoldville. 7/11: Microscope work all day. 7/12: Finish up 233 blood samples taken in Monrovia. Malaria incidence Krutown is 74 percent; Vaitown, 64 percent; St. Theresa School (elite) 20 percent. 7/14: Drums all night again for second day in a row. 7/21: Complete our survey of 1,000 children.

On July 22, Gwen's fortieth birthday, they packed up their lab equipment and microscopes and set out for Lambaréné, even though Schweitzer was not there. After arriving in Leopoldville, they crossed immediately to Brazzaville, only to discover that the plane to Lambaréné had already left and the next one wasn't due for a week. With time on their hands, they took a car ride down the banks of the Congo River to see the huge rapids below Brazzaville, ending up at the Hotel Metropole for some dancing. ("Not too gay," Larry reported. "We have to walk a couple of miles in the sand. No taxis.") They spent a day with George Carpenter, whose Congo Press "LECO" in Brazzaville published biblical translations and schoolbooks in African dialects. Later the Mellons sent a $5,000 donation.

When they learned that a small launch was leaving for Lambaréné the following day, they switched plans. Boarding the boat at 5 A.M., they found it crowded with lumbermen and a few missionaries bound for their posts. It took twelve hours to negotiate the Ogowe, a big river with dangerous currents. Word of their arrival had miraculously been received, and they were met at Lambaréné by a pirogue rowed by four lepers.

"I am hurrying to write you a couple of words telling you that at last we have arrived at the hospital and to let you know of the great joy we feel to be here in Lambaréné," Mellon wrote Schweitzer on August 2, 1951. "I had a pretty good idea what the hospital would look like but two things struck me. The first was the wonderful calm which surrounds it, the second was its size."

There, as everywhere they went, the Mellons experienced by doing rather than watching. "Helped Dr. Naegele operate after breakfast," Larry noted the second day. "We do two hernias, one hydrocele and one 4-pound scrotum excision with hemicastration. Gwen sets up her microscope and works with Joseph and Dr. Percy. In the afternoon, we visit one of the three leper villages and make slides of nasal mucous and skin scrapings."

On their final day in Lambaréné, a Sunday, he and Gwen visited three leper villages before ending up at a Protestant mission for church services. That old mission held symbolic importance for them: It had been the site of Schweitzer's first hospital, and the sermon was in both Gabois and French. The next morning, upon their departure, the entire hospital staff assembled on the riverbank to wave them off.

Later, when Larry and Gwen were trying to decide what to send, they reflected that Lambaréné's conditions were shocking by U.S. standards. There were no screens in the operating room, for example, to keep out the flies. Larry had asked the doctor in charge whether he could send screening, but the reply was "No, not without asking Dr. Schweitzer." Not screens, not sheets, not anything. It had to do partly with why he wouldn't let the New York drug salesmen send him too many products, storage, but it was also related to his profound and sometimes problematic belief in "reverence for life," which extended to flies, mosquitoes, and even rats, which dined on the contents and containers of his pharmacy.

"He would get little boxes of medicine," says Gwen, "and mark what they contained on five sides—because of the ants."

Undaunted by Schweitzer's peculiarities, the Mellons never ceased being attentive to what they knew was needed. They went ahead and sent the wire screening and many other useful things over the years, as the following effusion from Schweitzer attests:

I received [all] the precious items [you sent] to the hospital. I was completely overcome by your generosity towards my work. What a help this cloth will be! When I see the native members of my staff walking around in rags, I imagine their faces when we dress them in the pants and shirts that we are getting from you! I can already picture their astonishment. They are paid very modestly compared to the natives employed by other European companies here. Thus I am particularly pleased to be able to give them decent clothing, thanks to you.[18]

Deeply moved by their Lambaréné visit, the Mellons looked forward to their European appointment with Schweitzer more than ever. From Africa, they flew to Lisbon ("World War II didn't hurt Portugal!" observed Larry) and thence to Paris, where they danced at the Scheherazade nightclub into the wee hours. Finally, on August 17, they arrived in Günsbach and found the way to Schweitzer's house, catching their first memorable glimpse of his shaggy head in the doorway. Gwen recalls some magical moments of that long-anticipated encounter:

It was a lovely house, very close to a country road. At lunch, the talk was very easy, nothing too philosophical. He tended to do most of the talking, but he gave other people a chance, and there were long silences, too. Not a lot of chatter. When Mrs. Schweitzer spoke, nobody else said a word.

In the afternoon, he and I went for a little walk and sat across the street on his woodpile. I commented on the size of it, and he said, "Always be sure you marry a man with a good wood pile." Any conversation with him was unpretentious and unpredictable. He said he liked my dress "because it has nice big pockets." Later he told us he was going over to the church to play the organ—"Come with me!"— and we did. He played a little Bach, beautifully, and Larry played for a while, too.

The day went perfectly. But Gwen had an uncomfortable little problem she could no longer keep to herself:

I picked something up in Lambaréné and didn't notice it until we got to Günsbach. I'd gone to Africa with just lightweight leather moccasins, easy to pack, washed them every night, kept them clean. They said, "In Africa, you absolutely must wear socks," but I didn't have any, and so I didn't. I thought it would be enough to keep the shoes very clean. But in Günsbach, I noticed this huge blister on my big toe.

At times like that, it was good to be married to a doctor, or at least to a second-year med student.

"Larry looked at it and opened it up and out came this long, ugly parasite, all coiled up, called a Guineaworm. Awful-looking thing!"

Podiatry crisis solved, the Mellons and Erica Anderson, who had just arrived, were taken around the next day by Schweitzer's faithful Emma Hausknecht. They visited his birthplace at nearby Kaysersberg, the chapel where his father used to preach, and the old Riquewihr medieval fortress with its torture tower and a church containing an organ installed by Schweitzer, who enjoyed building and restoring as well as playing the "king of instruments." At dinner that night, Helene Schweitzer turned her attention to Gwen:

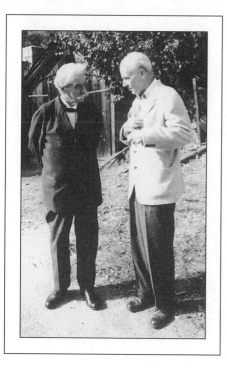

SCHWEITZER AND MELLON
IN GÜNSBACH

She said, "Mrs. Mellon, what part are you going to have in the hospital?" I said, "Mrs. Schweitzer, I have no idea yet, but I'm not worried." The next day she asked me the same thing again, "What part will *you* play?" I think it was a reflection of her own regret that she couldn't stay in Lambaréné because the climate there was bad for her TB. She was quite crippled by then, I think partly from a riding accident in her youth. She only went to Lambaréné periodically, for short

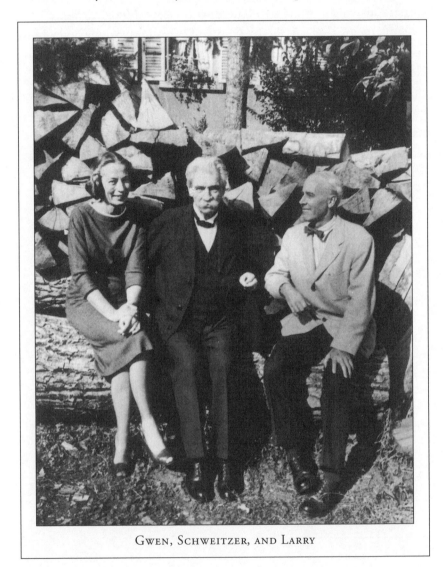

GWEN, SCHWEITZER, AND LARRY

stays, and felt bad about it. But the persistence of her question forced me to think about it.

The men continued their discussions of Lambaréné and Mellon's future project up to the moment of departure from Günsbach the next afternoon, August 21. "We walked down to the local station," Gwen recalls, "and this funny little wood-burning train came tooting up the valley. We got on and waved goodbye to Dr. Schweitzer from the window."

.   .   .

THE LAMBARÉNÉ AND GÜNSBACH pilgrimages had a powerful effect on the Mellons, whose search for a medical site of their own was now shifting into high gear. "We still have our sights set on Brazil," Larry wrote Schweitzer at one point, but he later ruled it out. The crucial process of locating the worst—meaning the best—place for a hospital was constantly preempted by the realities of medical school, where Larry was a very busy junior in the fall of 1951: "Sept. 17: Register at Tulane. Sept. 23: At hospital all afternoon doing lab work. Make a discovery! That if spinal fluid is not examined within a few minutes, yeast cells grow in it."

Always the quiet activist, he set about trying to get the junior class signed up as a group with a Blue Cross health plan. By the end of September he had succeeded, at rates that compare nostalgically with today's: $1.10 per month for a single man, $2.90 for a family, regardless of size.

As 1951 turned into 1952, Larry wasn't the only Mellon in college. He had been thrilled when his son, Billy, was accepted at Princeton the previous fall, and he was more thrilled to receive the school's *Nassau* literary review containing a story by Billy Mellon and high praise of it by English Professor A. R. Towers:

The display piece of the magazine is William Mellon's ambitious, vividly written, but somewhat disjointed story, "In the Event of Revolution," built upon a series of vignettes that effectively capture the ominous, lightning-streaked atmosphere of an unidentified Latin dictatorship. Mellon has a gift for hard, precise, descriptive writing that is yet (like Hemingway's best) strangely evocative. He can handle the revoltingly gruesome too without its degenerating into mere sensationalism.

Larry was further pleased that Billy would accompany him, Gwen, and the younger children on their first trip to Haiti, now in the planning stages, for Larry would research his thesis on tropical ulcers in fulfillment of a Tulane requirement. To transport all six of them and their gear, plus a mobile laboratory, Larry bought a four-wheel drive Dodge truck, also useful for navigating Haiti's narrow, muddy roads. He sent Schweitzer a snapshot of it (to "give you an idea of what we look like on wheels"), along with a flowchart of everyone's duties:

> Mrs. Mellon will act as chief lab technician. The oldest boy will be the courier and will obtain the necessary permits, contracts, etc. The second son will be in charge of driving the truck and its maintenance. The daughter (16 years old) takes charge of food supplies and cooking, while the youngest (who hopes to be a dentist one day) will help his sister with the dishes and his mother with the slides, etc. . . . One can always count on Americans to be fully organized![19]

In April, Gwen and Michael went shopping at Sears for camping equipment; Michael readied the new truck for shipment to Haiti, buying spare parts and installing new signal lights. In May, Larry ordered lab materials for taking blood and fecal specimens. A Miami newspaper heralded their departure on June 5: "Banker without ulcers [sic] is William Larimer (Gulf Oil) Mellon of Pittsburgh. . . . With his wife and the former captain of their 102-foot yacht, *Vagabondia*, he chose Joe's [Stone Crab restaurant] as his only stopover here en route to Haiti."

Research was the technical purpose of the Haitian trip. But their equally important, not-so-secret agenda was scouting a hospital site and discovering the unique people and customs of a culture that was completely new to them. They found early on that friends are made quickly in Haiti and that one always shakes hands upon meeting, lest insult be given. But according to protocol, *blancs,* white foreigners, must offer and extend a hand first. If not, the Haitians are impassive; if so, they brighten and respond instantly. The visitor must then adjust to the curious Haitian way of not clasping but just touching the hand, thumb up.

In Port-au-Prince, the charm and beauty of the people stunned the Mellons as much as did the poverty and disease—chains stronger than slavery's in a country with the lowest life expectancy and highest infant mortality in the hemisphere. The once-fertile island paradise with its fabulous mahogany forests was now deforested and eroded. Gone were the rich logwood, sugar, indigo, cocoa, coffee, and cotton industries. Malnutrition was as chronic as overpopulation. Two thousand people inhabited every square mile of tillable soil.

A Ministry of Health car conducted Larry on a tour of the Port-au-Prince medical school and government hospital. That night, he, Gwen and Billy went to the posh suburb of Pétionville, where they danced and met President Paul Magloire at the Cabane Choucoune, where good food and good *mereng* music abounded. The *mereng* was a popular Haitian dance, its rhythmic style similar to a French minuet. Big, round Cabane Choucoune with its high thatched roof was the most fashionable place to do it, and the president could often be found there on Saturday nights.

"People would wait in their homes, dressed and ready to go, their cars ready to roll," says Gwen. "When they heard the sound of the President's siren, they would race to follow it to secure space at his nightclub of choice for the evening." Getting a good table there had its disadvantages, however: The music and food were great, but you couldn't leave before the President, who liked to dance until three or four in the morning.[20]

A day or so later, the Mellons were introduced to Dr. François Duvalier, director of the Ministry of Health's landmark and highly successful *pian* program.

"*Pian* is the word for yaws," explains Gwen, "and it was a wonderful program. Everybody got a massive shot of penicillin and, almost overnight, there was no more yaws.* It cleared up syphilis at the same time. For a long time there was no syphilis in Haiti, until people started going to the States. It made Dr. Duvalier very popular and was a good basis for his political support later on."

The Mellons visited many experimental yaws and tropical-ulcer clinics, she recalls, "and Dr. Duvalier always went with us. In those days, he was very accessible, and we got to know him pretty well. He was absolutely the blackest man I ever saw, so black he was almost blue. He had a weak-fish handshake, very friendly, nothing terribly interesting about him. But he always received Larry and me with great dignity." When they saw him in later years, Dr. Duvalier always asked what happened to the little *blanc* boy who handed out the jelly beans with each prick of a finger at those clinics, referring to Ian.[21]

After securing letters from the Service Interamericain de Santé Publique and drivers' licenses allowing them to circulate in the interior, the Mellons left Port-au-Prince and traveled widely throughout the country, periodically checking in with the local police to say who they were and what they were doing. "That was important," says Gwen. "There was very little traffic in those days, and if you disappeared for any reason, they could track you that way." The Haitian army had given them permission to stay at regional army châtelets along the way and even provided them with a personal guard for portions of the journey.

When they arrived at the city of Port-de-Paix and inquired about a place to camp, they were escorted to a dance hall to spend the night. It had a roof and running water, luxurious by Haitian standards, and was located at the edge of a beach with beautiful, soft black sand and such crystal clear water that one could see down to the ocean floor.

Continuing on deeper into the countryside, they discovered that Haitian life begins extremely early. By the first light of dawn, women were already moving briskly up and down the paths on their way to

*Yaws is an infectious tropical disease primarily afflicting children, characterized by disfiguring, raspberry-like ulcers and eruptions of the skin. It is nonvenereal but caused by a spirochete bacteria that is closely related to the agent of syphilis.

market, carrying heavy baskets on their heads, often without even one hand to steady the perfectly balanced loads. It was fascinating to observe what the Mellons' friend Hal Krizan called "The Walking Tables":

It is often too dark [in the morning] to make out objects or people until they are close. So at first you only see a table against the light of the street lamp or sky. As it gets closer, you see that it's as tall as you. Then you see a person under it. . . .

The table and maybe a stool represent nearly all the personal property of the market lady's business. The commodities of her business, food, clothes, trinkets, etc. are piled on top of the walking table. . . . Some carry suitcases on their heads, opened to display the trinkets, cigarettes, etc. Fruit ladies dispense fresh fruit from large baskets on their heads. A lady with oranges will reach up to take an orange for the customer, peel it in one continuous peeling, put the peeling back in the basket for a secondary use, give the peeled orange to the customer, make change, then move on to the next sale, all without taking the basket from her head.

Much of the goods in Haiti move on the heads of the people. Women can carry 100 pound sacks of grain long distances in hilly, rocky terrain. They need help to lift the load up and down from their heads, but in between it's sheer individual strength and determination. . . .

Try an exercise. Put a heavy book on your head. Make it easier by building a "nest" out of a dishrag or hand towel. Walk around. Step up and down on a stool. Sit down, stand up. If the book falls, you have spilled your family's dinner.[22]

. . .

BACK IN PORT-AU-PRINCE, Larry's forwarded mail included his latest marks from Tulane: "Everything passed okay, but the shock is, 125th in a class of 128." They set out next in the Dodge truck for Léogâne, Cayes and the beautiful southern coastal town of Jacmel, where *La Nouvelle*, the local paper, reported:

We have just received the visit of Dr. and Mrs. Mellon. These amiable and distinguished personalities are traveling with their four children on vacation from the United States. . . . He will this year finish his studies at Tulane University and is going to pursue his studies in tropical diseases. . . . Dr. Mellon speaks French to perfection. He has rare courtesy and he seems agreeably impressed by the beauties of this country.

It was fascinating that even remote little Jacmel—in the Haiti of 1952—was attuned to "society." But for Larry, the trip was all business. Aside from his tropical-ulcer research, he helped conduct an important malaria survey, the grim results of which he reported to the Haitian government on July 15: 75 percent of the school children he'd tested had positive smears. Some consolation was that many of them "supported" the disease, meaning they could live without necessarily developing malaria.

In August, the Mellons drove back north to Port-de-Paix and then to Cap-Haïtien, the beautiful northern coastal city, Haiti's second largest, which had retained far more of its French colonial look and ambience than Port-au-Prince. The densely populated valley nearby "is delightful and might make a good clinic site," Larry noted. He and his whole family rode horses on difficult trails high up to the monumental Citadel, built in 1820 to house 5,000 men by King Henri Christophe—truly one of the man-made wonders of the world. It took two and a half hours each way, during which Ian found cannonballs and the remnants of an old flintlock rifle from Haitian struggles of yore.

Later, they traveled ninety rugged miles northwest of Port-au-Prince to the middle of Haiti for a look at the Artibonite Valley and some abandoned Standard Fruit Company buildings in a village called Deschapelles. But if that area made any big first impression on Larry, he failed to note it in his diary.

Of more immediate interest was the state visit to Haiti of Nicaragua's dictator-president, Anastasio Somoza, and the round of official events in his honor held by Haitian President Magloire in Port-au-Prince. The

Mellons cared nothing about Somoza, but they cared a lot about Magloire, whose approval was needed for any potential hospital project in Haiti. Their friend Dr. Élie Villard had spoken to Magloire and obtained an invitation for the Mellons to attend the president's August 23 gala for Somoza in Pétionville. Magloire's residence there, "La Boule," was a sprawling estate, gorgeously situated in the hills. Gwen would not soon forget the event:

> Somoza had come with his full army band, so needless to say Magloire's band was there, too, and all his officers, who were also beautiful dancers. The music started up and everyone danced. There was a buffet piled sky-high with food and when they announced "Dinner is served!" everybody leapt on it. By the time Larry and I got there, there wasn't a single bean left. We didn't know anybody and pretty soon we were ready to go, but Élie said, "You can't leave before the President." The dais was as big as a football field and the receiving line miles long. When we finally got up to him, Larry said, "Mr. President, I want to ask your permission to build a hospital in Haiti." Magloire said, "That's very nice, but this is no place to discuss it. You're holding up the line. I'll see you tomorrow morning."

Magloire was not present, however, when the Mellons arrived at the presidential palace the next morning. In his absence, they discussed their medical project with Dr. Duvalier, who suggested a location in Haiti's pine forest. Larry politely indicated his preference for the Artibonite Valley, based on the existing Standard plantation buildings there and on the simple grounds of *need*. A healthy ratio of doctors to population is 1 to 2,000. In Haiti overall, it was 1 to 10,000. But in the Artibonite—Haiti's rural mid-section, halfway between Port-au-Prince and Cap-Haïtien—it was much worse. That 600-square-mile area with 185,000 people contained not a single doctor in private practice and only two small government clinics.

Soon after, the Mellons got their audience with Magloire (and his wife) at the presidential palace, where they laid out their proposal for a hospital in Deschapelles, contingent on the availability of Standard Fruit's land and buildings there. When they finished, the president replied: "I'll tell you, this is the way it works here in Haiti: If Mrs. Magloire is for it, you'll get the green light. If not, you don't. If she is for it, write a brief proposal, and I'll run it through the Congress and turn it into law."[23]

All eyes turned to the first lady. Mrs. Magloire nodded approval.

Gwen and Larry left for New Orleans the next day.

.   .   .

A MOMENTOUS DECISION had been made, at least on the Mellons' part. "We now know Haiti better than 99 percent of Haitians," Mellon wrote Schweitzer, "since we systematically criss-crossed it from stem to stern." The need was in Haiti, and it was there they wanted to build their hospital. But a huge number of legal, financial, and logistical details had to be worked out, not least of which was the government's formal approval. Magloire had been receptive. But the type of foreign-supported, nonprofit institution Mellon was proposing would require legislative consent, and Haitian politics was a complex quagmire. Without knowing or needing to know any specifics, Schweitzer later warned Larry—in no-nonsense, Realpolitik terms—to be careful:

> I believe that Haiti, because of its relations with the United States, will give you greater guarantees of liberty than any South or Central American country.
>
> [But] I am very worried by the fact that you gave the impression that eventually you would give your hospital to the Republic of Haiti. If I were you, I would have said nothing of this. I admit that they probably won't go so far as to poison you if you don't give up the hospital when they want it, but they will be tempted to exert pressure on you in order to get control of their promised inheritance if they feel that they have been kept waiting too long. You have no idea what will become of your work when the Haitians run it as their own.[24]

In between classes during his senior year at Tulane, Larry was negotiating to acquire the Standard Fruit property but had to revise his strategy when his cash offer of $10,000 was rejected. This and other key elements of the scheme would take months to sort out, and much of the leg work was left to his wife.

First, Gwen and her sister Kathleen were dispatched to New York to gather information on hospital construction costs. Next he enlisted her to execute his plan, approved by Duvalier, to recruit five Haitian nursing students for training in the United States and subsequent service at his yet-to-be-built hospital in Haiti. By November 10, 1952, five days after Dwight Eisenhower's election as U.S. president, arrangements for that were in place. Gwen's next assignment was to find second-hand typewriters and hearing aids for the deaf and mute youngsters at Sister Joan Margaret's Episcopal School for Handicapped Children in Port-au-Prince.

Larry's diary entry of November 16 illustrates the two worlds they were straddling during a visit of their friend Scott Lockwood: "Scott, Gwen and I complete map of Deschapelles. Practice suture tying on Gwen and Scott after supper."

In December, he delivered his first baby (the mother was a seventeen-year-old Charity Hospital patient), to be followed by many more. As 1953 began, he was working on his tropical-ulcer thesis and Gwen was busy "collecting information on schools of nursing for colored girls" in preparation for the five Haitian students. They arrived in Miami that February and were whisked directly to the Harlem YWCA in New York, one of the few American cities then with nursing schools enlightened enough to admit Negroes.

April brought two giant steps forward: In Haiti, President Magloire agreed to make the Deschapelles property available for a hospital, while in Harrisburg, Pennsylvania, the charter for the nonprofit corporation that would serve as conduit for Mellon funding of the hospital was formally approved: In honor of Gwen, it would bear her surname and be called the Grant Foundation

Larry had also made up his mind and informed Dr. Schweitzer about another significant appellation:

My wife and I have decided that the name for this hospital should be "The Hospital Albert Schweitzer," if you have no objections. This decision stems from the fact that the idea of devoting ourselves to the dark-skinned race was not our own but has its origins in your work in Gabon. . . . With your permission we would like our work to remain linked in some way to the brother-institution situated in a corner of another continent—one which illuminated our path.[25]

Schweitzer's warm response, received in May: "Let me tell you how touched I am that your hospital should bear my name. I am truly moved, more than I can say, by this mark of friendship. I wish you all the best in your work. The beginnings will be difficult. But you are courageous."[26]

A few days later, Larry read his long-in-the-making "Diagnosis of Chronic Tropical Ulcer" at the senior scientific conference, and on May 19 he took his last medical exam at Tulane.

It was, God knew, cause for celebration. A bevy of family and friends arrived for Larry's med-school graduation on June 2 and the elegant fête for 185 that followed, featuring dinner and dancing to the Papa Celestin orchestra.

"Everybody came, including all his professors," Gwen said. "When I was dancing with Max Lapham, the dean, I said, 'I was so scared . . .,' and he said, '*You* were scared? *I* was more scared!' The other students originally viewed Larry as very odd and called him 'Grandpa' because of his bifocals, but they ended up electing him president of his class. It was lovely. "

Lovely, but not quite over. Larry now had to prepare for his state board exams to get a license to practice medicine in Louisiana. Assuming that went well, there was still the little matter of his residency obligation.

For the moment, however, those matters were put on the back burner in favor of a pressing appointment, much dreaded by Gwen, in New York. She and Larry were due there on June 14 for a reception at Emory Ross' home in honor of their Haitian nurses, whom the Mellons would meet for the first time. The reception wasn't what worried Gwen. It was the fact that Larry had agreed to join Ross's Disciples of Christ Church on Park Avenue at Eight-fifth Street, and that the whole family was slated to undergo its total-immersion baptismal rite.

"Dr. Ross was a minister there as well as a wonderful friend of ours and of Dr. Schweitzer's, and he was so anxious for us to join the church," she says. "Larry agreed to it as a favor to him, but we were so embarrassed. We didn't handle it very well, I'm afraid. They put bathing caps on our heads and the worst thing was, they had a kind of two-way mirror for the congregation to watch. Oh, God, when I saw Ian in his socks—it was terrible, but we went through with it."

Two days later, recovered from the trauma of conversion, they flew to Port-au-Prince, where Larry and Dr. Élie Villard called on President Magloire at the National Palace and were assured that the Haitian assembly would pass the bill concerning the Mellons' hospital. The next several days were spent inspecting Deschapelles one more time to be certain it was the best site. They came away satisfied.

Back in Port-au-Prince, the Mellons were introduced to a colorful, influential figure in the Haiti of that day: Episcopal Bishop C. Alfred Vogeli. They discussed with him the possibility of obtaining Anglican nursing sisters for their hospital, but it never worked out. Bishop Vogeli's primary interest was neither medicine nor religion, but Haitian art, and he was one of its earliest and most vital benefactors.

"He wore highly tailored robes and exquisite black suits—a very doggy guy," as Gwen remembers him. "He used to go to all the parties with an entourage of young priests, like a flock of black birds—young, charming and socially popular. He was quite open about his homosexuality."

Too open, it seems. Bishop Vogeli and San Francisco art historian, DeWitt Peters were the fathers of serious interest in Haitian art and mentors of the first great artists at Haiti's Centre d'Art, which Peters founded. Vogeli commissioned them to paint a fabulous set of murals at the Episcopal cathedral in Port-au-Prince and was devoted to them. But the homosexual controversy split the Haitian art scene then and for many years thereafter.

"Those murals were brand new when I first got there," Gwen said.

"He'd built the church and very few came. It was pretty much for foreigners, and there weren't a lot of Episcopalians in Port-au-Prince. The Haitians didn't come either, and he was discouraged. It was a beautiful church but it was never filled, so he said, 'I'll turn it over to you artists. You decorate it. I'm going away for the summer. I'll pay for the scaffolding and the paint.' And when he came back, there it was."

Gwen was intrigued, but Larry was interested in neither Bishop Vogeli nor Haitian art. On leaving for New Orleans, he wrote in his diary: "Gwen and I consider that we have completed a successful trip, and that Hospital Albert Schweitzer is in the process of becoming a reality." With a few sporadic exceptions, that was his last entry for a year. The hospital residency would occupy almost every waking moment.

To Schweitzer he wrote:

My life is beginning to feel the responsibility and a little of the stress of being a doctor and almost a missionary. Without a doubt, fatigue will follow. I'm expecting it, without regret. My heart is so full of joy and gratitude for having the example of your life and work, and for the possibility that, in one way or another, I may be allowed to share a small part of the load. . . .

Whenever I am angry—something which happens all too often— I am ashamed for a long time afterward. One day in December while I was working in the emergency room a big Black man came in. He had been superficially stabbed in the leg with a knife. As I was washing the wound I noticed that he was slightly drunk, and when I started to inject him with a needle containing Procaine, he became incensed and told me so. After awhile . . . I could stand it no longer. I shook him hard by the shoulders and ordered him to leave the hospital—not without adding a few words seldom heard coming from the mouth of a gentleman or an ecclesiastic! My shame was such that on leaving the hospital that evening I sought out the patient's wife and apologized and asked her to send me her husband in the morning— which she did, and I managed to sew him up without incident.

Each time I feel anger rising up I think of this man and the wrong

I did him. This is not a "confession," Doctor Schweitzer, but an indication that in wishing to cultivate the seeds of your work, I am struggling to sharpen [and] develop a "clear conscience," if ever that is possible. . . .

That which I have become since 1948 is certainly preferable to that which I was before. All the same, I dare say there is still a long road ahead before I become the man I hope to be.[27]

What exactly did he hope to be?

"To understand why Larry went to Haiti," says Ian Rawson, his younger stepson, "we first have to understand why he went to Arizona, what took him from a life of luxury in Pittsburgh to the simple life of a cowboy. . . . He was happy there, with concrete problems such as where to put a fence or drill a well or how to organize a roundup. But after he married Mother and picked up three new kids, he got more domesticated and, in turn, more restless. That *Life* article triggered a hair-shirt syndrome and made him think about whether he, too, had any right to be comfortable when others were suffering. So he made the decision to take himself to the edge a second time, learn new skills, test the limits of his competence."

Albert Schweitzer had received a Nobel Peace Prize the previous fall. William Larimer Mellon Jr., notwithstanding his lofty correspondence with the Nobel laureate and the president of Haiti, was a lowly intern on call at a poor folks' hospital in New Orleans. He had asked Gwen to take over his diary, and she dutifully did so. Her 1953 Christmas entry summed up their paradoxical life: "Opened presents at 5:30 before Larry leaves for ambulance duty in the A.M."

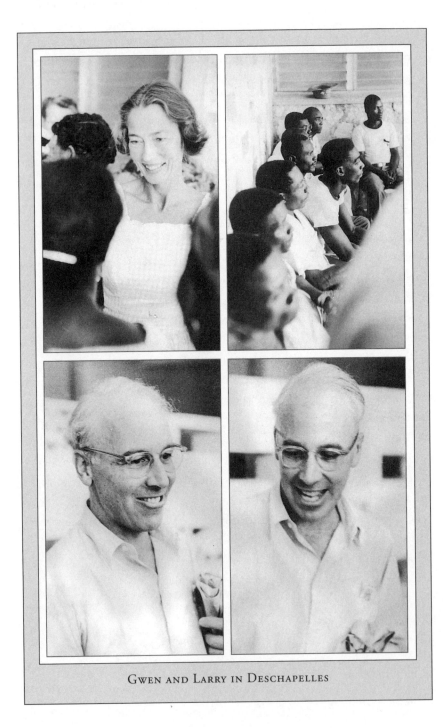

GWEN AND LARRY IN DESCHAPELLES

CHAPTER 4

PRESTO
Miracle-Working

CREOLE, HAITI'S DISTINCTIVELY singsong language, is as refreshing as the Haitians themselves. "Bo' jou', Blanc!" the children yell at the rare white face they encounter. Final consonants are rare in this Afro-French patois, which has a biblical quality rich in archaisms left over from Napoleonic buccaneer days. Its charming corruptions include *ti* for "petite." *Kokioko* is "cock-a-doodle-do." Only in recent decades has Creole been written, in simplified French phonetics: *Enfomasyon* is the word for "information." Puzzle out *kowalisyon* on an election poster and discover it's "coalition." *Thialy* is as close as Creole gets to "Charlie," since there is generally no letter R: One says *goodes* and *pwogwam,* not "gourdes" or "program." The word *oui* is drawled out long and broad to sound like "weigh."

Even with a minuscule vocabulary, a rollicking good time is to be had in this bantering dialect. If someone suddenly turns and says, *Cric?* it means he's got a riddle or joke to tell you, and if you answer *Crac!,* he'll tell it.

The teller of this tale has taken pains until now to stay out of it, for the simple reason that the events predated his observations of them or Haiti. Chronology and the narrator having now caught up with each other—and consistency being the last refuge of the unimaginative—the author now begs leave to wander into the narrative from time to time, promising to do so sparingly.

It's easy to fall in love not just with the language but with all of Haiti, including its falling-apartness and inefficiency, a celebration of the poetic over the functional. Nothing quite works the way it should in Haiti, but the most ubiquitous phrase is *pas de problème!*, regardless of whether there's really a *problème*—which there usually is.

In the crowded streets of the capital, for example, a flat tire is fixed by prying it off, putting it on an old truck piston welded to a bar, then pouring in some gasoline and setting fire to it. This melts the hole shut and fuses the tire to the rim—more or less. Often as not the thing explodes, providing an element of suspense that explains why a throng gathers to gawk at the process. It turns into a surreal event and an impromptu commercial opportunity: Some of the curious onlookers are street vendors attempting to sell other curious onlookers such unlikely products as cement—*by the cup*.

More organized commerce is conducted downtown at the legendary Iron Market, Port-au-Prince's huge, Arab-style bazaar. One side is devoted to food. The other is a kaleidoscopic maze of specialty booths peddling voodoo supplies, oil paintings and carved grotesqueries for tourists, suitcases made out of flattened beer cans, discount-drugstore products pilfered from the docks, steel sculptures cut from oil drums— you name it.

"In Haiti, everything's recycled," says my guide Guillaume as we wind through a labyrinth of stalls jammed with haggling buyers and sellers. In this rough-and-tumble scene, people shout *"Ey, blanc!"* and give you an instant nickname—"Jean Lennon" in my case, thanks to the wire-rimmed granny glasses. They give their children delightful names, as well. Gwen knows a pair of brothers named Hydrogène and Oxygène. And Guillaume knows the Haitian towns of Limonade and Marmelade.

Having forgotten our watches, we ask six vendors for the time and get six wildly different answers, according to what they think we want to hear. On this, my first mystifying trip to Haiti, I am such an inept American shopper that one merchant takes pity and helpfully advises me how to bargain ("I say 50, you say 25, then we go back and forward!"). We finally come to terms on a liquor bottle with a coffin and skull and crossbones inside, used to invoke Baron Samedi, the voodoo Spirit of Death. Later at the hotel, Guillaume catches me eyeing it nervously and says, "Don't worry, it's not *charged*. It takes a voodoo ceremony with the priestesses to do that. What you have there is like a Sony Walkman without the batteries."

This is brilliant techno-reassurance for a Yankee loaded down with the standard, horrific preconceptions of voodoo, the Duvaliers' Tonton Macoutes terrorist police, and the crushing poverty. It's a country where then-President Prosper Avril doesn't quite live up to his name ("Prosperous April"). Port-au-Prince is dirty to the point of filthy, yet most of its proud, self-respecting people and their children look immaculate.

"Yes," muses Guillaume. "I wonder how clean New York would be if they stopped collecting garbage and shut off the water."

Guillaume's wisdom is a many-splendored thing and includes unsentimental instructions on handling the beggars by whom *blanc* tourists are besieged: Keep a roll of quarters in your pocket and be discriminating. "There's a 50-center," he says, pointing out a legless man nearby. "But that one over there is just a 25-center—no amputations. . . ."

We make our way through Port-au-Prince along thoroughfares with such unlikely names as Avenue John Brown ("Lalue"), Avenue Martin Luther King ("Nazon"), and Haile Selassie and Harry Truman streets, whose busy intersections are often devoid of traffic signals. They are jammed with "tap-taps"—vans converted into buses, so named (depending on which etymology you believe) for the sound their old diesel engines make or for the way people hail them by knocking on the sides to make them stop. Each one is fancifully painted in red, yellow, and blue from hood to hubcaps and labeled with its own religious or thematic name—"Rambo," "Tabernacle de Jesus Christ," "Amour Maternelle," "Miami Vice," "Cool Baby," "Love Jehovah," "Computer Love". . . .

We pass the "God Is Good Bar" and stop in at the Hotel Oloffson, where intellectuals and assorted jet-setters gather, and where you can get terrific hot pumpkin soup. This was the setting for Graham Greene's *The Comedians*, and there this day, as if on cue, is the legendary Aubelin

Jolicoeur, energetically table-hopping and schmoozing with the foreigners in his dapper cravat and three-piece suit.*

It is *Ra-Ra* time, and at dusk there is much dancing and craziness in the streets of Port-au-Prince. The revelers are gearing up for Carnival and consuming a great deal of *clairin*, Haiti's raw white rum. A kind of dangerous exhilaration fills the air and tends to unnerve *blanc* visitors. I notice that the U.S. Embassy is surrounded by six-foot concrete block walls topped with big spirals of concertina wire to guard Ambassador Brunson McKinley, grandson of President William, snugly tucked away inside.

Nothing guarded the native citizens of Port-au-Prince at night except the silhouettes of 1,200 varieties of palm and frangipani trees. Haitians take it for granted, but their perfect tropical weather and the island's unique flora and fauna provide endlessly amazing delights.

For my part, I am mesmerized by the *zandolites*, graceful little lizards, that everywhere crisscross one's path. Indoors on floors and walls, they often pause to raise their heads, watch the human activity, and stare you down. Some have their own "reserved" places atop certain lampshades and picture frames. Others rest on window slats in the hot afternoon hours, from which stations they serve the useful purpose of reducing the number of flies. Their outdoor relatives, the tree chameleons, try to elude or hide from you by turning gorgeous shades of fluorescent green. They disturb no one, and no one disturbs them. One soon learns to adjust to the critters who are part of Haitian daily life, to cooperate rather than exterminate.

By coming to the aid of a bird or even an insect, said Albert Schweitzer, he was "doing nothing more than trying to pay a part of the forever-renewed debt of man to beast." When anyone caught a bee and released it outdoors, he said, "I always think that an angel whispers to the good Lord that one of his creatures has been saved."[1] Amidst the noise of putting up a building, Schweitzer's keen ears could catch the faint sound of

---

*Jolicoeur was Graham Greene's model for the colorful character "Petitpierre" in *The Comedians.* He is known as "Mr. Haiti," the country's senior journalist for *Le Nouvelliste* in Port-au-Prince, who dared to speak out against the abuses of the Duvaliers and lived to tell of it.

an animal in distress: He once insisted that his workmen rip open a newly-built wall to locate a kitten who had been trapped behind it. She was named Sizi and—liberated from entombment—lived gratefully with Schweitzer for the next 20 years.

Schweitzer would probably disapprove of my overzealous affection for the *zandolites*: I am determined to catch and bring one home to my son (totally illegal). Late one night I spend a frantic hour in the attempt, crashing and banging and chasing several around my room. But they are much too speedy, dashing away and glancing back to mock me in the attempt.

I eventually give up in favor of a calmer enterprise: waiting for the sunrise. Jacques Roumain described the dewy trees at dawn as "all shiny

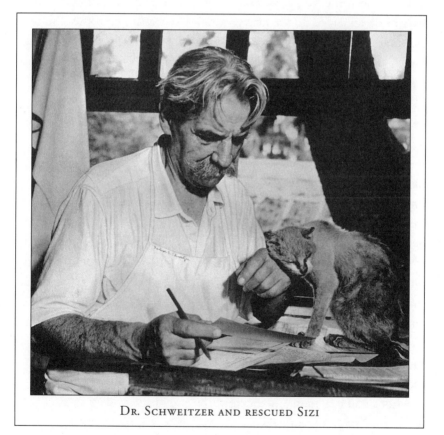

DR. SCHWEITZER AND RESCUED SIZI

and moist—like foam from the sun." My long insomniac anticipation of it is soothed by a soundtrack of drums from a nearby voodoo ceremony and a perfect view from my window of the Haitian moon, so bright one must squint to look at it. From this tropical angle of latitude and longitude, the man-in-the-moon looks Japanese, his craters framing two slanted eyes connected by one long eyebrow for Kabuki effect.

Glancing over at that voodoo bottle, I wonder if maybe the man-in-the-moon is Baron Samedi tonight.

．　　．　　．

"IF WORK WERE a good thing, the rich would have grabbed it all up long ago," writes Jacques Roumain in *Gouverneurs de la Rosée* ("Masters of the Dew"), the first great Haitian novel. "In Heaven, of course they have black angels to do the heavy work—like washing out the clouds or cleaning off the sun after a storm—while the white angels just sing like nightingales all day long, or else blow little trumpets like the pictures we see in church."

The abysmal state of public health in Haiti was a situation everyone had lamented for generations, but the Mellons were not ones to lament. They were ready to grab up some of the work.

That work could not begin in earnest, however, until Larry finished his internship. To his great relief, shortly after New Year's 1954, he was finally taken off ambulance duty and assigned to gynecology and obstetrics. It was a happier place to be, in every respect. He did his residency in the little town of Pineville, Louisiana, under his friend and former professor, Sonny Miller. One night when he was on call, Larry phoned to ask Miller's advice about a patient and was told, "Give her 10 million units of 45 penicillin." He went to the hospital pharmacy but could find no 45 penicillin, a type he'd never heard of. When he called back to clarify, Sonny again said, "Ten million units of 45 penicillin." It took several more futile searches for Larry to figure out that the "45" kind was in Miller's southern drawl, the "fortified" kind of penicillin.

Miller, still practicing medicine at the end of the millennium, chuckles at that memory and savors the tale of his initial out-of-class encounter with the pupil who was older than the professor:

The first time I approached Larry, I was a resident and teacher, and he was a student. I'd just come back from three years in the army in Japan, and I wanted to bring a Japanese boy I knew over here and put him through college. I'd gotten him a scholarship to LSU but needed about $3,000 to get him here, and I didn't have a nickel in those days.

So one morning at breakfast at the hospital, I asked Larry, "Do you by any chance know anybody that would help me get a young Japanese student over here to get educated? I got him a scholarship but I don't have the money to get him here." Larry said, "Yeah, I'll give you the name of somebody to call," and he wrote down somebody's name and number. I called the guy the next day and he said, "No problem, we'll send you $3,000 right away." I could hardly believe it.

Larry never told me, but I later found out how it was done. He had called the man at a foundation in New York and said, "If Dr. Miller calls you for some money, just give it to him and I'll take care of it."

The boy came over here and went through school and graduated and had a brilliant career here and in Japan.[2]

That spring of 1954, architect Jack King arrived in New Orleans with blueprints and a complete scale model of the hospital. But a vital legal matter had not yet been resolved. Mellon's proposed charter called for the Haitian government to grant the hospital the rent-free site and fifteen residential out-buildings on Standard Fruit's former banana plantation at Deschapelles, plus water rights, tax exemptions for equipment and supplies, and a 100-acre farm. For some reason, the agreement drafted by Georges Léger, a Haitian lawyer, contained a twenty-five-year limitation.

When Larry discovered that, he stopped the music and dispatched Gwen to Haiti to change it. Indeed, most of the delicate political legwork fell to her. More traditional wives of that day might have been daunted by the prospect of negotiating sensitive matters with the head of a foreign country, but Gwen Mellon was not among them. By temperament and background, she was an excellent choice for diplomatic messenger. Like her husband, she understood from the start that they would always be guests in Haiti and would have to conduct themselves as such.

Armed with Larry's documents and instructions, she went to Port-au-Prince, where she and Léger were ushered in to see the president. Her terse notation in Larry's diary said it all: "We arrive with maps and know what we want." The 25-year restriction had to go, she told Magloire. But nothing happens quickly in Haiti. This was just the first of many presidential sessions.

"Magloire called me in one day and said, 'Exactly how long can you stay, Mrs. Mellon?' I said, 'As long as it takes to rewrite the contract—I can wait two weeks, but that's all.'"

He met her deadline, but the amended agreement still had to be presented to the legislature. "Dr. Mellon was not a man who went in with a lot of demands," says Bill Dunn, "but he wanted to create a legal environment in which he could function."

Mellon remembered and adhered doggedly ever after to Schweitzer's advice in the letter Jack Beau brought back from Africa: "Independence is of foremost importance if you wish to do something worthwhile and do it well. You must be resigned to all sorts of sacrifices, but you should avoid sacrificing your independence. I myself lead a very hard life. But I find the energy to carry on precisely because I have kept my independence—having found it, I couldn't give it up."[3]

The Mellons finally got the two crucial concessions they needed from the government: authority to use the Standard Fruit property for as long as the hospital existed, and a waiver of import taxes on things brought in for hospital use. "Dr. Mellon stuck to that arrangement to a T'" says Dunn. "Anything brought in for personal use, such as Mrs. Mellon's car, he always paid duty on. He never overstepped those boundaries."

The founding of the hospital was approved by the Haitian legislature in 1954, with a second finalizing action in 1955. In addition to her critical Port-au-Prince negotiations that trip, Gwen spent many days in Deschapelles going over the property and water surveys to determine what additional residential structures and land the hospital operation would need. It was a tired, sore-footed woman who departed Haiti on April 13, but a very successful one.

The challenges to come would be even more daunting. Larry came to Haiti only once or twice over the next twelve months. Gwen would almost singlehandedly supervise construction of the hospital building and 50,000-gallon water tower, the laying of three kilometers of pipes, and installation of three diesel engines for electricity. The cost was $2 million plus another $1.5 million for staff housing, furniture, surgical

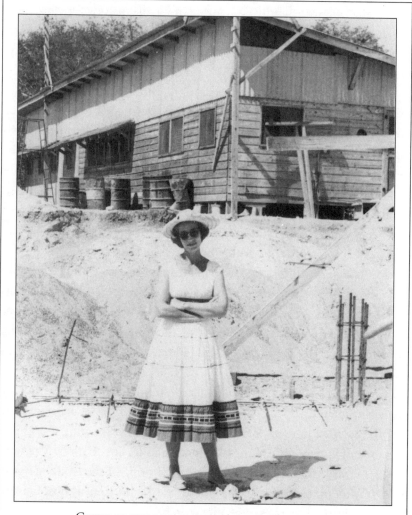

GWEN IN CHARGE AT THE CONSTRUCTION SITE

and lab equipment, pharmacy stock, laundry facilities, and other needs—all funded by the Grant Foundation. The hospital "cost dearly," Larry wrote Dr. Schweitzer. "It is my luck that my forebears earned some money, otherwise I would be on my way to jail!"[4]

Among the first necessities for foreigners living and working in Haiti was the need to master Creole. One might think the Mellons had a head start by virtue of living in Louisiana. Not so. Though both fluent in French, "We were hardly even aware of Creole in New Orleans," says Gwen. "I couldn't pick it up significantly until I came down to St. Marc during the construction period and had 100 percent exposure, twenty-four hours a day."

Linguistics were easy compared to logistics. Getting to Port-au-Prince in the mid-1950s was tricky, and to Deschapelles, even trickier. Gwen would head for Miami, stay overnight, then leave the next morning for Nassau and Havana, where she'd spend another night. Early the next morning, she would board another flight to Haiti. Planes did not fly at night. Once in Port-au-Prince, she could look forward to a grueling four-hour car ride north on bad roads to Deschapelles.

That was her itinerary at the end of June for the most solemn occasion of the project thus far. And where was the founder?

"My last night duty as a Charity Hospital intern—bring all books and clothes home from my room at hospital," wrote Larry on June 25, his first diary entry in eleven months. He was stuck in New Orleans with medical obligations on the day of the hospital's ground-breaking in Haiti—his birthday, June 26, 1954. But, as always, he kept close tabs on everything.

"Gwen moves first shovelful of earth from hospital site yesterday while workmen sprinkle clairin on the ground and throw picks into the air," he recorded June 27. Clairin, the strong sugar-cane rum, was as important in Haitian custom for propitiation as for inebriation. The next day, upon receiving a report on the initial clearing of the land, he noted his "great disappointment to learn that brush and trees at hospital site have been burned. Large trees badly scorched!"

It was the practical, not the scenic, damage that bothered him. But

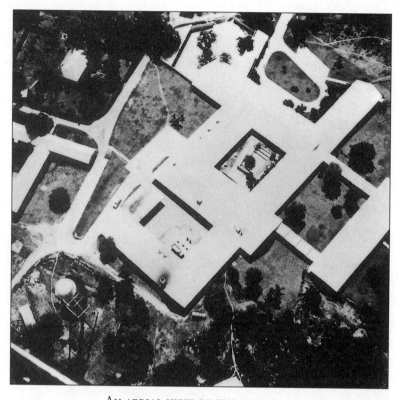

AN AERIAL VIEW OF THE HOSPITAL

he would make the best of it in repair. Among the countless details to which Larry gave long-distance attention was the arrangement of the hospital's central courtyard. Schweitzer had advised: "Don't plant any trees that won't produce fruit, something good for the people. There are enough pretty trees already—don't waste your time. Put in trees that give something back." Mellon now ordered new avocado, almond, cherry, breadfruit, and mango trees to be planted in the HAS courtyard. They thrived and remain to this day.

By September, most of the foundation was dug and the forms ready for concrete. In late October, Larry and Gwen went to Arizona, staying long enough to work in an operating room together for the first time, at Lawrence Hospital in Cottonwood, and for Larry to drive to Prescott on November 2, after performing surgery that morning, "to vote a straight Republican ticket." He was, after all, always a Mellon at heart.

He pasado muchos años pero no tengo miedo, "I am very old but not afraid," he confided in Spanish mode to his diary later that month, reflecting on the advanced age at which he would be starting his medical career. Simultaneously, he was immersed in writing his hospital dedication speech.

In December, he went to Haiti, stopping in Port-au-Prince to deliver medicine samples to Sister Joan Margaret before going on to Deschapelles for the formal laying of L'Hôpital Schweitzer's cornerstone. It took place at high noon on December 11, 1954, in the shadeless heat.

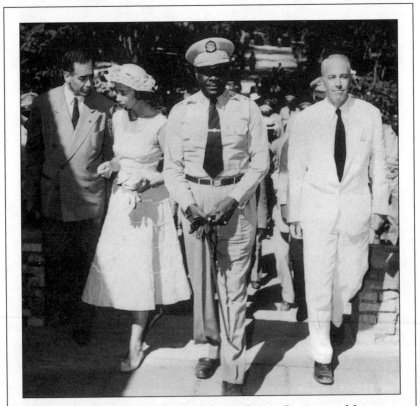

MINISTER OF PROTOCOL DANIEL THÉARD, GWEN, PRESIDENT MAGLOIRE, AND LARRY ON DEDICATION DAY, DECEMBER 11, 1954

Larry Mellon, Emory Ross, and Roger Dorsainville, Haitian secretary of state for public health officiated, in the presence of President Paul Magloire and his elite guard. "Local people came to make us seem like a crowd," says Gwen.* Larry's dedication exercise was delivered in flawless French:

> We are gathered on these premises not only for the dedication of a hospital but also to pay tribute to a person who inspired this work, one of the great minds of our day . . . Dr. Albert Schweitzer. It is because of his Christian goodness, his hard work and his intelligence that we perceive the reasons for which each of us is morally obliged to act in the service of humanity, to aid every life that suffers, to prolong life to the extent that we are able and to protect the life of our neighbor. . . .
>
> The aims of Albert Schweitzer Hospital are essentially three. First and most important is treatment of the sick from Deschapelles and neighboring areas of the Artibonite Valley. Second comes that of inviting foreign specialists from various branches of medicine to visit Haiti and encouraging Haitian doctors and qualified students to attend demonstrations of operative techniques. . . . Finally, the hospital staff must seek to foster interest and a sense of responsibility in members of the community, especially among the young, for solving public health problems and spreading information about hygiene and other aspects of disease prevention.
>
> It will be a policy of Hôpital Albert Schweitzer to engage Haitians whose character and training show them competent to perform a given job. If plans materialize, we hope to live to see L'Hôpital Albert Schweitzer owned and operated efficiently and on a sound financial basis by persons of Haitian nationality.
>
> Without doctors, nurses, technicians and staff consecrated to the service of humanity, this hospital will fall short of our expectations. A modern building complete with diagnostic and therapeutic equipment is not a hospital although it may represent a useful tool in a

*Other dignitaries included M. Zephirin, secretary of state for exterior relations; Luke Prophète, secretary of state for finance; Daniel Théard, chef du protocol; Monsignor Robert Evèque de Gonaïves; Milton Barall, American charge d'affaires; and representatives of the Haitian military and rural development organizations.

beautiful shell. Even when staffed with trained medical personnel, such an institution might be a dismal failure unworthy of the name "hospital." Besides buildings with men and women, hospitals require food and medicine administered with insight and love, all the qualities which make up *ethics*.

To this task my wife and I humbly dedicate ourselves. May the spark of "reverence for life" which came to us from across the Atlantic Ocean continue to burn until it has consumed us with real and deep concern for every living creature that suffers.

Ross, a good friend both to Schweitzer and the Mellons, delivered a soaring benediction that combined homily with homage:

From without come great forces, enormous influences. But in the final analysis, it is only from within that the heart is moved, the soul acts, man changes. . . . If progress in human affairs is accomplished, it is by this miracle in the hearts of men, this change in individuals, this new formation of intelligence and this new direction of mind.

We are united here today in the atmosphere of such a miracle, of an interior miracle of the mind and the soul, which can be stimulated from the exterior but which man must complete himself from the inside . . .

In the Southwest of the United States, in the state of Arizona, a 37-year-old man read [an] article. He, like many other Americans, had never heard of Albert Schweitzer. The *Life* article moved him. The influence from outside acted in combination with the accumulated influences of his entire past. Inside, new ideas came to light. . . .

The [result] we are seeing today is spiritual contact taking place across an ocean, thanks to an illustrated article: the birth of a new idea in a new place, the acquisition of new talents for a new profession, the dedication of a man to new goals in a new place.

The inspirational event was unmarred by a small diplomatic crisis that had arisen beforehand: The rivalrous Roman Catholic bishop said he would refuse to attend the dedication if Episcopal Bishop Vogeli were there, too. The Mellons' decision to forego the controversial Vogeli in favor of the conservative Catholic cleric turned out to be tactically wise. "At the ceremony," Gwen recalls, "the bishop said four Sisters of Charity—two nurses, a lab technician and their housekeeper—were en route to Haiti, but that the work arranged for them had fallen through. Did we want them? And that's how we got our fine Catholic sisters. They stayed about ten years."

After the dedication, everyone repaired to the United Fruit Company clubhouse for refreshments. Four huge trays, each with a cubic yard of sandwiches, had been prepared and were carried in to the party through the elite-guard soldiers lining both sides of the path. The trays made it safely, but not a single sandwich survived the gauntlet. Larry scrambled to find a bottle of Scotch and some potato chips for Magloire. "The president did not even look at the chips, but thought the Scotch was great," Gwen recalled. "He was charming and affable and acted as if he had had a full meal."[5]

Larry later confessed that, as he and Gwen stood under the broiling sun that day, the mind-boggling reality of so many people with so many needs began to sink in: "Our minds jumped from one idea to another— pure water for the villages, inoculations, surgery, nutritious foods, a chance to learn how to sign one's name, relief from bone-shaking chills and fatal fevers. Although it was exciting to know that we could be of service, it was frustrating to realize that everything could not be done in one day. Where should we begin?"[6]

Thomas "Buddy" Evans, Larry's former colleague and co-creator of the famous orange Gulf sign, had flown in from Pittsburgh to see this odd place and his friend's odd project for himself. "Larry," he said, "you're never going to get yourself out of this one."[7] It was true in every sense.

.   .   .

ALBERT SCHWEITZER turned 80 on January 14, 1955. Larry Mellon received a letter from him just a few days later.

"Dear friend, dear brother: Thank you so much for your good letter of December 15th, in which you describe the laying of the cornerstone of the hospital that bears my name. . . . Let me tell you, once again, how touched I am that you wish to name your hospital after me. I took good note of the fact that the cornerstone is marked 'AS.'"

In his reply, Larry, back in Louisiana, lamented "the long hours my internship demands. This week, for example, I am working nights at the maternity clinic—from 6 P.M. until 8 A.M., almost without time to sit down since the deliveries come so fast. Yesterday I delivered eight black babies in 14 hours. Tomorrow I begin my day shift (8 A.M. to 6 P.M.) which will give me four more hours at home, but in changing from the night to the day shift I will have to work 24 hours straight since it is impossible to find another intern to fill the gap. This will give you an idea of the shortage of young doctors here."[8]

Not unlike in Lambaréné. But of many extraordinary bonds between the two men, medicine was only the most obvious. Music and the people of Africa, often intertwined, were their other mutual abiding interests.

"Perhaps the greatness of the colored race lies in its faith, which has to be stronger, at least in America," Larry wrote that month. He was delving more deeply into the black world and recharging his own spiritual batteries through music these days: "Benny Goodman's records inspire me to limber up my fingers. Clarinet practice on Negro spirituals all afternoon . . . Jan. 2, Sunday: Quiet day at home. Various people stopped by to try out our new piano and we play Negro spirituals and old jazz songs . . . Jan. 6: Acquire an oboe and manage to learn its scale at the cost of several blisters of the mucous membrane of my upper lip . . . My oboe gives me great pleasure and I practice as much as I can."

Outside the Mellon home, the attitude toward blacks in New Orleans was not so enlightened. In March, Haitian consul Pierre Clemenceau phoned to say four or five Haitian businessmen had been invited to an economic conference, quite late—in the hope they couldn't make it. They accepted anyway and were on their way, but no New Orleans hotel would put them up. "Gwen and I gladly offer our house," Larry wrote in his diary.

But it wasn't so simple. With Larry at the hospital and Gwen working, too, they had to find time to squire the Haitians to their meetings because no taxi would pick them up. Worn out, they eventually rented a limo to ferry them to and fro.

"But one day, one of them missed the car," Gwen remembers. "He had gone off to find a florist shop—to buy flowers for me. It took him a long time to choose, and by the time he came out with his flowers, the car was gone and he couldn't get a taxi. The flower shop owner finally gave him a ride home in the delivery car. Another time I asked one of them, 'How did you get along today? Did you have a good lunch?' He said, 'Well, it was all right, but we didn't really get a chance to talk with anybody. They put us in a separate dining room alone.'"

The next day before their departure, "Gwen gives a grand farewell dinner party for our Haitian friends," Larry recorded.

She described it as "the fanciest dinner party I ever gave—silver, china, glass—but I had a hard time getting enough people to come to fill the table. There was the Haitian consul, and a Frenchman with his wife, and a couple visitors from the East who were staying in downtown New Orleans. Only about six came. When they were all getting ready to leave, I said to this couple, 'Would you mind dropping so-and-so off on your way downtown?' The wife said, 'I will not ride in a car with a Negro.' It was terrible."

Hispanics fared no better in New Orleans. One night, Larry invited a med-student friend and his Costa Rican wife to dinner at their club. The next morning, Gwen's phone started ringing with irate calls—*Mrs. Mellon, what do you think you're doing? What do you mean, bringing a black person to the country club?* "I said, 'She's not black, she's Costa Rican, not that it makes any difference.' We never walked into that place again."

How did Larry react to such racist incidents? Did he ever have any confrontations with the people involved?

"No," she replies, "one doesn't. After all, what does that prove? What you're doing proves how you feel. You don't have to say a thing. You just keep building."

.   .   .

WHICH IS WHAT they were doing, literally, in Haiti. Larry was busy as ever at the hospital in New Orleans (and learning to read the New Testament in Greek, on the side), but in April, around spring break, he found a few days for a quick inspection trip to Deschapelles. Typically, even on a tight schedule, he had time for other worthy projects. In Miami, he and two associates were met by an artificial limb maker whom they'd engaged to set up a brace shop in Port-au-Prince. Once in Haiti, Larry duly delivered some braces to St. Vincent's School before driving on to meet Gwen and the hospital construction chiefs in St. Marc.

Colorful, bustling St. Marc was an active seaport and the Mellons' temporary headquarters during the completion of their home in Deschapelles. On this occasion, Gwen was concerned about a shipment of slate for the stone floors of their house. They'd ordered it long before in Europe and it had finally arrived from Marseilles, but during unloading onto the dock, one of the huge crates slipped through and fell into the harbor. "We'll grapple for it," said Larry, but he was told to forget the idea; the harbor was so deep, it could not possibly be reached.*

At Deschapelles, Larry found "great activity on construction of the hospital and of our house. The nursing wing and mechanical area are already under roof."

The most beautiful buildings on the fifty-acre campus, were the eight stone homes left from Standard Fruit's heyday. Once fixed up by Gwen, they would house the chief hospital administrators and medical directors. ("I put wonderful flowering bushes in front of all the houses," says Gwen, "but the goats ate them.") The plantation company's spacious clubhouse, complete with large communal swimming pool in front, would serve as the public health office. Nurses' residences and a chicken-production area were still in the planning. Later would come ceramics, carpentry, and weaving shops, and a boutique where the wares would be sold.

Back in New Orleans, Larry recorded "busy days at 301 Northline."

*The story is interesting for comparison with the current state of St. Marc: Except as an arrival point for contraband and departure point for refugees, it is an almost completely inactive seaport. The once "bottomless" harbor, unattended for decades, is now so full of sludge that only flat-bottom boats can easily maneuver in and out.

He had lengthy discussions with Emory Ross on the religious aspect of Hôpital Albert Schweitzer (HAS), finally deciding "to keep it nondenominational and avoid assigning nursing supervision to any religious group." On May 5, the movers arrived to collect the first consignment of their household goods for Haiti. But now there arose a new problem, resulting from the increasing number of newspaper and magazine articles that had appeared:

"Swamped with fan mail. Letters asking for jobs and sending good wishes continue to pour in. Now spend from 4 to 6 hours answering them. Every time it begins to look like I'm caught up, another wave hits me. Another 20 personal letters today."

To the end of his life, Larry was never comfortable with celebrity, nor as adept at handling it as his mentor in Africa. Fame had been a burden to Albert Schweitzer, too, but the contrast between how they dealt with it was clear from Erica Anderson's observations in Lambaréné:

Late at night, Schweitzer was buried deep in answering his mail, his eyes alert with humor. 'I'm having a fine time with my mail tonight,' he declared. 'You've no idea of the requests I get. Here now is a gentleman in America who wants a gorilla and inquires if I could sell him one. He would also like some wire netting for caging the gorilla and says I'm supposed to have the best wire netting in the world. Now, where on earth could he have heard that? The strange part of it is that it's true. I know a nice old man in Strasbourg who makes the wire netting for me in any design and strength I wish.'

Another letter had arrived from a little girl in Germany. "I would like to come and visit you and play with the children at your hospital," she wrote. "But I know that when I grow up, you will be dead." Schweitzer laughed and remarked to Anderson, "She has sentiment, that child, hasn't she? But she is a realist. She shall have an answer."

With less amusement, Larry plugged away at his own mail and the demands on his time: "Much coming and going of friends to say goodbye, French lessons, medical callers, movers and packers," he noted.

Somehow, he also managed to complete twenty hours of Arabic instruction with Dr. Mahdi Murtadha of Baghdad and to finish reading both
The Life of Goethe and Dimner's *The Art of Thinking*. Then, on June 4,
he reached "the acme of success, the ne plus ultra of the professional
man—a gastric ulcer."

Ordered to take time off, he took to his bed exhausted and lay there
for two weeks. He asked Gwen to get him Beethoven's Pastorale Symphony, which, in between Maalox feedings, he played over and over on
the phonograph. "Am thoroughly enjoying my 'illness,'" he wrote,
"taking full advantage of protection from callers and phone, and playing
the oboe a couple of times each day. The restful life is delicious and
would be ideal if it did not mean I will miss Billy's graduation from
Princeton."

The ulcer healed in time for father and son to be reunited on a lengthy
excursion through Central and South America. In Mexico City, they
bought guitars; in Panama, Bill caught a 125-pound sailfish. In Colombia, they made a thrilling climb up rough mountains to 13,000 feet and
visited a leprosarium in the town of Agua de Dios. By the end of July
they were in Havana, where Bill met his school friend Ruben Batista at
the Palacio Nacional and Larry found a stack of wires from Gwen asking
him to bring more needed items—bandages, pliers, saws—when he and
Bill joined her and the younger children in Haiti the next day.

"That was the summer *all* the kids were with us in St. Marc," Gwen
recalls, "—the most wonderful summer we had there. I used to worry
when we were in medical school, 'What's going to happen to the kids?'
Larry said, 'Don't worry, it's going to work out.' And it did. The older
boys had college, the younger kids went to boarding school, and they all
loved coming down to Haiti during the summers. It worked out very
well."

Jenifer remembers the social highlight of that final summer during
construction was going to the dance club—booming with those rhythmic *merengs*!—in nearby Grosse Roche:

> My mother's favorite exercise is dancing, and she was always sought
> after as a partner by a variety of wonderful dancers. When Larry fi-

nally joined us, Ian and I introduced him to all our St. Marc friends, and when Saturday came, we took him proudly to Grosse Roche. To her great dismay, my mother's long list of dancing partners totally disappeared. They would all come over, speak cordially, but none would dare ask Madame to dance now that her husband was here.[9]

Once that summer, Ian was stopped in St. Marc for some minor infraction and told to report to the big police station there. An official finally came to inscribe his name in The Book: "Et votre nom, Monsieur?" Ian Rawson, he replied, and helpfully began to spell it—"R (err), a (aah), w (doublevee) . . ."—at which point the inscriber held up his hand to stop, and wrote "Mr. R. A. Doublevee." To this day, Jenifer swears, "he is still inscribed in The Book as such."

Gwen's love of riding and exploring were infectious. She took long rides on her stud horse Confiance, visiting beaches and marketplaces. The kids never let her forget the time she saw a shop on the outskirts of St. Marc with an iron horse's head above the door and went in to inquire whether they rented or sold any that might be suitable for children. The staff was stunned and the basic answer was no: Their product was horse *meat*.

Larry dug right in upon arrival, hanging mosquito nets over the beds and building a privy for the yard boys in St. Marc. On the first of many visits to the hospital site, he assembled and thanked his 230 Haitian workers, who later celebrated with a dance in the newly finished chicken house. He consulted at length a man who was to become the most important non-medical member of his team, brilliant Haitian agronomist Gustave Ménager, and together they laid out plans for the HAS garden and poultry program. The last of August was spent deep in dung: "Ménager and I inspect five depots to find manure and mulch for hospital planting . . . Work of collecting manure at depositories at St. Marc begins. We gather four cubic meters."

.   .   .

LARRY MELLON'S DIARIES contain many entries about two amazing women whose tireless efforts on behalf of ailing Haitian children predated his own. The first, Sister Joan Margaret, made frequent appeals to the Mellons for transportation or special treatment in the United States on behalf of needy kids at L'École St. Vincent, her school for handicapped children in Port-au-Prince. The requests never went unanswered. "Gwen and I get three Haitian children at St. Barnabas home on Mulberry Street," Larry noted in New Orleans on one such occasion, "and take them to the Panama line boat where Sr. Joan was waiting to deliver them home."

The second heroic woman was Caroline Bradshaw, a remarkable Baptist missionary nurse who founded a children's convalescent facility at Pointe des Palmistes near the north coast city of Port-de-Paix. HAS also had a close working relationship with her.

"We had a fine surgeon from Jamaica, Dr. John Golding, who made periodic visits and did up to thirty hip and spinal operations a week on those little kids," says Gwen. "Then Caroline would come down in her red Land Rover, pick them up and keep them for long-term care; they'd often be in casts for a year. She had an eye clinic, an orthopedic clinic, a brace shop, a fine school, St. Vincent's, and facilities for deaf and blind children."

It was a hectic but exciting time for Larry and Gwen, getting to know the country, its medical needs, its cast of characters, and its many eccentricities. On one occasion that September, the Mellons received a Haitian reporter named Jean-Baptiste. Those were the good ol' days of journalism, and midway in his inspection he informed them, much to Larry's chagrin, that his newspaper articles always had to be paid for.

By October, the hospital generators were installed and work was accelerating sufficiently for Gwen and Larry to leave the supervision to subordinates for a while. They toured the famine-stricken south—a result of Hurricane Hazel—stopping three times to pull cars out of the mud, getting stuck themselves once, and picking up a boy just released from prison who was asleep on the roadside, faint from weakness and hunger.

From there, Larry went to Puerto Rico to see an experimental agricultural station that grew fruit particularly rich in vitamin C. He bought some seed and brought it back to Deschapelles, where he was "distressed to find half a dozen garden workmen leaning on their hoes" and his architect "intoxicated and unable to work." Reprimands delivered, he was taken by Gwen to a makeshift refugee center near Kenscoff, where they examined thirty young victims of the recent hurricane's devastation. Virtually all crops and trees in the south had been destroyed.

"I stayed to help out," says Gwen, "but there was no room, so I slept with the dearest old grandmother. We worked like dogs there. Every day, I drove the sickest kids down to the general hospital in Port and got them admitted. People kept pouring up, on foot, from Jacmel. It's a long walk for you and me [50 miles], but not for country people."

Meanwhile, it took Larry a week and a personal meeting with President Magloire to dislodge a government permit to import narcotics for the hospital. Nothing was easy. In Deschapelles, he was "constantly intercepted by workmen, visitors, and others with requests and problems. By nightfall, it's often hard to remember what you've accomplished, if anything."

The day after New Year's 1956, he, Gwen, and Ian visited a new orphanage at Cité Magloire, where they found sixty of the children suffering from malnutrition. The relationship between food and health was symbiotic and paramount in Haiti, and the Mellons knew it would be so at their hospital. Hence the importance of the groundwork Larry and Gustave Ménager had been laying to get a hospital farm into production. Some months earlier, Gwen and Jenifer had discovered an idle Standard Fruit farm, about 112 acres in Drouin, fourteen miles from Deschapelles. Larry bought it for $11,000. He and Ménager met with local farmers and agreed on a fifty-fifty sharecropping plan. An enormous amount of preparation work was needed, including cleaning out all the clogged irrigation canals. But by January, tomatoes, radishes, and eggplant were ready to be picked and the onions and beets were sprouting in their seedbeds.

The Haitian government had to formally approve the turnover of that farm land to HAS. It chose to do so with a belated ceremony in June 1956, when Larry was back in New Orleans nursing his ulcer. Haitians love "occasions," observes Gwen, who stayed behind to represent her husband:

The officials all came out from Port-au-Prince in black suits and ties for the tradition of riding around the whole acreage, which was big. But they didn't want to do it by car. They wanted to do it on horse-back. So with great difficulty, we got them all horses. They rode around, even though they were ill-equipped to be out riding, and when they got back, we signed the paper on the hood of somebody's car.

The Mellons celebrated their tenth wedding anniversary on the same February day when Larry made a rare diary entry in capital letters, after visiting with a wise obstetrician from Port-au-Prince: "Dr. [Yvonne] Sylvain suggests LIMITING PATIENTS TO REGION." That idea and the need for it—the maximum capacity and exhaustibility of his re-sources—had never occurred to him before. The awareness came at a very late stage, when hospital construction was nearly complete.

"She really impressed us with the importance of that," says Gwen, "and it was very smart. Prior to that we planned to take anybody. We never dreamed we'd get the influx we did in this sleepy little town from the surrounding area."

A benefit concert for the hospital took place on February 17 at Park Avenue Christian Church in New York, arranged by June Sardi, wife of Vincent Sardi Jr. The restaurateurs, good friends of the Mellons, were amateur musicians themselves and raised $1,000 with the event. There was music that night in Deschapelles, too: "Day spent assembling beds and uncrating furniture," Larry recorded. "Build three small tables out of scrap lumber. All hands are physically tired and ready for bed early. Find great peace and rest in practicing the flute an hour before supper."

Sitting down to the meal, he and Gwen suddenly heard loud wailing coming from the village and were informed that "Ti Bob, the son of Ti Corneille, just died." It was a harbinger of their future closeness to the people that they immediately left the table, went to visit, and helped prepare for the wake.

.   .   .

On the extra Leap Year day that February, Larry and Gwen left for Port-au-Prince before dawn to pick up 300 day-old chicks, just arrived by air freight from Pennsylvania, and were relieved to find only one casualty. They returned to Deschapelles for the hospital's first official staff meeting on March 2, 1956. A great deal of medical talent had been assembled, but the Rock of Gibraltar, Larry's greatest find at the outset, was Walborg L. Peterson, better known in Haiti as "Miss Pete," HAS' indomitable head nurse. Recruited through Larry's sister Peggy, she was one of the best medical administrators in America. Mellon thought so highly of "this treasure" that he not only cited her credentials but included her photo for Schweitzer:

> I had the good luck of engaging a highly qualified woman to fill the post of Chief Nurse. She has worked for Mass. General Hospital in Boston for the past twenty-nine years. She has been Head Nurse there this whole time [with the current title] Executive Assistant to the Director. I am enclosing a picture of her in her American Red Cross uniform which she wore in England from April 1941 to September 1942.[10]

From the day she arrived in 1955 to the day she left in 1977, Miss Pete was far more than just head nurse, even though she could never quite learn Creole. "There was no corner of the hospital that her bright eyes did not watch over," Gwen recalls. "She would arrive at the hospital before dawn in her crisp white uniform and dirty sneakers, go to her office, put on her Massachusetts General Hospital cap and pin, and change into clean shoes, ready for whatever the day would bring. No aspect of the hospital escaped her notice, from the adhesive tape on the walls to the conductivity of the OR floor. She made sure the nurses always wore their caps and had their uniforms buttoned. The suction machines, the oxygen tanks, and the blood pressure apparatus were all supervised by her and kept in perfect order. The laundry and Central Supply Room fell under her care. She kept the narcotics count, and patients gave her their money for safekeeping. On her own, she assumed responsibility for the eye and dental clinics, the library, and the staff's annual health exams.

With the help of Miss Pete and Dr. Loren "Yank" Chandler of San Francisco at the initial staff conference, nurses' contracts were set at $100 a month plus meals, housing, and laundry.

The pace was stepping up, along with the problems. "A very discouraging day at the hospital," Larry wrote on March 10. "Lumber is given away and the workmen carry it off as fast as they and their families can lay hands on it." He had also discovered his architect "in an alcoholic fog" once again and decided "it is necessary to sever business relations and finish the hospital job without him." Larry and Billy drove him forthwith to the Port-au-Prince airport, put him on a plane for Miami,

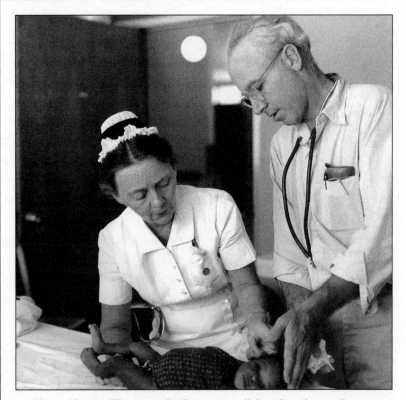

HEAD NURSE WALBORG L. PETERSON (MISS PETE) AND LARRY

and wired ahead for AA to meet and assist him there. They were back in St. Marc for supper, after the three-and-a-half-hour drive each way.

At least that problem had an end, unlike the ongoing dilemma of visitors and social duties. More and more dignitaries and journalists arrived, mixed in with curiosity seekers from Port-au-Prince, including Bishop Vogeli and DeWitt Peters, the art barons, to see what was going on. There were friends like the Sardis and others who truly wanted to help, but it was hard to tell the helpers from the gawkers. Olga Ditterling, whose family owned Shell Oil in the Dutch East Indies, arrived for a tour, and as Larry was showing her around, a huge Shell truck drove up with a load of gasoline.[11] In one forty-eight-hour period, the Mellons entertained the visiting heads of the Salvation Army and the Red Cross, President Magloire and his wife, and U.S. Ambassador Roy T. Davis.

The Mellons, in turn, were soon invited to dine with the Magloires at the presidential palace in Port-au-Prince. "Unable to refuse, we drove to the city," Gwen recalls. "After dinner, the men and women were separated. Among the ladies, I was lost and uncomfortable in local gossip. Among the gentlemen, Dr. Villard whispered to Larry, 'Now we play poker. The President likes to win.'"[12]

Back in Deschapelles, they were swamped with mail and visits resulting from a major article on the hospital by Henry La Cossitt in *Reader's Digest*, which had a worldwide circulation of twenty-one million in thirteen languages making the Mellons' project known globally.* "Most of day spent answering letters from doctors, nurses, agriculturalists, and others who have written after reading the article in *Reader's Digest*," Larry wrote. "So far no contribution of funds have resulted from it."

Gwen said he was disappointed, "but it was really his own fault. He didn't point out that there was a need. He just wanted it to sort of happen. At that point, it didn't look like we were going to need a lot of help, but it grew so fast and so expensive so quickly that we really did."

---

*The gentleman from *Reader's Digest* was nonplussed on the way to Deschapelles, Gwen recalls, after she and Larry picked him up at the Port-au-Prince airport: "He was admiring the ocean, and we stopped at a point by Kyona Beach. Nobody went near the ocean much in those days, but Larry said he was going swimming. So we went in, in our underwear, and Henry just giggled. He finally came in with us in his underwear but he never got over it. He thought it was so odd."

Like a newly elected president, Larry spent a lot of time with job-seekers, some of whom showed up unannounced. Many, even among the doctors, had to be weeded out and politely advised to go home, especially the drinkers.

In early May, Mrs. Sardi arrived (with her singing teacher) for a tour. Erica Anderson appeared the next day with Tom Morgan of *Look* magazine. Close on their heels came reporters from *The Montreal Star*, *The New York Daily News*, and two Florida papers, and the famous, Aubelin Jolicoeur of *Le Nouvelliste* in Port-au-Prince. Toward the end of the month, the Mellons held their first dinner party for the staff in their new home, and a few days later the HAS staff dining room was inaugurated with a full-course supper. In the fields at Drouin, there was great activity getting the rice and corn planted. Irrigation wasn't necessary, thanks to the heavy afternoon rains each day.

"Larry had said a few months before that the hospital would be opened on June 26," Gwen recalls. "People said, 'It will never be ready.' He said, 'You'll be ready. Whatever isn't ready, we'll do later.'"

Hôpital Albert Schweitzer opened on June 26, 1956, Mellon's forty-sixth birthday, two years to the day after ground-breaking. Its work—and the establishment of a routine—now began in earnest with a series of firsts entered in his diary in late June:

- First discussion and plans for dealing with TB in the Artibonite Valley. [TB patients presented a big problem because they could not be hospitalized with the general population.]
- First day of work for our three Haitian nurses, Mme. Cécile Dejois, Mme. Louise Remy and Mme. Elvire Boney [who had been recruited and subsidized at their New York nursing school by the Mellons].
- Examine the first clinic patient, Marcelles Brutus, who seems to have a gastric ulcer or gastritis—cannot check this clinical impression until we get x-ray working.
- Examine six employees and one bona fide patient, a four-year old with intestinal parasites and bronchitis and tonsillitis. Whole staff for dinner at our house, 24 strong.

- Mrs. Jacobs from Saut d'Eau comes into hospital to await her delivery. She is our first bed patient.

The real test would be their first outpatient clinic day at the beginning of July. The Mellons and the staff held their collective breath: Would anyone come?

"First out-patient clinic held at HAS today," Larry wrote. "See 62 patients and are forced to turn away 25 others at 5 P.M."

Would anyone come, indeed. They came in droves on that and every clinic day thereafter, two-thirds of them women and children. The average Haitian mother in her lifetime had twelve pregnancies and six surviving children, many of whom were afflicted in those days with the terrible problem of neonatal tetanus. Larry Mellon and his HAS team would soon tackle that head-on.

On the second clinic day, he saw forty-two patients and seventy on the third. "Started a ward and 24-hour nursing service for three malnourished babies," he noted after that. "The mothers said they'd have to return home to ask the fathers' permission to leave the babies. Only one did so. To my regret, the mothers of the sick babies we examined last Friday have not yet shown up to hospitalize them. It may take time to build up confidence."

Confidence as well as efficiency were soon achieved through the skilled hands of his nurses who, then and later, came from all over the world. "There was a tremendous strength," says HAS alumnus Peter Wright, "in having those wonderful nurses from Switzerland and Holland and Belgium, the likes of which you don't often see—really trained in a very rigorous way. They walked right into the wards, started IVs, and were willing to assume a great deal of responsibility."

In July, Larry was thrilled by the news that son Billy was the first in his class to do a solo flight at his Air Force flying school in Mission, Texas. On the other hand, the first voodoo ceremony that Gwen, Jenny, and Ian tried to attend did not come off so successfully: "They are discouraged by the recklessness of the mob on the trail and turn around before arriving at the Saut d'Eau waterfall," he wrote. Saut d'Eau was a very beautiful and important voodoo site.

At HAS, it was a month of more medical landmarks:

- 7/18: First death in HAS occurred today when 18-year-old Germaine Mergeno expired in the waiting room while her uncle was giving Jenny the particulars necessary to getting her admitted. Ian and I delivered the body to his home in Verrettes.
- 7/23: We see 99 outpatients today. Everyone is tired after a long day's work.
- 7/24: First blood transfusion given in HAS.
- 7/28: First spina bifida case.
- 7/31: First surgical operation performed today by Dr. Chandler on a baby for dermoid cyst of the sacral region.

In August, the first X rays were made, with good results. But the clinics were getting larger and more disorderly: "Having trouble keeping patients in line to get into the hospital," he reported. "Tried a system of numbers passed out as they arrive, but it didn't work. Number 50 was let in first." The doctors were called upon for more than just twelve-hour days: "I give blood to an anemic young mother who's here with a malnourished baby," he wrote. It was not the last time Larry Mellon gave pints of his own rare O-negative blood. The rewards were profoundly felt: "What joy, the greatest in all of medicine, I suppose—seeing patients leave the hospital well and happy! We discharged three bed patients, one adult, and two children, who came to us ten short days ago emaciated with starvation edema."

On clinic days, patients arrived on foot or on scrawny horses and mules. The animals enjoyed the shade of a roof that Larry had provided for them. "The hospital courtyard was then a parking lot for donkeys and horses," recalls Dr. Arthur Maimon, who first visited in 1956.* "We held outdoor TB clinics and preventive medicine and nutrition clinics there, which was a sort of holding area for the patients. There was a large water trough for the animals, but the patients liked to use it as a

---

*Dr. Maimon, whose medical career spans forty years, is a University of North Carolina professor emeritus and resident scholar in infectious diseases. He has returned some twenty-five times over the past four decades for short-term work stints.

bathtub. One poor guy had to sweep up the manure every day, and I want to tell you, on hot days, it was a challenge."

The numbers grew more staggering. "Dr. Verne Chaney starts and personally conducts the first 'screening clinic,'" Larry noted on August 20. "For the first time, every sick person who comes to HAS is at least seen by an MD. Verne screens 140, assigning them to future clinics." Two days later, at the second screening clinic, "Some 200 patients are seen and treated."

But Larry wasn't a "numbers man" at heart. Each patient with whom he came into contact moved him, often wrenchingly, as he confessed to his diary one night that month: "Turnbull brought me a Mr. Mahonne who is dying of pulmonary cancer. My function was to tell him his true condition. I slept very poorly after this, wondering whether I had really done right in being honest."

Larry was "a very gentle person—he had a great need to be gentle," says Dr. Maimon. "Concern for other people was a requirement he had.

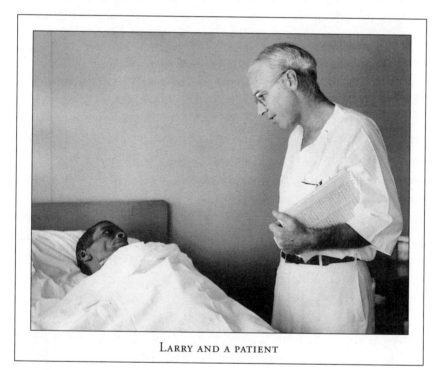

LARRY AND A PATIENT

If you were in his home, he'd say, 'Can I get you something? A glass of water?' He'd almost *wish* he could get you a glass of water, and you'd feel you were being waited on by someone who was very attuned to the nurturing of other people. He told us that in order to get along with the Haitians, the first thing to do is to ask them what they think they need, and let them know they shared in whatever you did. I worked in the clinics with him—an excellent physician, very perceptive. The patients I saw who'd been seeing him had withdrawal symptoms: They didn't want me, they wanted Dr. Mellon. Whatever he said was etched in granite as far as they were concerned. People became particularly attached to him because of his kindness."

Nobody doubted Gwen's kindness either, yet certain roles and duties of the enforcer fell to her. Then and now, many called it l'hôpital de Mme. Mellon (Madame Mellon's hospital) because she was the one who sat out front every day, recording the patients' names, checking appointments, and collecting the fees. The cost of being seen in the clinic—including examination, lab work, medication and food—was two gourdes (about forty cents), which was theoretically Haiti's minimum hourly wage at the time.

Larry determined the hospital's fee structures as thoughtfully as he did everything else. Charges were based on what was then the cost of a Haitian funeral—thirty dollars. If people would pay thirty dollars to bury a loved one, he reasoned, they should be willing to pay as much to save one. The average stay for a hospitalized patient was six days. Thirty dollars divided by six was $5, the daily fee for hospitalization at HAS. Fees were somewhat higher for patients from outside of the district, in a mild effort to discourage them.

It was hard for many to pay. Sometimes they did, sometimes they didn't. Often a bag of rice or fruit or some other item of barter was accepted instead of money. But payment was required on the theory that anything free is not highly valued.

.   .   .

NON-CLINIC DAYS were just as busy as clinic days. "Am contriving somehow to arrange to work Mondays, Wednesdays and Fridays in the outpatient department and to be free for farm building and office work the other days," Larry wrote.

On "days off," he could be seen digging ditches with the villagers or otherwise engaged in tasks not normally performed by practicing physicians. Jim Funk, a member of an Atlanta orthopedic group that volunteered annually from the hospital's inception, remembers his first encounter with Larry that summer: "After meeting the Mellons, we went to the Episcopal Seminary at Mont Rouis where there was a clubfoot clinic at a small pavilion on the beach. I have a memorable picture of Dr. Mellon with his hands deep in plaster of Paris, applying clubfoot casts together with Caroline Bradshaw."[13]

In October, the HAS farm celebrated its first major harvest of corn, rice, and bananas, but Larry was worried about expenses, which were skyrocketing. His payroll had grown to 173 and it was decided, at the annual meeting of the Grant Foundation, that costs should be cut by almost 50 percent. All foundation directors were present except Emory Ross, who was on his way back from Africa with the editor of *Saturday Review*, Norman Cousins. Cousins had previously visited Deschapelles and just published his account:

Why would a wealthy man give up everything and make such an enterprise his life? Dr. Mellon decided he didn't want to be a victim of his own wealth. He saw no reason why he should be condemned to a useless life because of it . . .

Parts of Haiti [and] the way of life [seem] almost indistinguishable from what is found in sections of French Equatorial Africa or the Congo. Indeed, in many ways the pattern of living is even more primitive than in Africa today. We traveled through villages where the wheel was nowhere to be seen. There were no carts, no wheelbarrows, not even a waterwheel. Some farmers had never seen a plow.

[Dr. Mellon felt] that the people in the vicinity of Dr. Schweitzer's hospital at Lambaréné were, if anything, perhaps better off than most of the people in this part of Haiti. It wasn't just a matter of poverty. He was thinking of the fact that the people in Haiti were brought to the island as slaves and are still displaced persons. All they had when they arrived was their African culture. They cling to it as it was. The cultural evolution that took place in Africa has not taken place here . . .

Larimer Mellon, like Albert Schweitzer, is in the business of creating a new image for the white man. In an age of blistering color-consciousness, this comes close to being the most important business in the world.[14]

Cousins and the Mellons had a burgeoning if eccentric friendship, as Gwen recalls:

He was a brilliant, friendly man, and there was quite a bond between him and Larry. In New York a few months earlier, he asked us to have dinner with him at the Lambs Club. He said, "Mrs. Mellon, you must be wanting to start a library at the hospital." I said yes, and he said, "I get so many books to review—come over and my secretary will let you in; take the ones you want, and then I'll pick you up for dinner."

So Larry and I and Ian and Jenny all went to Norman's office and looked through the books, and somebody knocked on the door and came in and sat down in another room. We didn't pay any attention to him, and he didn't pay any attention to us. I chose the books and then Norman came in and took us across the street to the Lambs Club, and this other man was right along with us.

When we sat down for dinner, this other man immediately leapt in on the subject of atomic energy and never stopped talking the whole time. We never had a chance to talk at all, and neither did Norman—and Norman Cousins wasn't somebody to be discounted in conversation. When he'd come to our house for dinner, he'd say, "Now, you listen to me, Gwen—" and then hold forth at length. But this other man really took over that night.

Norman listened politely and after dinner, outside on the street, he said to me, "Who is that guy?" I said, "I don't know." He said, "Wasn't he with you?" I said, "No, we never saw him before." We never did find out who the hell he was.

Except for Cousins and a few others, Larry had little truck with journalists. His diary contains several references to one George Barris of *Cosmopolitan* whose persistent interview requests were denied because Mellon felt *Cosmo* wasn't the "right" kind of publication. Once in Pétionville, Arthur Maimon ran into CBS's Mike Wallace, whose wife was Haitian: "I asked if he ever considered doing a *60 Minutes* program on HAS. He said he had, but that Larry had turned him down because he wanted to keep it low-key."

Gwen explains: "We thought a lot about who would see or read such pieces. A lot depended how the guy presented himself. A few years later, for example, Australian journalist Peter Michelmore hung around here for days, standing in the courtyard, while obviously Larry was in his office. Finally, Peter said, 'If he doesn't see me today, I'm going to leave.' So Larry finally saw him—and loved him. He was wonderful."*

The holiday season and the end of HAS' first calendar year were now approaching. On Thanksgiving 1956, Larry threw a staff party at which "everyone has a good time dancing to Deschapelles band." The next day, he and Dr. Gene Szutu played Handel and Telemann duets "for a couple of delightful hours in the p.m.," and soon after, the first Protestant prayer service was held in his home—with Mellon and Szutu playing the hymns. When sons Mike and Bill arrived in late December, Larry was thrilled "to have all our family together for Christmas. We sit up until midnight talking about the hospital and hearing about life in the U.S. Air Force." After Christmas Eve supper for the staff, Gwen and Ian passed out presents to the patients, and everyone attended a musical midnight mass in front of the hospital.

"Clinics are very small at this time of year," Larry wrote. "It seems as if much of illness is sublimated or forgotten when more pleasant activities are substituted." (A few lines later he recorded a less than pleasant activity: "Reprove Mike in front of the family for his shiftlessness and choice of friends.")

*Michelmore's resulting *Dr. Mellon of Haiti* (1964), published by Dodd, Mead & Co., was a lyrical portrait of the Mellons and their hospital, to which this author is indebted. Michelmore later gave permission for the Mellons to reprint it *gratis*, all profits going to support the HAS tuberculosis village, L'Escale.

But the spirit of Christmas, in addition to reproval, was alive and well at HAS. Ann Marie Judson reflected on the Yuletide that she, her surgeon husband John, and their young daughters spent in Deschapelles: "The day before Christmas we were besieged by continual knocks at the door by children asking for *ti cadeaux* (little gifts). By late afternoon I was exasperated by all these interruptions, and when I grumpily opened the door for yet another knock, there was Dr. Mellon standing in the doorway, holding two child-sized Haitian chairs with the names of our daughters painted on them. I certainly felt remorseful. Dr. Mellon not only bore the gifts of the chairs, but of calm and kindness."[15]

.   .   .

Hôpital Albert Schweitzer was and is the only hospital in Haiti to provide its patients with meals. Elsewhere, the relatives of the sick must bring in food. HAS' 116 beds would soon be holding some 2,500 inpatients a year. Many of those, and almost half of the hundreds of patients seen on clinic days, are children acutely ill with malnutrition and related diarrhea. Most have traveled, or been carried by their parents, a day or more on foot to get there.

Food, and the terrible lack of it, was at the root of the Haitians' poor health, and became the obsessive concern of those ministering to them. It is said that Eskimo languages contain twenty-four different words for "snow." In Haiti, an equivalent linguistic revelation lies in the dozen different Creole words and medical terms for "malnutrition" and "starvation." Most common are *kwashiorkor,* caused by lack of protein, and *marasmus,* from across-the-board caloric deprivation. This is endemic all year but worse in the rainy season, when food stocks are depleted. The condition itself is treatable by nourishment and oral serum, especially in the early stages, but mental and developmental damage can be lasting. Even when treated successfully, Haitian children usually return to the same circumstances and the vicious circle that produced the problem: Not enough food at home due to not enough income to buy it or farmland to produce it.[16]

Larry spoke of the problem with preacher's fire in a letter to his cousin, Jessie May Hill: "Our main diseases are malnutrition (which we consider a disease), and tuberculosis. So far Gwen and I have escaped them both, although I know in my heart that anybody who eats well in a country where there is starvation is a thief."[17]

The actual distribution of food was beyond the Mellons' capabilities, but the hospital's reputation for saving malnourished children spread quickly—bringing certain problems. Part of the HAS routine was the delivery of recovered children back to their parents, usually on their village market days. Since there is no such thing as an address in the impoverished Haitian countryside, staff members would often wander through the crowd, holding the child aloft in search of a relative who would recognize it. Sometimes none could be found.

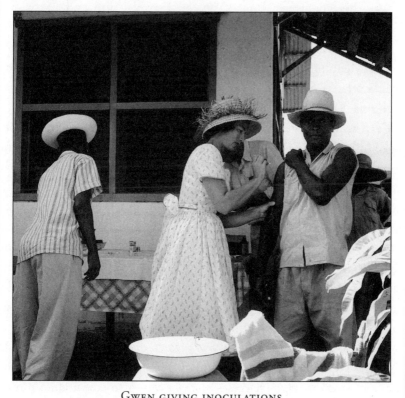

GWEN GIVING INOCULATIONS

Word of the good care at HAS brought another unwelcome result: Some well-to-do residents of Port-au-Price drove their cars to Deschapelles, changed into ragged clothes, and walked the final distance to HAS, seeking admittance as locals.

It also brought more celebrity visitors, including Dr. Karl Menninger, who was taken to visit HAS with his wife and daughter on January 8, 1957, by Dr. Louis Mars, Haiti's lone psychiatrist. Mars was a brilliant man who had worked with Menninger at his famed clinic in Kansas.

"Louis Mars didn't know what else to do with him," says Gwen. "It was not a charming visit. Dr. Menninger was a stuffy man, a little removed from reality, not someone who fit into our landscape easily. After he went back, he kept sending psychological articles—inappropriate things that had no application to us."

Was there no fascinating discussion between him and Larry, two founders of important institutions?

"No," she replies, "no bond."

The Menninger visit may have inspired a wry entry in Larry's diary two days later: A certain Mrs. Borden had stopped by "but didn't find me home. One can't be unlucky all the time."

Certain "drop-ins," on the other hand, were a godsend and were engaged on the spot. Snap decisions by Larry, on instinct at the spur of the moment, were infrequent but rarely wrong.

"He once hired a head surgeon over the telephone—Dorrien Venn," says Gwen. "Larry asked Erica about him in Port-au-Prince and went right in to call, got him on the phone in South Africa and said, 'My name is Larry Mellon, I run a hospital in Haiti, and I'd like very much if you would come and be my head surgeon.' Dorrien said, 'Well, this is unexpected,' and Larry said, 'I'm sure it is and I'm sure it's hard for you to decide, but I'll pay for your passage here, and if you don't like it, I'll pay your way back whenever you want.' Dorrien came and stayed six years."

None of Mellon's discoveries was greater or more beloved than Dr. Harold May, who appeared in January 1957 just to introduce himself and was asked to take charge—*immediately*—as medical chief during Larry's upcoming absence in New York.

"Larry was all set to take me there for a back operation," says Gwen, "when Hal May came by to visit and asked casually if there was a position open. Larry said, 'Yes, you can take my place.' Hal had the most beautiful look on his face. You could tell right away he was a marvelous man. Larry instantly sized him up and asked him to stay." May's story and subsequent intimate involvement with the Mellons are extraordinary.

A brilliant Harvard student (class of '47) and one of the first African-American graduates of Harvard Medical School ('51), Hal May had read Schweitzer's *Out of My Life and Thought* in college. What most impressed him, he reflects years later, was that Schweitzer "used every bit of Albert Schweitzer—all that he was and was able to express, in theology, medicine and music. I wanted to make sure that all of ME was expressed, too."

May had a deep desire to become a medical missionary. His father was a minister and presiding elder of the AME Zion Church in Auburn, New York. *Père* and *fils* agreed there were plenty of doctors in the United States and that his skills would be more urgently needed somewhere else. Hal would have time to ponder where during his two-and-a-half-year surgical residency at Massachusetts General Hospital in Boston. But there was a serious problem: In med school, he had noticed that his vision was getting poorer. It was now getting much worse. The diagnosis was corneal ulcers.

"In the dorm at Mass General, when I took out the contact lenses, my buddies had to lead me to the dining room—I was literally blind. I told the chief of surgery that I felt I should resign, but he wouldn't accept my resignation. 'We'll see that you get your corneal transplants,' he said."

In 1956, that relatively new procedure required a lengthy healing and recovery period, for which May went home to Auburn. There, his father read to him a lot, including a *Reader's Digest* piece about a patrician-physician, inspired by Lambaréné, who was starting a hospital in Haiti. Though intrigued, May did not feel strongly drawn to that project. His calling was different, more theological than social.

"Schweitzer talked about the white man's burden," Hal May explains, "and he had to help to shoulder this. I didn't. I was called to help, but I felt whatever I did would be so limited unless it was not just me doing it but God doing it with me and through me. That's when I started to live, literally, by faith rather than by sight. I looked beyond Schweitzer to God to guide me. That was a shaping experience. I never once prayed that I would see. I prayed that His will would be done in my life. I wanted to learn tropical medicine. If I could see, I would be a surgeon, but if not, I would be a minister."

As part of his recuperation, May's parents took him for a lengthy stay on Jamaica, where they had been born and where they hoped he might practice. But in Jamaica, Hal kept hearing about a more poverty-stricken and doctor-deprived country on a nearby island to the northeast. He made arrangements to visit Haiti at Christmas of 1956. It was precisely during another upheaval in that tumultuous place: The day May was to arrive, President Paul Magloire, friend of the Mellons and their hospital, was deposed in a coup leading to the dictatorship of François Duvalier.

"I was on the first plane that landed after the revolution," May remembers. "As it banked over Port-au-Prince, I knew this was where I was supposed to be. I just sensed somehow this was it. It wasn't a question of whether, just where. So I went exploring to find the place, and would know when I came to it."

May toured the country with other medical missionaries but did not find what he was seeking until he met Caroline Bradshaw, who said she was taking some ailing kids to Deschapelles the next day. Did he want to come along? He did. The Hôpital Albert Schweitzer that Hal May first saw with still-sore eyes was then barely six months old, and the visitor was taken immediately to meet the founder:

Larry said, "Look, two [of only five] doctors are leaving tomorrow." One of them was Larry himself, to be with Gwen for an operation in New York. "Would you be willing to help out here?" It was so clear: This was it. But I didn't say yes right away.

I said, "My reason for being there isn't quite the same as yours. You're here because of Dr. Schweitzer. I'm not. It goes beyond that for me—my guiding force is not Schweitzer but what God can do." I was up front. "If I'm here, that's why." I'm not a religious nut. I would be there as a physician, but not *just* as a physician, because the spiritual is at our core. We can treat the body but sometimes the problems are at the core.

And Larry said, "There's scope. There's room for that here." He welcomed that.

Larry indeed left the next morning, turning over the reins to a man he'd just met, sized up, and instinctively trusted. May shouldered the responsibility immediately—"It felt wonderful and very natural"—and he stayed for six months, until going back to have his second operation and finish his residency. Hooked on Haiti, May returned in 1960 and was chief of surgery at HAS for the next dozen years. He carried a full load as a physician there and, once his eyes healed, as a surgeon, "only I was a little slower than the others."

Dr. Maimon smiles at the recollection that "Hal was a great doctor but had a habit of exceeding the usual time limitations in surgery—by a long shot. Larry used to say that when Hal closed a wound, half of it would be healed by the time the other half had been sutured. That was so typical of Larry, to put everything in a light fashion and never be condemning."

Larry poked a bit of fun at Hal but highly valued his competence and mellow temperament, relying on him more and more for the day-to-day administrative duties to which his own temperament was less inclined. Frank Lepreau, later HAS chief of surgery himself, recalls Larry's distaste for regular staff-review meetings. Such sessions, says Lepreau, were usually conducted outdoors on a bench: "Larry would have a couple pieces of paper and make a decision in about five minutes. Then I'd go back to the clinic and he'd go off into the countryside." May's adept assumption of duties freed Larry to devote more time to community development projects, his other increasingly important agenda.

May had his own supra-medical agenda, as he acknowledged from the start, and actively pursued it. He helped organize adult literacy and Bible-study programs for the Haitians. Most important, says Gwen, "Hal founded the first religious services on campus." She and her husband attended regularly for reasons of convenience as well as conviction: The first Sunday morning services, for the Americans and HAS employees, were held in the Mellons' living room. Once a little chapel was obtained, an evening service in Creole for the Haitians was added. Attendance at both observances grew significantly and, although he was not ordained, Hal May became the community's ecumenical pastor:

> Saturday I would go up into the hills to start thinking about my message and work through the night to come up with a Sunday sermon. There were sharp divisions between Catholics and Protestants then, but we would have Christmas Eve mass with the sermon in French, then I'd give it in English, so the Protestants started coming to the Catholic service and vice versa. We formed a choir and held a Palm Sunday service on the tennis court where the Catholic sisters sang along with our Protestant chorus and the Haitians, who all love to sing—50 or 60 people, all races and religions, singing together. It was really thrilling and inspirational to be there.

Something—or, rather, someone—even more inspirational entered May's life then: Shortly after returning to Haiti full time in January 1960, he met and fell in love with a Mennonite nurse, Agnes Martens. Hal and Aggie were married in Deschapelles in April and celebrated their fortieth anniversary with the millennium.

.   .   .

DURING THEIR TIME in New York before Gwen's operation in 1960, the Mellons indulged in cultural delights unavailable in Haiti. They took Jenny to see *My Fair Lady*, followed by dinner at Sardi's. The next day they attended the opening of the Schweitzer documentary by Erica Anderson and Jerome Hills and then, accompanied by Larry's sister

Peggy Hitchcock, visited the new Salvador Dali exhibition. "Dali was there," Gwen remembers, "and you could hardly get in the door. He had just done that wonderful big canvas, 'The Crucifixion,' which was on exhibit. Contrary to his reputation, he didn't seem wild at all. He was very civil."

And what was Larry's opinion of Dali and his art?

"I don't know," she replies. "Larry wasn't much of an aficionado."

He pretended to be one the next night, following a banquet they attended with Peggy Hitchcock in honor of the refugee work of Archduke Otto van Hapsburg. At the table next to theirs was cousin Ailsa Mellon Bruce, who invited them back to her apartment after dinner to view her fabulous art collection.

"She had unbelievably beautiful paintings, as everyone knows," says Gwen, "all over her house. I remembered one of them from years before and said, 'Where is the Toulouse-Lautrec woman in the big hat?' She said, 'Go look in the closet.' You had to go through them like a deck of cards in there, but there it was.

"Ailsa had another whole apartment in New York just to store her paintings in. She was a strange, difficult woman, scared to death of everything. She was afraid to go out on the streets of New York because once she looked down and saw holes and sewers and she felt she would fall through. She had a very cloistered childhood in Pittsburgh. Her husband David Bruce was a brilliant guy, ambassador to France, England, and Russia. He did a beautiful job everywhere, the epitome of how an ambassador should behave."

Larry couldn't wait to take his leave of Ailsa. There were Mellons and there were Mellons, and he was more comfortable with his own sisters. Rachel, ten years older, was an inwardly very religious person who had been sensitive from the beginning to his reasons for establishing the hospital and to the philosophy behind it. Over the years, she has supported the hospital generously and often visited Deschapelles.

"Rachel would always be very quiet and listen and enjoy being alone here," says Gwen fondly. "She loved the house, got up late, walked about and spoke to everybody. Everyone loved her for herself, and because she looked so much like Larry."

Peggy, who died November 8, 1998, at the age of ninety-seven, always preferred a faster pace than Haiti offered. Her direct involvement with HAS was less active, but she and her children were likewise faithful supporters, proud of the hospital's accomplishments.

Among Larry's siblings, the greatest contrast was between him and his brother. In the early days of the hospital, HAS mail came through a post-office box in St. Marc. Matthew Mellon's post cards to Larry would arrive there with such messages as, "Are you still taking care of those niggers?" More than once, Larry asked him not to write such things on an open card. In response Matthew replied, "I didn't know they could read." Michelmore, the author, summed him up in *Dr. Mellon of Haiti:*

> Matthew Mellon had been idling away the years, strolling the deck of his yacht, dabbling in archaeology, building an estate in Jamaica and villas in Europe. When someone once suggested he must be pleased about Larry's medical work, Matthew had raised an eyebrow and said matter-of-factly: "I'm not at all in sympathy. He's keeping alive the wrong kind of people. The money is misspent. It would be better used to help poor white people."
>
> Perhaps to confirm his views about "undependable French niggers," Matthew traveled to Deschapelles to see how his brother was doing. He stayed only three days. "Dreadful place, Haiti," he said cheerfully. "And that Larry—he's chasing a dream." But a few months after his visit, Matthew transferred $15,000 to the Grant Foundation so that the dreamer could keep on dreaming. Better than anyone, he knew that stories of Larry Mellon's reserve wealth were a fable, because most of his family inheritance was tied up in trust funds for the children. Without outside contributions, the hospital would go broke.[18]

Larry and Gwen came back to Haiti from that particular New York trip with a cello, a guitar—and an aluminum leg. (Two of the three items had been promised to the St. Marc Symphony for a concert at the hospital.) Soon after, they had to return to New York's Presbyterian

Hospital for Gwen's second multiple-disk operation, a five-hour procedure, followed by a three-hour operation to fuse three lumbar vertebrae and sacrum. They returned by boat to Port-au-Prince, where they were met by Miss Pete and a station wagon equipped with mattress and cushions for Gwen on the grueling drive north to Deschapelles. "How glad we are to get home again," wrote Larry. "Hospital is beautiful."

It was significant that he and Gwen both unequivocally regarded Haiti as home now. While she recuperated, Larry plunged back into work. "The chicken houses are neat and operating," he reported, "although they sustained a loss of 60 percent of the pullets by disease." Neither that nor any other setback derailed him: "When one's principal joy is in systematically overcoming difficulty, life takes on a satisfying serenity. The rate of progress, like perfection itself, is a relative thing and is not of primary importance."

On a beautiful Sunday morning in September, Larry took a new phonograph and records to play for his patients in the wards. "They loved it," Gwen recalls, and he did it often in the future. The following Sunday, September 22, 1957, was presidential election day in Haiti. The only candidates on the ballot were Dr. François Duvalier and Sen. Louis Dejoie. Duvalier's victory brought ominous rumors, and Mellon called a staff meeting to address the uneasiness and stress his position that the work of HAS "must continue full steam ahead regardless of developments."

The U.S. Embassy was advising Americans to leave Haiti. The Mellons held tight, though faced with a related political crisis of their own. Verne Chaney, one of their doctors, had performed an autopsy in Port-au-Prince on a man who had reportedly been abused and killed by the Haitian army. Larry Mellon felt Chaney had no right to practice outside the hospital and that it was a bad political move. Chaney took strong exception. When subsequent discussions failed to change his mind, Mellon discharged him. "His attitude toward his responsibilities and his example are incompatible with our program at Hospital Albert Schweitzer," Larry wrote. "Sending him away isn't pleasant or easy." It was a classic example of Mellon's desire to avoid political entanglements, and also of his strictness.

"I remember another time Dr. Mellon got angry," recalls Dr. Lucien Rousseau. "A new expatriate doctor came to the hospital, but the second or third day he didn't wake up in the morning. His door was closed and there was water coming under it. There seemed to be a flood in the house. Someone went in and found him asleep on the floor, drunk. Dr. Mellon was really mad and dismissed him that day. No appeal. If he said 'yes,' you could count on it. If he said 'no,' that was it—the end."

A more comical instance of Larry's impact as disciplinarian occurred when he learned some employees were pilfering food and supplies from the hospital and taking them home.

"The thievery problem was always there," says Dr. Lepreau, "but people were getting stickier fingers than usual, and so he figured he better check. The bus to St. Marc was taking the employees home for the weekend, and he picked that day to personally check it. So he went to a particular point, stopped the bus in the middle of the road, climbed on and walked down the aisle. The minute he set foot on that bus, things started flying out the windows on all sides—towels, soap, all sorts of things. I was standing outside and saw it. It was remarkable! Larry did what he thought needed to be done, no matter what. If he thought the bus needed to be checked, he was going to check it.

"One reason why the Haitians trusted him was that he treated them and foreigners alike, in contrast to most expatriate missionaries, who were always a little more lenient toward Haitians. Larry didn't tolerate misdeeds on the part of anybody. That had a good general effect. If a foreigner did something improper, his response was, 'There's a car leaving for Port-au-Prince in the morning,' which meant you'd better be on it. 'There's a car leaving for P-a-P tomorrow' became a byword for 'You're gone.' Fired."

Larry felt any dismissal should take place quickly and the person should leave immediately. "It sometimes seemed harsh," says Bill Dunn, "but as I watched it play out, I felt there was a great deal of practical wisdom in that: In a small, tight community, a person who is not 'on board' can become a very destructive influence."

It was nevertheless hard for Mellon or Lepreau to "correct" anyone for whom they had great affection—such as Dr. Florence "Skeets" Marshall, the first HAS pediatrician and a tremendously conscientious one, as Dr. Lepreau recalls:

> There were so many people who needed care but had to be turned away—it was very trying and difficult, beginning with the screening on the front steps. The clinics led by Skeets were running late—like 'til 11 at night. It was too much for her, psychologically and physically. It meant keeping an x-ray technician around and everyone was getting upset. But it's almost impossible to tell a good doctor to stop taking care of sick patients. Larry said, "We have to cut those hours down," but he turned the problem over to me and I didn't know how to do it. I tried to tell Skeets, but it was like hitting a brick wall.
>
> She's a Quaker and so am I, and I decided, "I've tried everything

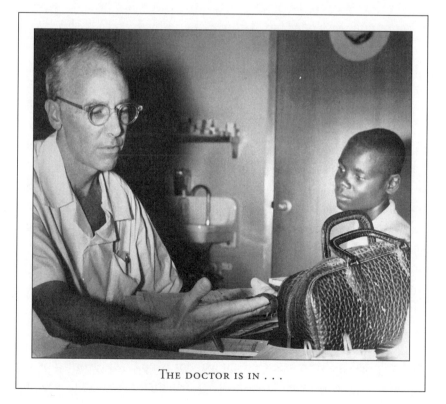

THE DOCTOR IS IN . . .

else, I'm gonna try the Quaker approach." So one night I went over and sat in a chair in the corner, and she sat in the other corner, like a boxing match. I suggested [doing the screenings in under five minutes] and then waited it out. I sat and she sat—we both just sat there silent for 30 minutes. I decided, "Lepreau, you sit there with your mouth shut, just sit it out." She probably decided the same thing: "I'm gonna sit it out no matter what that SOB does." And then I got up and said, "See ya."

In about a week, the clinics started to get shorter, and we got over that crisis. It was an application of Larry's management style.

To give Dr. Marshall equal time:

I remember one dispute [with Lepreau] over a kid from out of district. The kid and the mother were behind me when he and I were confronting each other out in front of the hospital, which is where we would screen people. He told me, "You just have to send these people (from out of district) away." I turned around and I picked up this limp child and handed it to him. It fell over his arm like a towel. And that took care of that.[19]

Both in Arizona and Haiti, Larry "had to learn new skills to be self-reliant," says his stepson Ian Rawson, "and he had to find a small group of dependable partners. In Arizona, they were mostly cowboys like himself, whom he could count on to do their work without a lot of fuss." At HAS, one of the people Larry counted on was the comptroller-accountant, Gérard de Vastey. When he was arrested during the Duvalier period, Dr. Mellon went straight to the lock-up. "Put me in jail instead," he said to the authorities. "I can't run the hospital without him."

They let de Vastey go.

"Larry rarely told other people what to do," Ian continues. "This probably led to frustrations on the part of people who worked at the hospital, but he assumed other people knew their jobs as well as he did and didn't need to be given specific instructions. When corrections were necessary, he approached a problem in a way to preserve the dignity of others.

"At one time in the late '70s several physicians were unhappy with the way the hospital was operating and created a general feeling of internal unrest and conflict. Larry monitored the problem for a while, and then went to one of the regular staff meetings and asked for a few minutes at the beginning. He spoke gently but with force about the reasons for the hospital's existence and reminded the physicians to focus on the needs of the patients and of each other. He said he recognized it was hard to work in an area of great need with limited resources, but that the work would not get done unless everyone treated each other with respect and empathy. He thanked them for the time, and left. It didn't solve the problem entirely, but he set some ground rules for the way stresses should be expressed, and that brief speech was remembered long after the principals were gone."

Bill Dunn describes Larry as "a very precise decision-maker. I always tried to make sure he had all the information, because he could be triggered into decision-making very quickly, and it was important that he have all the facts. He always wanted to implement a decision as fast as possible. Some procrastinate the implementation. Not Dr. Mellon." In Dunn's view, that attitude was related to Larry's insistence on doing things "by the book," whether the book was tax law or his own ethical principles:

One time, all of a sudden, we had no water at the hospital. We looked into it quickly—obviously it was an emergency—and found that the pipe that brought the main water supply from the hill south of the hospital had been broken. So we sent a crew up and mended it immediately.

Next day, same thing—no water, pipe broken. Repaired it. Third day, same thing. Now we began to get suspicious. I went up with the crew and found a group of local people from the village near the spring, standing around watching. I engaged them in conversation and said I hoped it wouldn't happen again. They let me know in a roundabout way it probably *would* happen again. I said okay, let's get to the bottom of this: Do you have a grievance? They said, "Yes—you've taken this spring, which is on our doorstep, and carried it all the way down to the hospital, and now our animals don't have anything to drink."

I went back to the hospital and told Dr. Mellon the story. He listened carefully and didn't have to think on it a bit. He said, "Bill, those people have a good point. Let's get them a fountain." Just like that: "Let's take care of the problem."

So we went back up the next day, talked to the folks, made plans with them to tap into the line at a place where they could get their horses down to the ravine, water their livestock, get drinking water, and let the women wash their clothes. He heard a need and responded immediately.

.   .   .

NOT ALL PROBLEMS were so easily solved. The biggest in Haiti's Artibonite Valley was tetanus, the number one killer of Haitian newborns, due largely to the custom of rubbing mud, dung, or charcoal on freshly cut umbilical cords.

"It's a terrible disease," says Gwen. "The kids go rigid, and you have to feed them by tube. It's treatable, but it takes somebody watching all the time because they can get in a spasm and can't breathe. We used to have dozens of them, a whole room full of tetanus babies. We lost quite a few, but a lot of them survived. Those who do are often extremely healthy because they've been well fed and cared for, and there are no sequelae, no mental things. They're good kids."

Skeets Marshall remembers the neonatal tetanus ward being so full that "at times there were two babies in a crib. We would save better than 50 percent of them. Newborn tetanus is almost never seen in the United States."

The conventional wisdom among epidemiologists in those days was that tetanus immunization should be provided only to mothers who came for prenatal care. The doctors who held that view, for the most part, had not been in the field long enough to learn that in countries such as Haiti, most mothers did not show up for prenatal care or, if they did, it was usually too late in their pregnancies to get the benefit of the vaccine. The medical world now knows better, thanks to the Mellons, who were determined to immunize every woman in the Artibonite Valley against tetanus, not just pregnant women. But any such incredibly ambitious outreach program required great internal planning and development.

"Larry and I just decided mutually that the hospital should have a public health department," Dr. Lepreau remembers. "I was not really a public health guy, but they had me out there riding a bicycle making house calls in the valley. So if the medical director does it, then everyone on the staff has to do it." Going out into the countryside changed his whole outlook, and that of the other HAS physicians, "just like a house call in the U.S.: You can find out after five minutes in the home what you could never find out in an office visit."

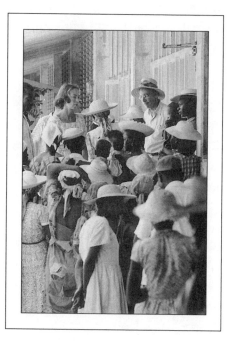

VISITING DAY

The dynamic, unprecedented effort was initiated and held together for years by a remarkable husband-and-wife team.

"It went by steps," says Warren Berggren, who with his wife, Dr. Gretchen Berggren, headed the HAS public health program in late '60s and early '70s. "The first work was done on pregnant women, but it was later learned that you did not have to give the injections during pregnancy. You could immunize a woman and for the next five years, any babies she had would be protected. That brought a much more efficient way to deliver protection: Instead of waiting for the women to be pregnant, we would vaccinate them all. But the women were not terribly interested in coming to the hospital to get immunization. They didn't see the point of it. It was a little insulting to them to suggest that something they weren't doing was causing the death of these children. You can't suggest to a parent that he or she might be the cause of a child's death. This was an unacceptable message. So we took it out of the hospital and put it into the community."

The task of immunizing *everyone* was staggering, and the only way to accomplish it was to meet the women on their own turf, at dawn in the marketplaces. Anything that works well in rural Haiti begins early in the day. It was said of Larry that he ate breakfast by the light of the luminescent dial on his wristwatch.[20]

"Our teams would arrive at 5 a.m. and find that many of the market women would have slept there overnight so they could get good spots the next morning," says Gretchen Berggren. "Government teams would get there about 11 or 12 when it was hot, and there wasn't enough shade or places to sit. They'd miss the window of opportunity, which is at dawn, when Haitians are up and moving around, especially on market days.

"We had a fantastic rate of return, compared with most countries where it's about 40 percent for the second dose. WHO [the UN's World Health Organization] said if a woman has two doses before she delivers, it's 85 percent protection. But Warren said from the beginning that wasn't good enough and that we needed to give two to three more boosters to provide lifetime immunity."

They wanted success, and they got it. The message was being passed by women among themselves: Get your tetanus shots before you have your baby. Nowadays, the process is still referred to as "marketplace immunization" and is recommended by the World Health Organization. But in terms of social mobilization, HAS' methods in the tetanus campaign had applications far beyond tetanus, as Gretchen Berggren explains:

> One thing we hadn't thought about but soon saw was that there were missed opportunities—women who came to the hospital for other reasons but weren't immunized against tetanus. So our nurses checked every mother who came in [for anything] to see if she had her immunization, and if not, she got it before she left the hospital. This happens in the States, too: A kid comes in with a bad cold and someone notes that he didn't have his polio shot, for example. Those opportunities are crucial not to miss.

Equally important was the education of midwives, some 175 of them, begun by Larry Mellon and Dr. Lucien Rousseau. It was the first traditional midwife-training program in the western hemisphere, teaching proper delivery techniques, cord-cutting, and avoidance of contamination. Around the same time, UNICEF and the Pan-American Health Organization (PAHO) initiated a program to supply midwives with equipment boxes containing a plastic apron for delivery, clean sheets, and other materials, many of which the midwives had difficulty using.

"You can't just give her one set of tools," says Gretchen Berggren. "You've got to keep giving her soap, brushes, and clean umbilical-cord ties. These were expendable supplies that had to be constantly resupplied."

When that UN project was discontinued, HAS was one of few hospitals in the world to keep it alive by providing its own Traditional Birth Attendant supplies. Dr. Rousseau and his wife created new boxes with simplified equipment. They had discovered that giving the midwives scissors, for example, was not only nonproductive, it was dangerous.

The scissors were used for hair-cutting and other things and were soon unsterile. How to convince people to boil them for twenty minutes? Traditional birth attendants do not have watches. In their eyes, as soon as steam rises, the water is ready. And once the scissors are boiled, how do you get them out of the water still sterile?

Dr. Rousseau found a simple, cost-effective alternative: a small paper kit containing a surgical pack, sterile razor blades, umbilical-cord tie, belly band and two safety pins—the whole kit wrapped in paper, used for the baby to lie on. And he took up all the old scissors.

"Deschapelles doesn't often get credit for it," says Gretchen Berggren, "but it's now accepted worldwide. It's called 'the clean cord-cut kit.' Lucien Rousseau was the first doctor to introduce it, in 1960 or so. So HAS not only continued the TBA training program started by the World Health Organization, but modified it in a very practical way."

Rousseau practiced as an obstetrician in Haiti before going to the United States to study anesthesiology and do a residency at Brooklyn's Jewish Hospital. He worked as an anesthesiologist at HAS from 1960 to 1966. His wife, Renée, a nurse-specialist in child care, worked in the pediatrics department, running the *femmes sages* (midwives) program.

A key aid in the process of preventing tetanus was an educational film in Creole, made in 1960 by the Rev. Lloyd Shirer, his wife, Margaret, and Billy Mellon with local people as stars. Shirer took the film throughout the countryside with a station wagon and a motion-picture truck, and screened it in the villages. Among other things, the movie pointed out that the midwives were not at fault.*[21]

"Usually, she did her job well," says Gretchen Berggren. "She's washed her hands, cut the cord properly, used sterile instruments, dressed the umbilical cord stump properly. Then here comes Granny or Auntie from next door to unwind the belly band and put some dirty old charcoal—or spider webs or candle wax or dung or burnt straw, all sorts of things—on

---

*Shirer joined the Mellons in 1959 and started a community-development program that covered eight villages on a meager budget of $30,000. They made two other excellent short movies of their own, one on prevention of tetanus in babies and the other on the raising of pigs.

the cord. The TBAs said, 'Look, we're not the only ones interacting with these umbilical cords.' So the script of the film said, '*Non, grandmère, don't do that! We don't need another tetanus baby.' And it flashes back to what the film begins with, a little coffin being carried to the cemetery. It was very effective, and it's been translated into English and Spanish and shown everywhere."

Even after most women in the valley learned about tetanus prevention, they often came to the hospital for cord care anyhow, wrapping their babies in a banana leaf and a towel, placenta and all, for the cord to be "professionally" cut.

"I would say a good 20 percent of them have cord care at the hospital," says Dr. Berggren. "Many think you have to cut the cord right away, but you really don't. So much emphasis is on cutting the cord, but

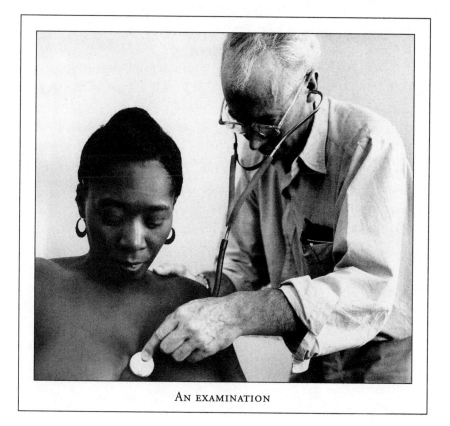

AN EXAMINATION

the TBA's first reaction after the baby is born should be to make sure the airway is open—help the child to breathe. We said, 'Don't worry about the cord-cut first.'"

In Haiti, after a child is born, it is crucial to ask if the parents want the placenta. Mountain folks in particular always do, and they bury the placenta in or near their homes.

"That's terribly important," says Dr. Berggren. "Most people, in rural Haiti especially, know where their placenta is buried. When we were trying to limit our patients to within the district, we were told, 'Don't ask them where they're from, ask where their placenta is buried, because they won't lie about that.' The placenta is considered the seat of nourishment of the baby. It represents the spirit of the mother and baby together, deserving of very special treatment. It's a spiritual belief."

Soon enough, the tetanus rate in the twenty-three villages nearest the hospital fell to nearly zero, an enormous achievement and one of the great miracles of HAS. "In a year's time, the whole thing had rolled back," says Gwen. Yet as word of that spread through the country, there was a baffling follow-up development, which Dr. Berggren likes to pose in her medical classes:

"I say to students, 'What do you think is happening? The more midwives we trained, the more tetanus cases came in.' You'd be surprised how long it takes them to figure it out: It wasn't that there was more tetanus in the district, but that the tetanus was coming from farther and farther away. The point is, looking at hospital statistics doesn't help very much unless you understand the broader community from which people come."

As noted, the Mellons had established the policy of keeping their operations strictly within the district. It wasn't an easy decision, but when Larry saw that most of the tetanus was coming from outside, he permitted a broad expansion of the boundaries.

"That was a pretty nervy thing to do," recalls Warren Berggren, "and sure enough, with crowds of 2,000 or more gathering in the outlying towns, it got into the newspapers in Port-au-Prince and we got a letter from the minister of health saying, 'Why are you immunizing people out there?' I replied that tetanus was the most frequent cause for admission to the hospital, that we'd been able to diminish it, but that the cases were now coming from outside the district and we were taking advantage of the large crowds in marketplaces in order to do immunizations there. They never bothered us after that."

One of the biggest clinics took place at the large Catholic church in Petite Riviére where, on market day, the courtyard in front of the church was packed with 4,000 people. Gretchen Berggren recalls it vividly:

I wanted to get a picture of this because it was really quite a scene, people crowding to get in for their immunizations. Women were losing their shoes in the melee, so they'd take them off and hold them above their heads. The French Catholic priest there had been very kind to allow us to use the church, and I asked if he'd take me up to the bell tower to get that wonderful shot of the women holding their shoes above their heads. So we climbed up with my camera, and while we were up there he said, "You usually vaccinate children, why are you vaccinating women?"

So I explained to him all about how the mother's antibodies protect the newborn—more than he ever wanted to know about tetanus. I said, "Look at those women: There's hardly one of them that hasn't lost at least one baby to tetanus, and many of them have lost half their babies to it." I had done 2,000 birth histories by then and knew what I was talking about.

He looked at me and said, "Well, life doesn't mean that much to them. They're so used to seeing death." I was appalled. I said, "You don't know what it's like to have your breasts filled with milk and to have that baby be unable to take your breast that's swollen and sore because he can't open his mouth." I gave him a lecture on Schweitzer and the idea of respect for life. I told him a mother never forgets the death of a tetanus baby. Studies in many cultures show that if a baby survives long enough to get tetanus, the mother never forgets in her pregnancy history to tell you about it. It's real human suffering.

You would never have heard that from a Haitian priest. They know what children mean in this society. This was a Frenchman. Maybe he learned something. But I must say, he was wonderful to allow this huge mob in the churchyard.

HAS mobile immunization teams eventually inoculated some 114,000 child-bearing women and newborns a year, and the Berggrens had the satisfaction of seeing neonatal tetanus virtually eradicated in the area they served. Their tireless consciousness-raising efforts were successful closer to home, too, as Gretchen recalls:

> One year we took our two little kids to the Christmas Eve ceremony on the HAS tennis court in Deschapelles. Mary rode in on a donkey and Joseph was there and the nasty innkeeper turned them away. They finally went to this humble little animal shed, where Jesus is born. At that point, my four-year-old sang out at the top of her lungs, "Is that baby Jesus in there?" I said, "Shhh!" Then she said very loudly, "Who cut the cord? And why didn't Jesus get tetanus?"

.   .   .

CONTRARY TO THE ASSUMPTION of many, the old Haitian custom of rubbing dung or other tainted substances on umbilical cords was a folk remedy and not a voodoo superstition. But voodoo did, and does, have a relation to certain medical problems in Haiti, particularly in regard to children.

HAS doctors discovered, for example, that there was a rather high incidence of twins in Haiti, and that, for voodoo-related reasons, Haitians do not regard twins a good phenomenon. Often the stronger of the two is fed first, and the second is far more likely to die. Beyond that, twins signify twice the amount of responsibility and medical problems. "A twin birth is usually complicated," Gwen observes, "even in the States."

There are medical implications to certain other voodoo beliefs and rituals, particularly those involving the passing of children over fire. "We take care of the burns," says Gwen, "but we don't tell people not to do things. We wouldn't dream of that. It's a religion of Haiti and we're not going to tell them not to do it. If epileptic children have a seizure, they can roll into an open fire and get burned. But it's hard to tell if they're epileptics or if they've been through some ceremony. You don't ask, and you're not told."

Dr. Marcella Caldi-Scalcini, a HAS doctor, added:

> We see a lot of burned children from ceremonies where they throw children across the fire. Burns are related to voodoo. It's impossible that they happen accidentally. We had an American director who used to go and try to investigate those things, but he couldn't break the wall of silence.
>
> I went once or twice to see a *bocor* (voodoo doctor) because a patient of mine was seeing him, and I wanted to find out what kind of doctor he was. So I went to visit him, and he truly was a good, intelligent man. Some *bocors* are quite good with folk medicine. Most of our patients come to us after they have tried the local traditional medicine.

Indeed, most Haitians consult their voodoo healers before visiting the hospital. Only arrogant Westerners use or put stock in the term "witch doctor." In Haiti, the meshing of voodoo with Catholicism is paralleled by the meshing of voodoo and medicine, and there is more cooperation than conflict between the two. Voodoo priest-healers come in two forms—*bocors*, who deal mostly in salves and mixtures, and *houngans*, whose practice is similar but more mystical.

"All medicine is trial and error," says Gwen. "We see the voodoo remedies in such highly synthesized form that they're often unrecognizable, but it's largely based on plants and other things that grow. There are good and bad voodoo doctors, and they're very expensive."

Once when Larry was walking past the house of a *bocor* who lived in his neighborhood, the man called to him in greeting and said, "Have you noticed that when people arrive in Deschapelles by camion, they stop at my place first before they go to your hospital?" Larry replied,

"No, I'm usually not this far down the road when the camion arrives."
The *bocor* said, "Well, you should know that they come to my place
first, and that's why they don't have any money when they get to your
place—I get it all."

Larry was always respectful toward this canny group of professionals.
He preferred to call them "leaf"—not "witch"—doctors and he recognized their contributions:

> These leaf doctors have borne most of the burden of country medi-
> cine since French colonial days. [They] know how to treat malaria
> and average cuts and pains. I've seen a broken leg perfectly set by a
> *bocor*. And they understand the psychiatric problems here better than
> we do.[22]

There is no such thing as a mental hospital in Haiti, though there are
as many mentally disturbed people—plagued by "evil spirits"—there as
anywhere else. Voodoo healers often tend to them. Like most other hospitals in Haiti, HAS has no psychiatric unit. When such cases arose, Dr.
Mellon often referred the mentally and emotionally afflicted to their *bocors*, knowing that their functions were similar to those of a psychiatrist—or of any wise man who simply understood his people.

CHAPTER 5

MODERATO
"Go to the People"

L ARRY MELLON, no less than the *bocors*, was also a wise man who understood his people. In Haiti, one of his earliest and most profound insights was that medicine alone could make only a dent in the underlying Haitian dilemma: to cure and then return people to the same environment that produced the disease did not much help them in the long run.

Accordingly, Dr. Mellon only "doctored" full-time for about three years in Haiti. After that he turned the bulk of his attention to creating an array of service projects that were ambitious to the point of gargantuan. Thenceforth, if you wanted to find Larry Mellon, you went outdoors, and often a long way.

"Once the hospital was well established," he later told Bill Dunn, "I saw that other people could do the doctoring and that what was really needed was work in the field." Dunn irreverently replied, "Come on, Larry, don't give me that. You're just a cowboy at heart and you couldn't stand being indoors." Mellon smiled and said, "Yes, that's probably true."

Bill Dunn studied and admired Larry's habits for years:

"Dr. Mellon had great ideas. He could visualize and he could plan. But he hated administrative paperwork. The documentation of things bored him. Consequently, he designed his life to be out in the field much of the time. He would stop in the business office, where he had a little desk. People would put checks there for him to sign the evening

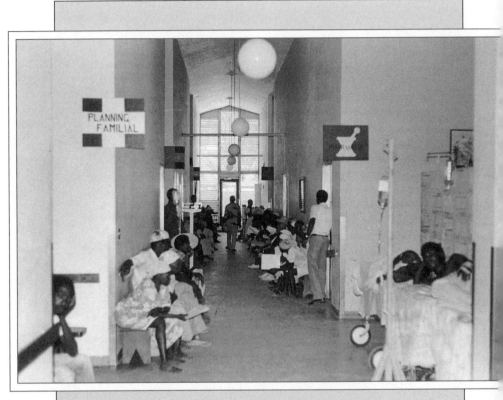

The waiting room

before. He would come in before anybody else, sign the checks, and be out of the hospital before the day shift came to work. He'd be available in the late afternoon at home if people needed him, but basically, he left the administration to Mrs. Mellon and to the rest of the administrative folks in the hospital."

In his most strenuous years, from the late '50s to early '80s, Mellon's daily routine consisted of visiting the hospital by 6:30 A.M., spending as little time as possible there with the managerial chores he loathed, and then getting out. To him, life was "out there," working on an irrigation project, calling on the sewing centers, figuring out the carpenters' problems, deciding whether to put in a pipeline from this spring to that community.

"In those days, there weren't as many vehicles around," Dunn recalls. "The appearance of a car was a big event, and the presence of Dr. Mellon was always a welcome sight. I remember two sounds very vividly. One was kind of a chant. As he drove along those miserable roads, people would all recognize him and holler, 'Doc, Doc, Doc!' as he went by. People would yell and wave and he would always wave back and be friendly. Often he'd stop to visit. Sometimes that 'Doc, Doc!' had a more urgent tone when someone needed transportation to the hospital. Sick people would wait along the road and his old jeep would be jammed with them when he got back in the afternoon, making a loop in front of the hospital to disgorge everyone he'd picked up along the way."

Art Bergner, a longtime HAS physician, often accompanied Larry on those rounds, as Bergner's wife, Renée, also an HAS doctor, remembers:

Larry didn't tolerate too many people for too long. He was a loner, but he let Art drive a lot, in part because Art didn't ask him any questions. Art would ask him about the people or Haitian culture but never anything personal. In driving around, Art learned a lot about him. But he never figured out the criteria for how Larry knew whom to help or not help on the road—whom he would pick up and whom he would drive right by. Where to stop and ask what he could do and where not to—was it was totally intuitive? How did he figure out who should be helped directly? Larry was at that time the one-man out-reach program.[1]

That second sound Bill Dunn always remembered was Dr. Mellon's car horn, which he used to call together the community meetings: "He would tell a group of people he'd be out to meet them at 10 Monday morning. But come 10 o'clock, nobody would gather. They would wait for the sound of his horn and then they'd emerge from all kinds of places. Within a few minutes, everyone would be there and the meeting could begin. It was an effective way of getting a meeting started: People didn't have to sit around and wait for him, nor did he have to wait for them. When he blew the horn, people knew it was time to assemble."

Larry set the pattern and the rhythm of life for the whole HAS staff. He never took food with him when he went into the countryside, out of sensitivity to the Haitians who had little food and didn't eat till late afternoon. "I don't remember him even carrying water," says Dunn. "He went out with what supplies and tools he'd need for the day's work, and that was it."

The day's work was always intense for, by 1959, the HAS community development program had begun feverish activity. On the campus and at the HAS outreach centers, literacy, health, sewing, carpentry, homemaking, and child care were taught.

"He started teaching young girls basic health," says Gwen. "He said it was the first step in development, and he was right. It was all part of the public-health picture. When we first came, they didn't read or write or even sew. Our classes taught the girls how to dress and speak and behave. It was important especially for those who didn't go to the regular school."

That school, L'École La Providence, was the brainchild and labor of love of Harold May, and therein lies a tale he can tell best:

I had volunteered for the Air force before I was 18 in 1945, while I was in college, and had flight training in Tuskeegee, Alabama, where the black airmen were instructed during WWII. Tuskeegee had trained ex-slaves and helped them develop skills to live a productive life once they won their freedom. When I saw the poverty, the need in Haiti, it seemed to me they needed the same kind of access to this development, to learn skills they didn't have. I said from the beginning that what Haiti needed was Tuskeegees.

[By 1962], from passing the plate at the HAS church services Sunday after Sunday, we had $4,500. What was the best investment of it? Some said we should have a primary school for hospital employees. I

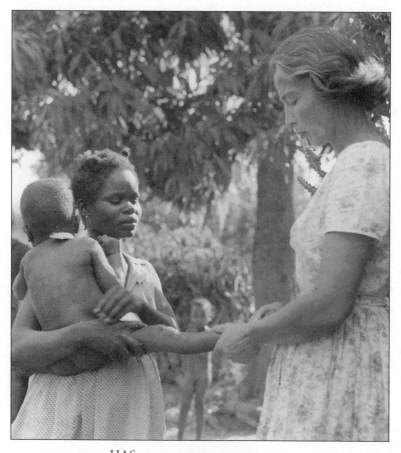

HAS COMMUNITY DEVELOPMENT

thought it should be for all children of the community. So we started the school.

You have to start at the beginning, not in the middle, and decide if you're going for quality or quantity. There would be room for seventy-five children, five to seven years old, kindergarten and first grade. I was thinking in terms of a long-range, not a one- or two-year plan. Haiti took from 1804 to get into this condition and won't be corrected in two years or five or ten. You have to prepare those who'll be leading the next generation. Think in terms of multiplying, rather than addition. Each of those seventy-five you'll invest enough in so they'll affect life in their community. It shouldn't be given to them, they must share the responsibility. Haitian friends said charge eighty cents a month, most can pay that. But they should either pay something or provide some service so they'll have the respect of sharing the responsibility and contributing.

The parents, who couldn't read or write, took a keen interest. We were thrilled to see them march up their kids to register them. *Seven hundred fifty children came.* We could only accept seventy-five, so that was hard. Those accepted had to go back into the courtyards and teach other kids. And they did it. They couldn't get the impression they were better than the others. They had to share it.[2]

.   .   .

DOZENS OF sanitation projects were initiated. Old wells were collared and new ones dug for the clean cooking and bathing water that had not been obtainable for generations. Latrines were built—Dr. Mellon always among the laborers—along with new dams and irrigation canals. As a result of Larry's keen interest in, and self-taught knowledge about, water, crops would flourish in places where they had never succeeded before.

The Peligre Dam, built by a Haitian government agency called the Organization for Development of the Artibonite Valley (ODVA), provided water all over the floor of the Artibonite. ODVA had the responsibility for keeping the dams and canals clean and water levels up and for creating secondary canals in an area embracing the whole valley down to the sea. But ODVA was riddled with political conflicts and corruption and was out of money. Its apathetic employees went unpaid, its equipment was in disrepair, and the water in its undredged canals barely moved. There was a huge restoration job to be done, and the government wasn't doing it. Larry Mellon was in no position to do so, either. But on a smaller scale, he did what he could, initiating dam and irrigation projects at a higher elevation above the existing rice fields. Never mind that he had no engineering degree.

"Neither had the Romans when they built their aqueducts," he once observed.

In the early '60s, Larry and Gwen visited Italy, where Michael Rawson was then studying. Knowing their interest in archeology, he

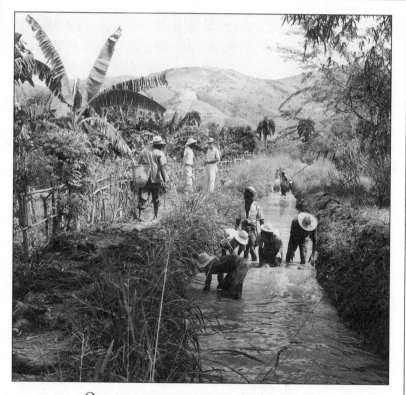

ONE OF DOZENS OF SANITATION PROJECTS

arranged for them to visit the excavated Etruscan tombs at Tarquinia. The ancient burial sites captivated them, but the real highlight for Larry was in the nearby wheat fields, where he inspected some new elevated irrigation flumes. Fifty-foot U-shaped concrete sections, joined and caulked at their pedestals to maintain a continuous level and conduct water from various collection sites to adjacent fields in the dry summer.

"We took photos and made measurements of the flume sections," recalls Michael, who thought no more of it until six months later on his next trip to Haiti, when he visited a dam site on the Tapion River, where Larry had been working to provide irrigation for new bean fields on rocky slopes above Liancourt. There, Michael was stunned to see several kilometers of familiar-looking raised flumes carrying water from the thirty-five-foot-high dam to the now-thriving bean plots.

In that short time, "Larry had designed and built the forms using local lumber, somehow acquired the rods and cement, and poured the concrete dalles in the HAS schoolyard," Michael said. "The transporta-

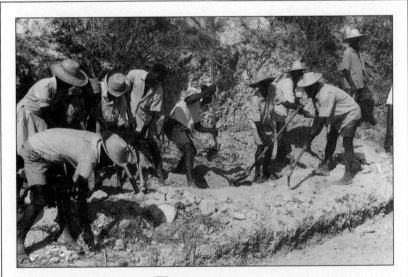

WELLS BEING DUG
Old wells were collared and new ones dug for the clean cooking and bathing water that had not been obtainable for generations.

tion of the sections, weighing several tons each, over rough trails, and their installation on the pedestals fabricated at the dam site was in itself a major logistics feat made possible through the teamwork of the local farmers and HAS's Mennonite volunteers. Larry worked side by side with dozens of laborers to install them, providing a water source for years to come. It was a classic example of his ability to adapt an idea to the local materials and available talent in Deschapelles, and to solve the problem at hand."[3]

Larry had carefully calculated the height of the pedestals versus the depth of the trenches, lowering the pillars into position by ropes. "He went down every day to make sure the levels were right," says Gwen. "They had to cut through a high hill to keep it going in a straight direction—all of it by hand, of course. No tractors or bulldozers. It was a beautiful thing to see, and our young Mennonite boys deserved a lot of the credit for it."

The Mennonites were among the most valuable of the "available talent" pool then in Deschapelles. In that era, many young Mennonites came to HAS in lieu of military service. They were a coterie of young men gung-ho to work in community development, especially on the canals and other irrigation projects.

"The Mennonites were farm boys from Pennsylvania, Kansas, and all over," says Gwen. "When they were brand new here, Larry said, 'I have a good project for you. A man over in Ti Rivière wants to build an *asile* [old folks home]. Here's some cement.' He put a wonderful boy named Jim Shirz in charge, and they went away and did it. They had the independence. Solid people. There are many different Mennonites. Some are very withdrawn. When we started, we had quite a large group of them who all lived in the same house. The girls were lab technicians and nurses. They'd stay in the house, eat together, never go out after hours. Very strict. But that seemed to change here. Both the men and the women became tremendously involved with the Haitians."

Among many other things, the Mennonite Central Committee initiated a major reforestation project for the region, planting 20,000 seedlings and then distributing them to the people later that year. There were all sorts of fruit trees—"anything we could think of," says Gwen, "to get the kids to collect seeds and plant them in the little bags and make compost. It's wonderful. The door is open for them."

Larry had taken to heart Schweitzer's advice to plant only trees that produce edible fruit. He followed up on an irrigation project at the poor town of Valereux, for example, by staying to plant beans. After the Mennonites left Deschapelles, Gwen Mellon personally took over the seedling project for several years before turning it over to her helpmate, Anny Frédérique, the daughter of HAS ophthalmologist Dr. Gérard Frédérique. Anny supervised the spring planting and also ran various grafting projects. One of them spliced new varieties of mango onto existing trees to make them produce five different kinds of fruit and, since grafted trees produce in one-fourth the time, quicken productivity.

·   ·   ·

URBANE, SOFT-SPOKEN Dr. Lucien Rousseau leans back in a chair in his Port-au-Prince living room and reflects on the phenomenon he and his wife witnessed over thirty years, and on the man behind it.

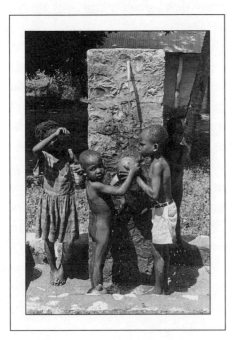

TINY BENEFICIARIES
OF CLEAN WATER

"What surprised us when we became close to him," says Dr. Rousseau, "was that a man like Dr. Mellon, so wealthy, had made a choice to come to Haiti. He could have done so many things in so many other places. But that simple life in the country, giving health to Haitians, meant more to him than anything else. The people were in misery, suffering from all kinds of dreadful diseases. He was moved by that.

"But he was concerned also about their way of life. He saw that putting more and more money into the hospital, getting more and more doctors and modern equipment, wouldn't solve the problem. He realized something very important: That curing the disease is fine, but if you go to the cause of the disease, it's much better. That's what gave him the idea of the community development projects. He became interested in all those ways to improve living conditions because, by doing so, he could treat the cause of the diseases and there would be fewer sick people."

What struck the Rousseaus even more than *what* Larry did was *how* he did it, Madame Rousseau says: "Dr. Mellon was always ready to give himself for others, and he behaved the same way toward anyone he happened to meet in a difficult situation. On the road, he would stop his jeep to help a peasant with his donkey. If he saw somebody's car broken down, he would stop and do something to help. This simplicity of his character made him somebody with a great heart and soul."

Lucien Rousseau continues: "He treated everyone he worked with so respectfully, not just the chief of the hospital. Dr. Mellon would talk to every orderly or low-level employee or peasant with the same respect that he would give the administrator or chief surgeon. That's one of the things that always astonished us and that we most admired. People remember him not only as a good doctor but mainly as a man with a large and generous heart—someone who was concerned about people as human beings. The role he played in the valley had a very wide scope."

A very wide scope, indeed. A comprehensive account of HAS community projects over the years would fill volumes, but among the highlights were the bakery, the production of bricks, tiles and brooms, and a wide range of farm, livestock, and veterinary activities. All were initiated by Larry and his colleagues with one thing in common: the innovative use of indigenous human and material resources.

The bakery at nearby Liancourt, for example, began with a single local woman, who had six children and no way to make a living. She baked 150 loaves at a time for the hospital. Dr. Mellon would take her flour in the back of his jeep, which was also loaded with wood for her fire, and haul the newly baked bread back to the hospital.

"I grew up in the little village of Borel, three or four miles north of Deschapelles," says Pastor André Sonnal, former HAS chaplain and director of community relations, "and as a boy I got to know Dr. and Mrs. Mellon and used to go with him in his Land Rover to the bakery. People would stop him along his way home, just for the pleasure of buying bread from him."

Dr. Art Maimon accompanied Larry on one such bread run to Liancourt and asked to buy a few loaves for himself: "I said, 'Here, I'll pay you,' and he said drily, 'Never mind. I'll just charge it off to advertising.'"

The bakery functioned nicely for years but, like many other projects, eventually fell victim to a failure to adapt.

"The baker was a very good, proud woman and it was good bread,"

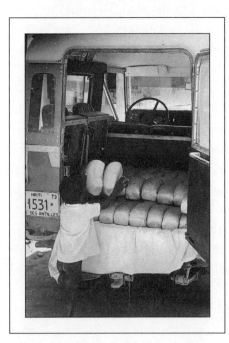

NEWLY BAKED BREAD
LARRY WOULD HAUL BACK
TO THE HOSPITAL

Gwen recalls. "She did very well, built herself a nice house. But when we closed the hospital dining room, we didn't need 150 loaves anymore, just half that. She said, 'I can't just make seventy-five loaves. I use all this wood and I can't afford it.' We said we'd try to take the 150 loaves and put half of them in the freezer, but bread doesn't freeze well and people in the kitchen complained that hers was twice as expensive as the local bread. She wasn't willing to lower her price. So we had to find another small baker in Verrettes whose wife delivered it each day on foot. I felt bad about it. If she had made an effort, we would have found a way to continue it."

.   .   .

THE HAS brick- and tile-making operations were classic instances of Larry's pragmatic resourcefulness. He had discovered large clay deposits by the Artibonite River and was determined to exploit them. Bill Dunn recalls the day he arrived in 1973 to provide administrative help:

"I got here, and the first morning, he picked me up and said, 'Why don't you go out in the country with me? We'll just talk today.' I said fine, and we talked, and finally I said, 'Well, where do you want me to start? I'm ready to go.' He said, 'You've got to straighten out that brick-making operation.' I said, 'What are you talking about? I'm a hospital administrator.' He said, 'You'll do okay. You'll figure it out.' And I did. That was my first project, and we got to the bottom of it. We straightened out the brick operation."

The manufacture of roofing and floor tiles came about as a result of one of Gwen's and Larry's visits to Mexico, where they observed a family of tile-making artisans and learned the process from them. Back home, in turn, the Mellons taught their new skill to the Haitians. The results were beautiful and of sufficiently high quality that the leading architectural firm in Port-au-Prince regularly purchased HAS tiles for use in posh new resorts and restaurants in the capital city. But in the long run, despite the popularity of the product, the operation had to be discontinued due to fuel and transportation problems.

Broom-making presented a different set of challenges which, as so often, could be surmounted temporarily but not permanently. In the first place, brooms required a special stiff straw similar to cane that had to be imported until Dr. Mellon acquired seeds from abroad and began raising it on the hospital farm. But the broom corn didn't grow well in Haiti, due to the lack of wind. "When straw grows in windy places, it's better and stronger," explains Gus Ménager, the HAS agronomist.

They got the operation running, but there were other problems—one a bit macabre. One of the broom workers was a faithful HAS hand named Aristomene Jacques, known to all as Ti Blanc (Little White) because he was very light-skinned. Ti Blanc had a sixth finger on his left hand, "hanging by a thread," Gwen recalls. "The machine operator who came down to train them said, 'No way—I won't have anything to do with him unless he gets rid of that finger.' Ti Blanc said, 'But it's a sign of my heritage!' He was very proud of it. The trainer said, 'Then you can't get the job,' and so Ti Blanc ended up having the damn thing cut off."

A more conventional problem was the broom handle. You could grow the straw, but for the handle you needed wood, which was scarce and expensive in Haiti. Larry tried to tell people to save the handles and bring them back, but wood still had to be imported, which pushed the broom's cost higher than its five-dollar selling price.

The chronic lumber problem throughout Haiti was due to deforestation, plus the fact that in the tropics, the life of a lumber tree is limited. If not harvested by a certain point, it gets hollow in the middle and the resulting planks tend to split. The longer-range dilemma is that two or three trees must be planted for every one cut down; failure to replace and replenish is at the heart of the shortage. The magnificent wood used in the interiors of the Standard Fruit houses on the HAS campus, for example, was all mahogany. In the '20s, there were still plenty of such trees in Haiti. But nobody replanted them, then or later, and the mahogany forests are now entirely gone.

In the end, the HAS broom operation, too small and expensive to sustain a profit, had to be discontinued.

More lasting were the construction projects that occupied an enormous amount of Larry Mellon's time and energy. Through the years, he helped countless Haitians build new homes and communal buildings in what is known as the "rammed-earth" process.

"You decide where you're going to put the walls of the house," Gwen explains, "and you dig a ditch and put hard stone material in it, to get a good base. You set up plywood walls and join them at the top. Then you make a mixture of *touf* [powdered calcified rock with a small amount of cement and water] and pour it in. You keep the forms on quite a while until it dries. It's very good, simple and inexpensive. We have rammed-earth houses built many years ago that are still standing. People are crazy about concrete, which is more permanent but much more costly."

.   .   .

LARRY AND GWEN had a special concern for the mysterious mountain people of Terre Nette above Verrettes. They are descended from the *marrons*, runaway slaves and mulattoes who hid from the French in the hills and intermarried with Haiti's few remaining Indians, who were themselves in hiding. Some of them were involved in Haiti's independence struggle. Terre Nette is located in one of the most inaccessible and neglected areas served by HAS.

Gretchen Berggren's description is lyrical:

Market days found its farmers wending their way down the long mountains with heavy loads of produce on their heads or on their donkeys, headed for market places to sell what little excess they had been able to eke out from the rapidly eroding mountainsides. The women seemed especially thin and often carried malnourished tots in their arms; the men, too, seemed to wear the strain of centuries on their faces. Their way of speaking was different: they spoke in a *petite voix* [little voice] to show respect, which Haitian ethnologists identify as harking back to the time slaves were not allowed to address their masters in a normal tone.

Larry and Gwen rode horses or hiked to Terre Nette many times. Larry listened with inexhaustible patience to the peasants' stories.

Every trip brought a new heartbreaking tale: He had met a father on the way to HAS with an eight-day-old boy in tetanus spasms; a mother with a kwashiorkor child in her arms; a grandma with long-neglected TB who couldn't get down the mountain to the hospital. How could we reach these people? What would be the most meaningful help?[4]

Gus Ménager said a road into the area could open it up for agricultural development and enable community health workers to get into those mountainsides to immunize. Soon enough, a Caterpillar tractor driven by a Mennonite volunteer arrived on the scene. Ménager distributed shovels and picks while other Mennonites worked side by side with Terre Nette farmers to build the road. Larry, with his inerrant sense of grass-roots engineering, had laid it all out and was there to supervise.

On weekends during construction, Berggren and Gwen drove up the new road as far as it had progressed, then hiked the rest of the way up to Terre Nette. Once, they stopped to look down into the valley below, where the HAS water tower and shining roofs of the hospital could be seen. An elderly Haitian man approached and told Gwen she was looking at "Mme. Mellon's Hospital." She smiled and asked what that hospital meant to him.

"Ah," he replied, "it means we can finally have all the children we want!" Gwen liked to quote that gem whenever Berggren spoke of "a felt need for family planning" in the area.

When at last the day came to open the Terre Nette road, the politicians arrived on the scene, complete with dark glasses and guns on their belts, just in time to take credit for it. They paraded at the ceremony with a big sign they had brought: "The Duvalier Road," with comments below on the "generosity" of the government. Berggren felt a deep sense of rage: "The Duvalieristes had not spent one cent on this road, nor contributed any labor. I pointed to the sign as I slid into a seat by Dr. Mellon. He was quick to sense my emotion—and to save me. 'Look at that sign board,' he whispered. 'Don't you see it's made of cardboard?'"[5]

.   .   .

ONE DAY BEFORE the hospital was completed, Larry and Gwen were stopped on the road to Drouin by a man who asked them to see his wife. Lying on a straw mat, she was thin and wasted and breathing badly. It was all too evident that she had TB. There was little they could do for her. But each day as they passed, Larry brought her an egg. At that point in her illness, his concern and the daily egg were probably the very best medicines.[6]

It is estimated that as much as 10 percent of Haiti's population suffers from tuberculosis, or roughly 500,000 people. This staggering problem is made greater by the fact that, due to the nature of the disease, its victims can not mix with a general hospital population. As the tetanus immunization program was a crossover from medical to community-development work, so, in 1962, was the founding of the HAS TB village, L'Escale. Its creation was personally financed by four HAS Haitian physicians and later supported by the hospital itself and private gifts from the Rawson children and other benefactors. Today, L'Escale's six houses and 49 beds (nine of them for children) are always occupied and more than 1,000 cases of pulmonary tuberculosis treated there each year.

The need was for a community-based approach. Project workers had to do door-to-door follow-up and therapy with TB patients in the villages, where a big stigma was attached to the disease: People thought TB was incurable.

"One day Larry came up to the community health office with X rays of a tubercular patient's lesion, which he showed to everybody," Gretchen Berggen recalled. "We said, 'Did that man die?' He said, 'No, he didn't die at all. In fact, that man can carry a 100-pound cement bag and throw it around.' They were his *own* X rays! He'd had TB at one point and there was some scarring, but it was completely healed. Many are ashamed to admit TB and go into hiding. But here was Dr. Mellon with his own X rays."

Warren Berggren provides a good postscript to the story: "Larry was a very strong man, who kept in shape by the amount of work he did. I wouldn't have taken him on arm wrestling."

.   .   .

ANY ATTEMPT TO recount the enormous range of HAS farm, livestock, and veterinary activities might be subtitled, "The Gus Ménager Story." Ménager, as noted, was Larry's most important nonmedical "discovery" and cofounder of the HAS community-development team. He served at HAS for seventeen years (1954–1971) and held various high-level government posts afterward, including that of minister of agriculture from 1986 to 1988. He is a big, gregarious man with a brilliant mind that bubbles forth with knowledge, new ideas, and fond memories.

"In January 1957, Dr. Mellon came to me one day while I was putting in some beets," says Gus. "He wanted to participate in the job, and he took up a hoe. I was surprised. It's not usual for a doctor to do planting. I said to myself, 'He probably wants to show that I am not doing it properly.' I didn't think that he was having fun, and that he just *liked* doing it.

"He said we should raise as many kinds of vegetables as we could in all the places that could produce them for the hospital. So I organized some terraces and opened the irrigation canal, which was collapsed and

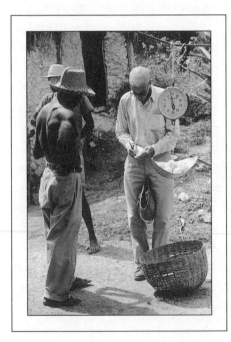

"LARRY SAID WE SHOULD RAISE
AS MANY KINDS OF VEGETABLES
AS WE COULD . . ."

abandoned for many years after the fruit company left. I said it would take money to restore, because it was a long way—six kilometers of canal—to the dam at Verrettes. He said, 'Let me think about it,' and the next morning he left me a note saying, 'Go ahead and put it in shape.'

"Originally, that canal had the capacity to irrigate more than 950 hectors [2,347 acres]. But the water was barely moving because it was so filled with sediment and weeds. In many places people had cut into it and multiplied the number of gates improperly. One man had a canal gate on his property, and we had to stop the water to repair it. But he didn't want his field even temporarily without use of the canal. He was powerful enough—he had a large family and prestige—that he stopped the work. When I told this to Dr. Mellon, he said, 'Go ahead and get the job done, because that man doesn't know how good it is for him. But be patient with him.'

"The next morning I went back and asked the man to recommend some people to hire to do the job. He said, 'I will send twenty-four men—how much will you pay?' I said three and a half gourdes, the average rate. But I didn't need twenty-four, only ten. He said, 'Okay, if you pay them five gourdes [$1] each.' So we agreed to it and he sent me the ten men, and they worked. Dr. Mellon later told me that was a good way to work it out—not harmful to anyone. So we managed to put it back into shape from the bridge up to the dam in Verrettes, which gave more water to all the farmers."

The process was typical of how Mellon and Ménager worked together on dozens of projects: Get an idea, discuss it, start in on it, work out the bugs, solve the problem.

"One of the most interesting times I shared with Dr. Mellon was on the beef farm," Ménager remembers.

He knew a lot about that from his ranch. We had a 100-acre farm nine miles from here, and I wanted to modify it into specialized production. I had thought about it very deeply. I said, "We can't buy good milk or clean meat here. It's not just a local thing, it's in the whole country. We can always buy rice and bananas cheaper than we can produce them, but we cannot buy eggs, milk and meat cheaper. We should raise them ourselves." He agreed, and so we imported some Holsteins for dairy. We started with local stock for beef and up-graded and crossbred them with Brahman and Zebu, to reinforce their resistance to flies and the heat, and we managed to put weight on them.

That dairy took about five years to produce sufficiently for the hospital—100 gallons of milk a day from twenty-four milking cows, which is about what Holsteins in New York State perform. We proved that the Holstein was capable of withstanding tropical condi-tions and producing about the same. It was successful, but the ani-mals consumed much more protein to produce that amount of milk here. I was trying to figure that out, and Dr. Mellon said, "I have a friend in Arizona I'll write to about that." One day he said, "Your milk bacteria count is only 500. Do you know that your milk is much purer than what is being sold in the U.S.?" I didn't know he was fol-lowing that. It was kind of a secret test.

Once he saw there was one cow that was exceptional, giving more than sixteen times her body weight—Louisa. He asked me why I named her Louisa, and I said, because her mother was a Haitian cow I purchased in the valley and bred with a Holstein. Aretha, the grand-mother, was bred to a brahma bull. I crossbred her to the Holstein, and that was how Louisa came about. My point is, he followed things so closely, he even knew the individual cows!

Larry prided himself on such knowledge and on the hospital's self-sufficiency: "We raise our own beef. We use the local tomatoes and onions and melons and carrots, and we make our own ice cream. We eat a lot of goat meat. We even have a special refrigerating room for garbage, otherwise it spoils before the hogs can eat it."[7]

The momentum was exhilarating, as Gus Ménager recalls:

I'll tell you, the hospital was really going in those days. Everything was more, more, more—more patients, more doctors, more food, more everything. I realized that I wouldn't be able to produce enough calves from the herd at the farm. I must find other sources to cross-breed, and the hospital did not have enough farmers or land to do this. I thought I'd better combine with the participation of the farmers around the area.

A creative plan was devised whereby HAS would buy a heifer and give it to a selected "outside" farmer on the condition that he breed it to the bulls at the farm and sell every calf to HAS at the fair market price. After seven calves (seven to eight years), the heifer would belong to the farmer. More than 100 cows were given out in that way, and HAS got the calves it needed to improve its herd. The method was affordable and had incentives to both sides.

"I don't know any other place with cooperative herds—cooperative working animal production—where it really worked," says Ménager. "Later, the hospital had to shrink its whole operation and get closer to the basic things. But we had the most beautiful dairy and beef herds in the country. I don't think there was one in the whole Caribbean to surpass it."

Ménager is proud to have sold the idea to Dr. Mellon in the first place. The beef project lasted nine years, from 1966 to 1975, a great experiment with a good record. A less successful experiment, on the other hand, was Larry's brainstorm of how to solve two problems at once, as his colleague recalls:

He came to me one day and said, "We have so many patients who do not pay their bills. Since they are farmers, why don't we utilize them on the farm in the vegetable garden? When they leave the hospital, we can hire them to do farming jobs to work off their bill." I said, "I'll try but I am not very optimistic, since they are convalescents who won't be able to work hard. I need people to work hard." But he was all for it, and he said what I often heard him say—"See what you can do."

I gave it a try but, first of all, they didn't show up. Second, they would send somebody to replace them, which was good in theory, but in practice those replacement people didn't want to work. They would show up for a day or so and then disappear. Pretty soon, we threw away the whole idea.

Julian Strauss, HAS's second veterinarian (1961–1963), was attracted to the hospital by the infectious idealism of the day. "It was the beginning of the Peace Corps," he recalls, "and I had that kind of vision young people had then." He brought his wife, child, veterinary skills and farm background to Haiti:

I went from one farm, my father's, to another, and I looked up to Dr. Mellon as my teacher and guide. He was a surrogate father figure. I saw him first and foremost as a cowboy and rancher. The Haitians

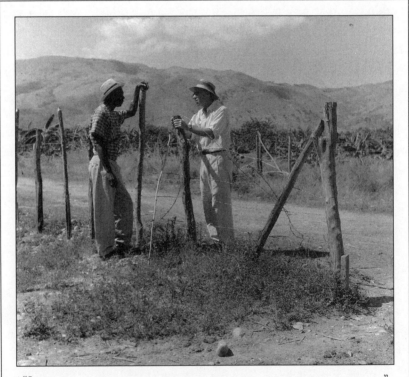

"I SAW HIM FIRST AND FOREMOST AS A COWBOY AND RANCHER . . ."

around him were farmers, as were he and I. He liked to solve problems as a farmer does: A farmer lives a long way from town and works
with whatever he has at hand. He improvises. And that's what we did.
He had his favorite communities and I had mine. He made friends
with a farmer contact person or village leader, and started to help
with some plan they had. I helped him with his projects and he
would help me with mine. It was always, how can we improve health
in one way or another?

He was a homey guy. He let me do whatever things I saw that
needed to be done. He never was discouraging or disparaging, never
critical about what you wanted to do. He always trusted you to find
some contribution to it as well.

He loved horses and was very concerned about the ones he saw
there. That was one reason he started a veterinary program there.
My main thing at first was to take care of the animals that came with
the patients. He felt so sorry for the horses tied to the trees in front of
the hospital. We would work on the back sores, the lame horses, the
skinny ones. Then we would go out to the homes and help with the
pigs and chickens and goats and other problems.[8]

Not everyone had such a positive experience with Mellon at HAS.
One of Strauss' ill-fated successors exemplified the fact that, even in
highly successful operations, unexpected problems could arise from unlikely sources—initiative, for one thing; surplus, for another.

During travel to the slaughterhouses, cows and pigs suffered many
bruises, and the quality of the meat affected. As a result, it was decided
to start butchering in Deschapelles, primarily for the hospital's kitchen.

"We made a 'kill floor'—just a cement slab with a pole to knock the
animal and then bleed it," Ménager recounts. "To bleed it fast, it was
necessary to hoist the animal. This is how the idea took form to build
the slaughterhouse, which I designed and built completely."

That was fine for hospital consumption, but not otherwise. Later, an
industrious young HAS vet began slaughtering surplus animals at Deschapelles for sale in Port-au-Prince, on the correct assumption that both

the weight and the meat quality would be higher that way. But Haitian law required all meat sold in the capital to be slaughtered there. When Larry Mellon found out about the violation, he was furious, and fired his vet on the spot. Appeals for clemency were rejected.

It seemed too severe. No second chance? He was trying to get more money for the hospital's benefit, after all. Wasn't the man only really guilty of overzealousness?

"It was very simple," says Gwen. "It's the law, you've broken it. Good-bye. He broke the law of Haiti, and that's the rule of the hospital. It's very clear, and everybody knows it."

.   .   .

AMONG LARRY'S MANY SKILLS, and fondest activities, the fine art of surveying ranked high from his Arizona days. In Deschapelles, says Ménager, "We did a great deal of surveying, and he taught me a lot about it because I had to map the farm and he found he could be confident in my accuracy. I was the only one to share that with him, except for Mrs.

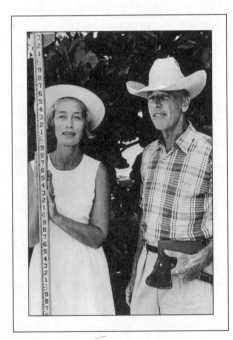

WHEN LARRY WANTED TO
TAP WATER FOR A COMMUNITY,
THE SURVEYING WAS *HIS* JOB.
NOBODY ELSE TOOK
THE TRIPOD.

Mellon. She usually held the stadia rod when he made the readings. He never got tired of it. When he wanted to tap water for a community, the surveying was *his* job. Nobody else took the tripod."

Indeed, Larry and Gwen Mellon were both expert surveyors, and his survey journal reveals the scope of their work in an incredibly meticulous series of measurements for countless new waterlines and fountains in and around Deschapelles. The journal contains thousands of figures, four columns for each project: (1) station number, where one plants the stick, (2) elevation, (3) distance, and (4) angles. With water, elevation is the most crucial factor: Are you going up or down? The nature of the beast is gravity.

Gwen speaks of the time Larry was determined to put in a waterline from points X to Y, with many hills and vales in between. No one believed it would work because of a huge uphill grade at the end where the pipeline was to emerge: The water would have to flow straight up. But due to accurate surveying, Larry knew the final uphill grade would be surmounted by the fact that the elevation where the water began was some fifty feet higher.

Larry began his survey journal in Arizona in 1946, long before he came to Haiti, with elaborate entries for well sites and water lines in such colorfully named places as Cross Mountain, South Prong, Badger Flats, and Wallapai's Eyebrow. He was so compulsively thorough that he even produced a fine-tuned survey of the family vegetable plot, with precise topographical variation and elevation of each row for irritation purposes. In New Orleans, he learned how to measure river currents, practicing on the mighty Mississippi, and made latitudinal observations of sunrises, declination at noon, and sunsets, for no other reason than that it interested him and that he knew how.

His first entries in Haiti concern the laying of pipes for the hospital and for the Mellons' home a few hundred yards away. The rest of the journal is occupied with massive sets of figures for community projects in Deschapelles and surrounding villages involving the springs and tributaries of the Artibonite River.

"The spring in the dry season will fill a 3-inch pipe," he wrote, for example, in 1961. "Elevation of spring 'Madame Rousseau' is undoubtedly higher than Drouin, but I have not yet measured it. Source Coupois lies further from Drouin, up a torturous ravine of perhaps 2½ km. Water rises out of a rocky wall in the canyon, 18 inches above the stream bed. Flow in the dry season probably would fill a 2-inch pipe. Elevation above Drouin must exceed 100 feet. Amazing." He next drew a precise map, followed by the notation: "Rough estimate required for the job is 3,500 feet of steel pipe, 3,890 feet of large plastic pipe, 4,752 feet of smaller plastic pipe."

Soon after, he scoped out a project at La Chapelle, where he set up his instruments and "measured 300-gallons-per-minute flow where the trail crosses the canyon below the source." In 1962, he lugged his tripod to the site of a proposed cotton depot and determined it would require exactly "5 loads of rock, 2 loads of 2-inch gravel, 5 loads of sand, one load of lime, 60 sacks of cement, and 7 iron bars, 20 feet by ½-inch." Next he was off to drain a culvert pond near Liancourt, so that a social center could be built. From there, to source Coquillot near Estrale, to bring water up through several forks of a steep canyon.

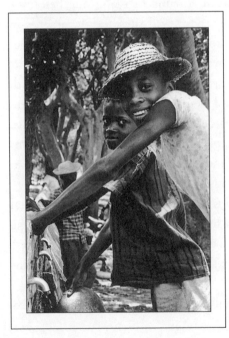

ONE OF THE RESULTS OF THE
MELLONS' WATER PROJECTS IN
THE ARTIBONITE VALLEY

The quantity and quality of water projects Larry initiated, supervised, and brought to fruition for the Artibonite Valley was immense. Pipelines, wells, fountains, and windmills were established at Savannah Roche, Petite Rivière, Anse Rouge, and countless other places. Always, he worked with and ate the same food as the workers and stayed until the work was finished.

By far the most important project was the Tapion Dam in April 1965, which made an enormous difference to the towns and villagers. It was Larry Mellon's greatest hydraulic achievement but, like many great achievements, full of great problems later.

"There were taps to the fountains and the system and people there every minute, day or night," said Ménager. "'Let the water run,' Dr. Mellon said. 'Don't try to close it down for part of the day,' which they were doing at first. 'Otherwise, people will always just break it.'"

Even so, people cut into the main line to divert the water to their own houses, a practice that still threatens the system's integrity. So, even more, does the lack of maintenance.

"The dam at Caneau needed repair but nobody was doing it," Mé-

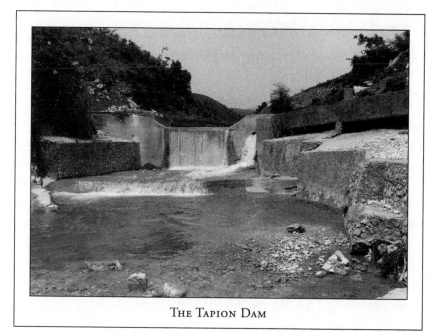

THE TAPION DAM

nager says. "It was the Duvalier government's job, but the local agents only interfered. I told Dr. Mellon if we didn't do something, the dam would collapse. The door was stuck in the mud and wouldn't raise up and down. So I bought a high-pressure water pump, and we tried to force water under the door to make it go up. It didn't work. Dr. Mellon said, 'Put some grease on it and maybe they can hoist it by hand.' So I bought the grease and got someone to do the greasing every week. He told me, 'Don't put that in the expenses of the farm—give me the bill, I'll take care of it personally.' He was very strict about accounting for anything not directly for the hospital."

At the HAS community development meetings each Saturday in Larry's cluttered office, he and the staff, plus the young Mennonites and the Haitians, would assemble to review what had been done the previous week and make plans for the coming one.

"The meetings were at 7 A.M. sharp," Gretchen Berggren recalls, "and Larry was never late. One by one we all arrived. Gus Ménager would be one of the first. He would have come all the way from St. Marc, over sometimes almost impassable roads. Gus was a well of information about everything, from chickens to pig-raising to the best seed for corn, rice or millet. With Dr. Mellon he would later bring into the valley a new strain of rice that would double the yield. Later, a cross of that strain would be named after his wife, 'riz Mme. Gus.'"

Larry and Gus would review the projects under way: a well to be dug, a water line to be repaired, a community council to form, a road to be built. Gretchen Berggen would bring requests from farmers in the villages. Dr. Mellon would ask if anyone had found an equivalent Creole proverb to "a stitch in time saves nine." For such moments did Gretchen look forward to those meetings:

"They revealed his deep-seated commitment to the development process but also the frustrations we felt in the face of Haiti's grinding poverty and the lack of future value orientation on the peasants' part. Dr. Mellon thought there must be a proverb that would help. Each Saturday someone would offer another one. He would shake his head, 'No, that's not it. . . . Haitians use proverbs to express what they think and feel. If we can find it, this proverb will help us introduce the idea of maintenance in a way they can understand.' I knew what he meant."

In her own home, Berggren's Haitian helpers would wait until supplies were gone before informing her. The day before, when there was still a little left, nothing would be said. A small leak in a pipe would grow until the fountain at the end of the line was dry. Only then would the problem be brought up.

"We never found the proverb," she says. "The closest we came was one from Haitian fishermen: 'A small hole in your net will lose little fish; if you don't repair it, you'll lose the big ones too!' Gus came up with that one; he knew the fishermen. But Dr. Mellon was still searching. Farmers in the valley were not familiar with nets; some of them had never seen the ocean . . . The search is still on, as far as I know."[9]

Ménager's knowledge of fishing led him and Larry to another ambitious project. Both the freshwater and the saltwater industries in Haiti were then in a state of decline. In former years, the off-shore shrimp beds had been rich, but the shrimp had almost completely disappeared due to pollution from soil erosion. Mud and clay overwhelmed the habitats, clogging up the fish's gills and suffocating them. There was nothing that could be done about the coastal ecology, but Larry and Ménager decided to try their hand at reviving inland fishing.

In the town of Sordeaux, they initiated a stocking project to put in eggs and develop five hectares of fish ponds. In the first year, everyone was enthusiastic and got small returns. They had to start guarding the ponds at night because people would come by and throw nets and steal fish. "We put pine branches in the water so the poachers' nets would get caught," Ménager recalled. "But we populated too fast, and there was not enough oxygen or feed. The fish started to die. We tried to feed them hormones so they would all come out one sex, to cut down overpopulation, but that is not natural or good in the long run, and eventually the project collapsed. Haiti won't solve the problem by fish-farming. It must restore natural conditions, get the water clean, and then we can have fish naturally as before. Our experiment did not work out, but we learned a lot from it."

After leaving HAS, Ménager was working as a specialist for U.S. Agency for International Development when the Haitian government asked him to negotiate a major farm-loan project with the World Bank—on three days' notice. He did it brilliantly, and it turned into a four-year job with the World Bank itself, during which he mastered international as well as Haitian agricultural management. He returned to USAID service from 1983 to 1986, and then became Haiti's first minister of agriculture in charge of both livestock and farming.

"Most of my training, I got at HAS," he reflects on a sunny day in Deschapelles, thirty-five years after his first encounter with the Mellons. "I could handle the pig situation for the whole country later because I practiced here. I understood how to manage the livestock division at the ministry of agriculture because we raised cattle at the hospital and developed the dairy barn there. Deschapelles was a microcosm. The work at HAS gave me the framework for everything I did beyond."

.   .   .

ALTHOUGH LARRY MELLON had been unable to find the perfect Haitian proverb for that stitch-in-time situation, he had a few potent mottoes of his own. One of them was, "Arms are cheap, but fingers are expensive." It was not a denigration of manual labor, always essential, but a recognition of the greater value to Haiti of skills that, once learned and cultivated, could bring new industries and income to the Artibonite Valley. Often Gwen headed up such efforts, some of which worked and many of which didn't—but all of which would at least be tried.

"We have some girls coming from Guatemala to teach weaving in Haiti [and] see how much we can do here with it," Larry noted in his diary at the time. Gwen remembers the attempt:

On one of our Central American trips, Larry had found a girl who was a very talented weaver and agreed to come down with some friends of hers to teach the Haitians. We spent days in Guatemala City getting her picture taken, passport, etc. She was to meet us at the airport the next day. We got there. The girl was there. So was her father. "I'm not going to let her go," he said. And that was the end of the whole thing.

Temporarily. Gwen later revived and modified the idea of a weaving operation, with a modicum of success. She also helped create and supervise three other HAS workshop industries—ceramics, carpentry, and art—that have survived and thrived to the end of this century:

> The word of mouth in Port-au-Prince was, "They make good furniture and ceramics in Deschapelles," and we are now well enough established that we get good orders from outside the district, even from the States. People from our shops have gone off and started their own. But here, they're subsidized, not really self-sufficient. They use our [HAS] electricity, our oil, our crates, which aren't factored into the selling price.

When Larry's niece Farley and her husband, Josh Whetzel, visited Deschappelles in 1962, a high point of their trip was accompanying Larry with a big pressure cooker to a nearby village to demonstrate how to can tomatoes—the principle of saving food for later. After all the local maids took a turn at stirring, Larry showed them how to put the cooked tomatoes in sealed jars and said to store the jars for three months. In all Haitian probability, the tomatoes were eaten the next day: Farley thinks Larry didn't expect a major breakthrough, but wanted to try anyway.[10]

Other ventures started by Larry and Gwen Mellon rose or fell without intending to turn a profit, notably their sewing and day-care centers. A little church in Petite Rivière provided space, as its aged pastor fondly recalled:

> Some ladies in our church and I built a *tonelle* [hut] of coconut leaves for girls to come and learn how to sew. We went to Dr. Mellon and the head of sewing at HAS and asked her to come and teach these twenty-five girls. Dr. Mellon took responsibility to keep this center

running and, after that, to make a place for babies in a canteen by the sewing center. Parents would bring their children from eight in the morning to three in the afternoon, and we would feed the children—day care. It worked for a good long time before we finally had to close it for financial reasons.

Before Dr. Mellon came along, said this pastor, "The land was dry, but the dam let us cultivate plantain, rice, beans, cabbage, carrots. It gave us riches. After the water came, we found the biggest, most beautiful banana to pick and had a party and presented it to Dr. Mellon. He was so pleased because it was 'his' water that helped us produce it. Once he said to me, 'When I am not here anymore, maybe you will remember me.' It was true. Dr. Mellon did so many things."

With all community outreach efforts, however, the key was to find a local Haitian leader who could follow through. "The minute that person was located," says Gwen, "Larry left the project." But often, no such man or woman could be found.

Warren Berggren remembers helping Mellon install a pipeline at Petite Rivière one day and suggesting a treatment plant was needed to assure enough water for future population growth:

Larry pointed to the water tower at Verrettes and said it was built by President Dumarsais Estimé, who was from this region, but when he was no longer in office, it stopped working. One day some hospital mechanics said, "Let's do something about it," and they loaded up tools and went up and in less than an hour, they had the pump apart and found a filter plugged with sand. They cleaned it out, polished it up, put it back together, put in fuel and cranked it up. Everyone was very happy. But by Friday of that week, it ran out of gas and hasn't pumped water since. His point was that gravity systems are better than anything more sophisticated.

Dr. Mellon's operative theory was "Keep it simple."

"We had the same problem with the windmill in Anse Rouge—a

beautiful thing," Gwen recalls. "Larry realized right away that nobody was going to grease it, so we used to go up twice a year with our intrepid plumber Yves, who would climb up and grease it himself. But after he stopped, nobody else took over."

Each year, a group of Harvard medical students came to spend several days at HAS and meet Dr. Mellon. "He was always very courteous and said, 'What would they like to hear about?'" Berggren recalls. "I'd say, 'community development,' and Larry would answer, 'Just take them out and show them some of the things that *don't* work, and then they'll begin to understand a little bit about it.' He was very much a disciple of Jimmy Yen."

A quote by Larry's friend Dr. Y. C. Yen, copied out in Mellon's own handwriting, still hangs in his study at home:

Go to the people.
Live among them.
Learn from them.
Love them.
Serve them.
Plan with them.
Start with what they know.
Build on what they have.

It was what Larry preached and practiced alike.

"We used to have little plays in which people would always be looking for Doc and be unable to find him, because he would always be out somewhere laying pipe," said Dr. Gérard Frédérique. "They would find Mrs. Mellon instead, as she was the one who was ever present for everybody. In the plays, Dr. Mellon always had a pipe wrench in his hands."[11]

That gentle parody was based on truth: Larry loved nothing more than working alongside the Haitians on an equal basis, in and out of the hospital.

"Those with high functions got no more attention than those with small jobs," said a longtime HAS employee, Antoine Véus. "He made no distinction. I was given a job in the Autopsy Room. He encouraged me by saying it was important. He always confirmed that my job was important. Sometimes people would remain ten days in the morgue without any relatives claiming them. When that happened, Doc would arrange to have them buried properly and often helped dig graves for the unclaimed dead himself."[12]

On those occasions, the deceased would be taken to the potter's field in Verrettes, accompanied by Pastor Bois and the Mellons. Maître Delinois would make the coffin out of waste strips of cardboard and wood. "Once, we arrived and the grave was too short for the coffin," Gwen recalls. "The gravediggers were asked to extend it, but refused unless paid more money. So Larry just jumped into the hole himself and started digging. Pretty soon the Magistrate appeared, and the gravediggers quickly took Larry's place. From that day on we never had a problem. The coffin was placed in the ground, Larry played his accordion, and we sang, 'Nearer My God to Thee.'"[13]

When Dr. Mellon was working in the hospital, he took night call on a regular rotation with all the other physicians. "He gave an example from the beginning," says "Bos" André Cassius, HAS maintenance chief and the Mellons' close friend. "As the people worked, Doc worked alongside. When we spent the night at Peligre together on a [water] project, he was the one who went to get food. Then he sat and ate with us, the same food, together. He always stayed until a project was finished."

A former HAS agronomist, Raphael Valéry, remembered the time Larry needed some sand for construction, and the hospital accountant said he had sand at home:

Dr. Mellon came with the jeep and two shovels, picked up the accountant and proceeded to his house in St. Marc. When they arrived, Doc took off his shirt. The accountant took off his shirt also. Doc began to shovel the sand into the jeep without saying anything. The accountant, realizing the second shovel was for him, did the same. The accountant became exhausted, and when he saw some people passing by, he suggested they give the men a job shoveling. Doc replied, "*Mon cher, nou jeunes garçons, nou kap travay.*" [My dear, we are young men, we can work.] The accountant finished the job alongside Doc, and was totally exhausted as Doc drove off in his jeep loaded with sand.[14]

.   .   .

"Doc" was exhilarated by *doing*, rather than pondering, in the little part of the world he could affect. From their earliest days in Haiti, he and Gwen conceptualized and initiated projects for the betterment of the Artibonite Valley. At the same time, they had an even rarer, complementary skill.

"One of the qualities I most admired in Dr. and Mrs. Mellon was their ability to kill an unsuccessful project—a unique ability to recognize when something wasn't working and to give it up," says Bill Dunn. "I saw this over and over again: Larry could see needs, come up with ideas of how to meet those needs, and get projects going—leather-tanning, tile-making, fish production, brick-making, dairy cattle, broom-making, sewing centers, on and on. He would try it, but if it didn't work or he wasn't satisfied with it, he closed it down, and that was the end of it. So long, no regrets. Many of them, in his mind, simply failed. In our minds, they probably would have been labeled 'successful,' especially if we'd had the proprietary interest of having started them. Most of us put so much of ourselves into something we start that, even when it isn't working, we drag it on and on."

The fish-stocking and tanning projects, for example, did not meet his expectations. The brick-making, on the other hand, was successful but faltered when turned over to the Haitian who'd been running it. "After the man made a bit of money," says Dunn, "he began spending his time in Port-au-Prince, not minding the brick operation, and pretty soon it folded. Dr. Mellon did not pump new life into it. He'd tried, made it a success, turned it over to somebody in the community—and then was done with it." The bakery was also a casualty of transition. But other HAS cottage industries endured, including Gwen's cotton-ginning and rug-weaving projects that thirty years later still supports many families, however meagerly.

"Cotton is very hard to raise because the goats eat it, but I'm holding tight to this, even though it's in enormous debt," Gwen says. "They pick it from spindly bushes planted by the French before the 1804 revolution. We buy the cotton in Desarmes and hand it out once a week to 32 crippled indigent people here to be cleaned. They bring back the seeds and clean cotton, and we give them five dollars. They're old people—mostly blind or crippled, with no relatives—who depend on that five dollars. They'd die if they didn't get it. It keeps them from starvation."

Dr. Peter Wright, who first came to HAS in 1974 as a young pediatrician specializing in infectious disease, considered the failed experiments just as important as the successful ones, in terms of an overall approach to community health care:

"At that point, Larry had moved his major focus to public health, his irrigation and other projects. I'd see him in the morning going off in the Land Rover and never knew quite what he was doing. I only knew he'd made the correct decision about how to have the greatest impact on

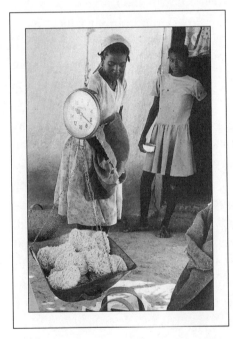

"Cotton is very hard to raise because the goats eat it . . ."

health, as he went around to the towns and monitored the water that he piped in. You'd walk up the hill behind the hospital and see those great pipes running down, and you'd realize that running a hospital wasn't just being a doctor and making sure there were enough antibiotics on hand."

Larry was not one to spend a lot of time discussing the feasibility of a project. Having given it some serious thought, stepson, Michael Rawson, testifies, "He started out in the Land Rover with a transit, range pole and one other unsuspecting person to begin surveying a pipeline to bring water from a spring high in the hills to a village along the road. Such a project was of course far more complicated, but it would progress from one stage to the next until completed. On most mornings we would find dozens of volunteers, chipping away at limestone benches and clearing trees to create a path for the pipeline. It was those volunteers who made the project a success, but it was Larry who convinced them it was feasible and that by their efforts, their village and their children would benefit many times over."

Dieutel Toussaint, a Liancourt funeral director, worked with Larry on various community-development projects before serving in the Haitian legislature for eleven years, 1969–1980. He remembers:

Dr. Mellon was interested in potable water for the valley. The water from the creeks that leeched into many of the wells was polluted. The first thing he did was to surround the wells with "collars" one meter high, so the polluted water couldn't seep in. When we worked together, I never saw the millionaire within him. He was always humble, more simple even than the country people.

He wanted to teach people about dying, for example. They would come here from 30 kilometers away to bury their relatives. Often they just wrapped the dead person in hay because they couldn't afford a coffin. When I asked him about this, he said, "That's fine. I and my wife will not be buried in a nice coffin, just a little box here in Haiti." When he said that, I laughed. I thought it was a joke. But that's exactly what happened.

It is said that no one knows a man better than his secretary. In that case, Marie-Thérèse Menos perhaps knew Larry best. A native of nearby St. Marc, she graduated from high school in June 1964 and was looking for a job in Port-au-Prince when her friend Gus Ménager told her the HAS business-office secretary had been badly injured in a car accident: "He asked if I could come to work," Menos said. "First I said no, but he kept asking, and finally I agreed to come and help out for a month just for the experience. That one month turned into twenty-nine years—all my life. I saw that the work Dr. Mellon was doing for us here was so fantastic. He left everything he had and came down here. So why couldn't I just stay and work here too?"

Larry relied heavily on Mme. Menos over the years, and she, in turn, was inspired by his way of dealing with people:

> Every single person, even a child of two who stopped and said, "Dr. Mellon?"—he spoke to them. When you talked with him, he always listened very carefully and paid attention to what you said. When you were done, Dr. Mellon never gave two answers. He took his time to listen to you, and he gave you one answer, and it was the right one.
>
> If he knew that an employee was taking advantage or using things from the franchise, he would get very mad. He said we were to follow the rules. If he ordered something for Mrs. Mellon as a gift, he paid the fees. He didn't want HAS to do anything against Haitian law. That's why he never had any trouble in Haiti, because he set the example. Once when we had to pay a patent—a kind of tax we have to pay every January—the hospital employees said they were not going to pay it. Dr. Mellon was angry. He said it was the law, and if they refused to pay the fee, he would pay it himself. Everybody was so surprised with that answer. He was really mad that day, and later, everybody paid. When he was angry, you knew it. Everybody felt it when Dr. Mellon was not happy.

But most of the time he was happy, having attained a state of "self-actualization" much like that of Dr. Schweitzer. "Life here is not so romantic as people think it is," Schweitzer once said. "To be a success in

Lambaréné, you must be a carpenter, a mechanic, a farmer, a boatman, a trader, as well as a physician and surgeon." His chief carpenter was once asked how often Schweitzer came to the site of a leper village then being built with his Nobel Peace Prize money. "Just once a day," the man replied, "but he stays all day."

Dr. Frank Lepreau, the former HAS medical director and chief of surgery, says that, in view of how Larry Mellon spent the bulk of his time, men like Gus Ménager and the Mennonites "were closer to Dr. Mellon than the hospital staff. There along the pipeline with shovel and jeep he was practicing the Schweitzer principles of personal service, teaching by example."

Today, there are more than 120 people employed in the HAS community health, development, and outreach programs—Larry Mellon's true metier.

"I think life tended to be simple for Dr. Mellon because he had the capacity to boil problems down to their lowest common denominator," says Bill Dunn. "I've tried to figure out how he was so good at this. One reason was that he was such an ethical person. The issue of right and wrong stood out so prominently for him that other issues such as finances and feelings took a back seat. I was always amazed, when I took a complex problem to him, how he would listen very carefully and, when I finished, restate the problem in such simple and succinct terms. I'd say to myself, 'Son of a gun, why couldn't I do that?' Once you did that, the solution often jumped out at you. It was a joy to work with him because of the way he would visualize a problem and the solutions that emerged from that."

·   ·   ·

THERE WAS ONE great community-development project at L'Hôpital Albert Schweitzer, however, whose visualization became more problematic and whose solution was less joyful, at least for Dr. Hal May: his beloved L'École La Providence. Each year from the school's inception, another grade had been added, a process which Hal felt should continue naturally.

"There was no reason why we should stop it as long as it was growing in a natural way," Dr. May recalls. "It was a wonderful complement to the hospital. You can't do one without the other. You could focus on health, but you can't really accomplish that without the other. So much of public health is education. Larry and Gwen and I were very close, and they knew from the beginning that was my dream."

On July 4, 1969, a teacher from Port-au-Prince arrived in Deschapelles and told May he was interested in working at the school. May thought he seemed a good candidate and wanted him to meet Larry, who was head of the HAS school committee. But when informed, Dr. Mellon said, "Why would we need him?" May answered that it was so the school could go to the next step: "We have six grades, the primary school is complete, it's time to move on to the secondary school." As far as he was concerned, there should be no stopping. Mellon's reply was chilling to him:

> Larry said, "Pal, it ain't in the cards." I said, "Larry, you know that's why I'm here." He said, "That's not why *I'm* here. We're not in the business of education. I came to focus on health." I said, "You can't do one without the other. But this is your hospital, you're the one who has to make that decision. I don't agree with it. The only right thing for me to do is, one year from now I'll leave."
>
> I was an independent. I wasn't really there for Dr. Schweitzer or Dr. Mellon. I felt God wanted me to be there. If Larry had other ideas, I would move on. A day or so later, I wrote a letter of resignation and asked Gwen and Aggie to be present as witnesses. We had quite a serious exchange in which I refused to accept his reasoning. Gwen and Aggie were in tears. I felt the approach I wanted us to follow was right for everybody, including the hospital. I said, "I will leave, but the school will continue."[15]

A showdown between two tough Christians was at hand. Mellon asked where the school would be. May said, "Where it is now." Larry said, "It can't be there because I need that land." May said, "That land isn't yours—we bought it with $4,500 of the church money." On his small HAS salary, Hal and Aggie had purchased additional small parcels of land in the name of the Grant Foundation.

"I was very strict in saying that if he wanted it, he would have to buy it," says Dr. May. "He had to do so, and we used that money to buy land in Verrettes so that the school could move there. It was unpleasant. We had been such close friends. It was a wrenching separation. I believe he was wrong, though I believe he was trying to be true to what he believed. But we were adversaries. My concern was to find a group that would take responsibility. I didn't want to leave the country without making sure somebody would keep the school open."

A Protestant mission agreed to do so, and May and Mellon signed an agreement transferring ownership to that tax-exempt institution in Verrettes. The school moved and continued to thrive, if not as fully as May had envisioned. "Things don't always work out exactly the way you hope," he muses today. "But you've got to persevere. You have to keep moving."

Was it not arbitrary and inconsistent of Larry Mellon to rule that education wasn't HAS's proper mission, while fostering a wide range of other ambitious, nonmedical community programs? "All I know," May concludes, "is it was something he strongly embraced as long as it was a primary school, as long as it was contained. But Larry couldn't envision it continuing to grow, and at that stage, he said no. His term was that he 'didn't want the tail wagging the dog.' I think perhaps it was a matter of control."

For Hal May, there was no hatred but there was a deep wound that took many years to heal. It would be seventeen years before he set foot in Deschapelles again.

.   .   .

AN INFINITELY DEEPER WOUND for Larimer Mellon the father, not the administrator, was a private one that could never fully heal. After Grace Rowley and Larry were divorced, his son Bill—William Larimer Mellon III—lived for the most part in Los Angeles with his mother. He was "a tragic boy," according to his aunt, Rachel Mellon Walton, who said that "Grace never bought him new clothes, his shoes were always too small," and in Beverly Hills he spent much of his youth "having to sit in beauty parlors waiting for her" and being mortified by his father's periodic appearances in dusty ranch clothes. "He never realized I was embarrassed," Bill said years later, "because he always did what he wanted to do, not what somebody else thought was proper."[16]

Perhaps there was too much melodrama in those judgments. Gwen recalls Billy as fun-loving and affectionate. In any case, once enrolled at St. Paul's School in Concord, New Hampshire, he began to come into his own, playing football and soccer and singing in the glee club. As a Princetonian, William Larimer Mellon III certainly enjoyed greater success than had William Larimer Mellon Jr. An English literature major, he conquered Princeton in proper four-year fashion. A significant change of address came at the end: Upon entering, he had given his residence as Beverly Hills. Upon graduating in 1955, he listed his home as New Orleans—a clear indication of his having gravitated away from his mother toward the life and love of his father.

After college, Bill spent two years in the Air Force, earning his wings while continuing, with difficulty, to work on his writing. He then spent several months traveling through Africa, recording programs for NBC Radio and meeting Albert Schweitzer in Lambaréné, before coming to Deschapelles to live with Larry and Gwen and fulfill a vow to finish his first novel before marrying his fiancée, LeGrand Council, an Episcopalian Sunday school teacher from Greenhill, Mississippi.

In Deschapelles, Bill put his communications skills to good use by helping Lloyd Shirer make HAS's seminal film on tetanus. He did indeed finish his book there and, indeed, married LeGrand in September 1959. Then he took her to Haiti where, together, they made a beautiful documentary on L'Hôpital Albert Schweitzer that is still shown and admired throughout the world.

But Bill Mellon's early literary success at Princeton did not assure fast entry into the professional publishing world, and he was not equipped to deal with its setbacks. Still searching for his niche, he and LeGrand moved to Cape Cod where he decided to follow his father's footsteps by entering Boston University as an undergraduate premed student in September 1963—very briefly.

"The marriage was troubled and a separation decided on," Gwen recalls. "Billy was offered a teaching position in Virginia. The night before his departure, he and LeGrand had a sad farewell dinner with much drinking. It was not alarming when morning came and the packed car and Billy were gone."

Not until the school called asking why he hadn't arrived was a search conducted and Bill found in his car on a backwoods road not far from home, in a spot where he often went to watch the sunrise when he couldn't sleep. He was dead, at thirty, from a lethal ingestion of sleeping pills and alcohol. It was a time before that combination was known to be fatal, and the family strongly believed the death was accidental.

"Larry asked to go alone to Cape Cod to Billy's funeral," says Gwen. "That was hard for me because Billy was one of my devoted children. At the funeral, Billy's mother asked him to thank me for having been such a good mother to her son."[17]

Larry and Grace and the tragic situation were beyond bitterness. It

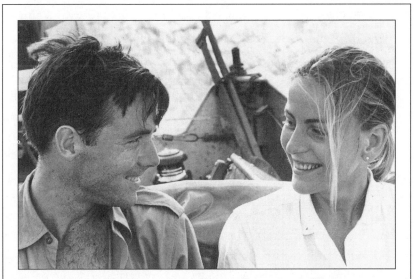

BILLY MELLON AND LEGRAND COUNCIL IN HAITI

had been twenty years since they had seen each other. They would never do so again.

Gwen, Larry, and the Mellon family would remain close to Bill's ebullient widow, LeGrand, for life. "Such a lovely person," says Rachel. "Whenever I see her, I like it! Gwennie loves her very much." LeGrand faithfully visited Deschapelles and assisted HAS in many ways, not least with her unique gift of laughter. "She continued to play music with Larry," says Gwen, "as she and Billy had done before."

Gwen continued to find solace in the letter Billy wrote May 31, 1953, upon his father's graduation from medical school:

> It seems to me the greatest thing in the world [is] that a person should find his life's work and be going in a straight line toward a goal. Without such, a person is just wandering and really can never prove anything monumental or hardly even worthwhile. In my opinion you've picked the best. I want you to know that I'm behind you all the way, and though I guess I haven't shown it outwardly, I would like to be part of whatever you're doing. That means everything in the world to me. However, you are not the only figure in the spotlight. Without Gwennie's love and help, I doubt if I would be writing this letter now. I sure envy you, Dad, for having found such a wife.

.   .   .   .

WHAT WAS IT about this wife and her complementary effect on the husband?

"Dr. and Mrs. Mellon were both fun to be around," says Dr. Gérard Frédérique. "They wanted everyone to enjoy the everyday gifts of life and felt sorry for those who could not." Husband and wife had that and much else in common, though their personalities were quite different— Gwen "the enforcer," Larry "the idea man." "Gwen was at the front desk making up charts and registering patients at 5 A.M. She often went to find out what happened to some child she'd seen the day before and was always impatient to get lab results and concerned that the patients be well treated. She was the nerve center of the hospital, and the one who communicated important questions back to Larry."

Jenifer calls her mother "the trouble shooter—the eyes and ears of the hospital, always aware of what was going on. Larry always had to focus on the big picture." As a contemporary woman, Gwen loved fashion and clothes and had her own personal mode, marked by stylish simplicity.

"One day Mrs. Mellon was going to help folks at the mission in Kenscoff," recalled Sister Joan Margaret. "She was wearing a lovely dress—not fancy, but on Mrs. Mellon it was elegant—and I had seen her buying the fabric in Petite Rivière. Someone made a comment, 'What an elegant dress! It is probably from some couturier in the U.S.' I replied, 'I think that Mrs. Mellon makes most of her own clothes.'"[18]

Indeed, after moving permanently to Haiti, Gwen honed her ability to rework clothes with an artistic eye to suit her everyday needs as well as special occasions in Deschapelles. But what charmed people more than her clothing was her quick mind and engaging manner, especially "after hours" at home.

"She is a great storyteller—stories about life on the ranch, early days of the hospital," recalls Sandra Wadley, director of the HAS pharmacy and acting administrator from 1988 to 1992. "She loves games—Scrabble, Rummicube, bridge. 'Oh, I just love to win!' She hates not getting good cards. She is drawn to strong, positive individuals, she admires strong people and is not much interested in 'unformed' people. She is not above disappointment in people."[19]

She also was not above laughter, as Jean Bellows, who spent six months at HAS with her physician-husband in 1970, recalled:

Imagine the splendid day when Mrs. Mellon graciously came to call on the new ophthalmologist's wife and sick baby, bearing flowers, fruit and kind words. Without warning, she sat on the gutted couch and went straight through to the floor. I went white and, mortified, waited to be expelled instantly from the country I was beginning to love. I did not yet know the true Mrs. Mellon, because, instead of banishing us, she calmly climbed out, despite her own bad back, laughed, and welcomed us again to Haiti—where anything can happen, and usually does.[20]

Lucien Rousseau recalls that, "At first, she appeared very strict. But throughout the years, she looked after so many details at the hospital—all the houses and all the new people coming to work. She did that in a very neat way. That's why we were all so full of admiration for her."

On a recent day in Deschapelles, she could be seen fixing up a new doctor's residence, attending to every detail from the curtains and linens to the paintings on the walls. "Everybody who comes here gets an attractive house," Gwen remarks. Yes, but does she have to do it all herself? Her withering glance says, "Only a man who would ask such a question." Her verbal reply is more polite: "I *enjoy* doing it. I want everybody to be happy and have their privacy, their own life, nice working conditions—simple but nice."

Her realm is internal as well as external. Says Marie-Thérèse Menos, Larry's secretary: "Mrs. Mellon is the one who took over inside the hospital. From the time I first worked with him, Dr. Mellon always said, 'Any complaints you have, any changes you want inside the hospital—see Mrs. Mellon.'"

It was Gwen, for instance, who fashioned a dark bulk-storage area into the handsome HAS library. She studied and redesigned the space

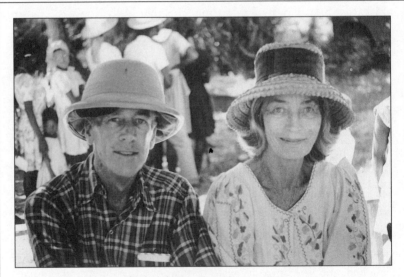

A PERFECT UNDERSTANDING

and supervised the carpentry shop's creation of fine wood paneling, doors, and furniture in 1969. The library was named in honor of Addison Vestal, the Mellon Securities tax expert and longtime financial troubleshooter for W. L. Mellon Sr. and Jr. alike. On opposing walls are Lester Bentley portraits of the Mellons. Close inspection reveals that the one of Gwen is truncated. Originally, it depicted Gwen holding one of her large, trademark floppy hats in her lap, but she had the hat cut off. Why? "Because my portrait was bigger than Larry's," she replies.

Gwen was the proverbial woman behind the man. "He was lucky to have her as a wife," says Dr. Marcella Scalcini. "She made it possible for him." Dr. Lucien Rousseau said: "Mrs. Mellon was always the perfect companion for Dr. Mellon. She understood his philosophy and the meaning of his work from the beginning."

In that, as in many other things, there is a strong temptation to draw parallels between Gwendolyn Grant Mellon and Helene Schweitzer-Breslau (1879–1957). Many such parallels exist between the two women, but so do many contrasts. *I Am His Wife*, a 1981 one-woman drama about Mrs. Schweitzer by Harold Watts and Lilly Lessing, moved Gwen deeply with a set of monologues that seemed to speak directly to her own experiences with Larry in Haiti. At the play's outset, Helene Schweitzer is pondering the request of an American publisher to write the story of her own life:

> Albert told his story more than twenty years ago in his book, *Out of My Life and Thought*. Suddenly, they want me to tell my story? . . . Certainly, there is a story to tell, but what is it? Should I try to discover it? Can I tell it after all those years so absorbed in Albert's life?

Helene's father was a learned history professor at the universities of Berlin and Strasbourg and a Jewish agnostic who'd had his children baptized as Christians. At twenty-two, Helene eagerly accepted a post as welfare worker for the City of Strasbourg, determined to improve the life of the poor, orphans, and unwed mothers particularly, in the days when that occupation was considered demeaning for a person of her background.

She met Schweitzer, a young clergyman-musician, in 1902 at a dinner party. His German was the Alsatian dialect at its worst, and she frankly told him that his ideas would sound better in good German. He smiled and invited her to help him.

The depth and complexity of his mind quickly earned her love and respect. He helped her raise money for a home for unwed mothers, and they found that they worked very successfully together. She gave up her career as a social worker while he studied medicine and worked in a hospital herself in order to become a nurse to serve with him.

In *I Am His Wife*, the character of Helene says, "My concerned parents thought that I had made his madness mine. I told them he made my madness his."

After a nine-year courtship, they were married in 1912. "What I love about you," Schweitzer told his bride, "is that you are Parisian in taste, German in spirit, and Jewish in intellect." In later years, she would often lament that her physical limitations and health had forced her to leave their hospital in Gabon and return to Europe. Even so, she continued to do what she could, accompanying her husband on his important fund-raising trip to America, serving as his interpreter, and working to overcome her shyness. They were always pressed for money, and she was instrumental in helping to establish the Albert Schweitzer Fellowship in America, which sustained the hospital in Lambaréné both during and after World War II.

In the Cold War era of the 1950s, when Schweitzer took his controversial position against nuclear weapons, she stood behind him 100 percent, defending his stance as a matter of philosophy, not politics. Privately, she wrestled with a certain resentment: Schweitzer was the Man of the Century, the press kept saying, but everyone neglected to mention her contribution to his work, including Schweitzer himself. In his autobiography, he devoted a total of two sentences to Helene: "My wife, suffering from poor health, could not accompany me this time to Africa. I will forever be grateful to her for her sacrifice."

She wondered, sadly, why he could not have said a bit more.

.   .   .

Gwen Mellon had similar reflections but no similar resentments. Her husband, unlike Helene's, was a constant source of positive reinforcement, and her health was robust. It was a different—if not yet "liberated"—era. She had American, not European, sensibilities and freedom of action. If Larry often gave her credit publicly and privately, which he did, it was because she deserved it. From Day One of their great enterprise, her responsibilities had been huge, and she would continue to deal with the life-and-death issues of HAS and the Haitian people for the next forty years.

Take presidential politics. Gwen's encounters with Haiti's heads of state over the years were in themselves riveting—beginning with Paul Magloire and François Duvalier. In the mid-1980s, she was called upon to receive and entertain General-President Henri Namphy on his state visit to Deschapelles. "It was supposed to be a nice quiet lunch for four," Gwen recalls, "but the president arrived with his full cabinet and an enormous entourage of soldiers and aides totaling almost 100."

Larry was ill that day, but his hostess performed brilliantly under duress. Marie-Thérèse Menos, whose family was friendly with Namphy says that when the chief of state got back to Port-au-Prince, "he told my brother, 'I never knew there were people like the Mellons living in the Artibonite Valley. They are a big gift to Haiti.'"

Martha Weinman Lear, the wife of visiting HAS surgeon Dr. Harold Lear, experienced a dramatic glimpse of Gwen Mellon in action on the very day of the Lears' arrival in Deschapelles:

The day was already fiercely hot as she drove the quarter-mile from her home to the hospital. The small market she passed had come to life with sunup; the women were crouched on their haunches chattering loudly, laying out neat rows of limes and melons, soap and matches, stirring over their charcoal fires bits of pork and strange gray and ocher porridges. She didn't take particular note of the peasant couple standing just ahead, waving her to a stop. As she drove slowly past them the woman cried, "Mama Mellon, Mama Mellon!" in great distress, and threw a bundle through the open window and into her lap. Gwen looked down and saw it was a very small baby, wrapped in rags.[21]

She took one look, recognized tetanus paralysis, rushed to the hospital and flung the child into the arms of the first doctor she saw. He worked hard but couldn't save it. And then Gwen Mellon, the pillar of strength, did something very rare. She broke down and sobbed: "It wasn't at all in character for me, but I couldn't stop myself. And those parents—you know what they did? *They* tried to comfort *me*. The woman kept patting my shoulder whispering, 'Mama Mellon, Mama Mellon. . . .'

"Well, then the problem was, how would these people get home with the body of their child? Caskets aren't allowed on the bus, and they lived a long way off, a two-day walk. So all we could think to do was wrap the body up to look like a bundle, and we drove the parents to the camion and told them, 'Just get on and sit there and don't say anything to anyone.'"

She could only give them the fare and hope they would not be discovered and thrown off with their tragic little load. It was but one of a thousand such days in her life at Deschapelles.

CHAPTER 6

SCHERZO
"Mon Pays Est L'Haïti"

DESCHAPELLES FOLKLORE was forever enriched the day a new nurse put on her bathing suit, went outside, and thought English—if repeated enough—would work with the villagers. "Where's the pool?" she kept asking. Finally, somebody brought her a hen.*

The poor woman just wanted a cool dip on her day off, a change of pace from ailing human to thriving Mother nature. Who could blame her? The flora and fauna of Haiti are to be savored, as is Haiti's second-largest and most beautiful city, Cap-Haïtien, the country's charming coastal vacation spot. Among its attractions are picture-perfect beaches, which the Mellons loved and frequented, notwithstanding the notorious undertow. "We once had a nurse who just arrived from the Philippines and took a beach trip with a group," says Gwen. "They only went into the water up to their knees and, with no warning, she was just washed away."

It was a rare tragedy. Most beach-blanket outings were happy and restorative for HAS' overworked staffers, especially when Dr. Mellon himself went along, as Dr. Marcella Scalcini remembers:

The first month I was here, we were understaffed and always on call. At one point, there were only two internists, myself and one other. Mrs. Mellon used to come at 9 P.M. to my office and say, "Marcella, you're still working?" I was so full of enthusiasm. Even when not on

Poule is the French and Creole word for chicken.

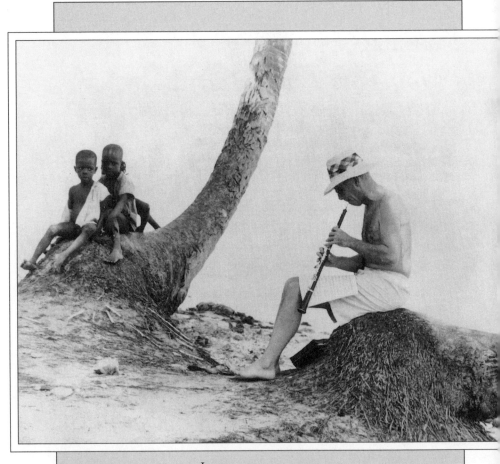

LARRY ON THE BEACH

call, I used to make rounds. Once Dr. Mellon said, "I want you to spend the weekend with us so they won't call you in from the hospital to make rounds."

So on a Saturday, we went to the beach. Mrs. Mellon and I were in bathing suits, but because [of a developing skin-cancer condition] Larry couldn't expose himself to the sun and went in wearing a tropical hat, his shirt, his bow tie and glasses. To see Dr. Mellon going into this wonderful sea like that! Then we went to eat lunch, and each time someone came up to Dr. Mellon, he would give a few coins. He said, "Marcella, don't do this in Deschapelles. You could go mad— they ask, ask, ask." But he himself, however, could never say no.

The next day, Sunday, he said, "Let's go to Petite Rivière in the Peugeot," his nice sedan. Whenever we saw any Haitians walking along the dusty road, sweating, he would stop to take them in. Later, sometimes Mrs. Mellon would find a patient lying outside the hospital and would bring him in and say, "Marcella, take a look at him." I would do so and would often find he was wearing a Brooks Brothers shirt that Dr. Mellon had given him.

No trek through internal Haiti lacks adventure. Gwen recalls one journey to the town of Labadie, which required crossing a big river by *bumba* (dugout canoe): "The river was high and a lot of people were in the boat, which had a bent bow. I thought, they can't get one more person on this thing—and then they loaded on a horse! I had my hand on the edge of it, and it was so low in the water that my fingers were wet. It was scary. All the time I kept thinking, 'Nobody in this boat can swim.' The horse bothered me most. But we made it. I asked somebody the other day, is that *bumba* with the bent nose still there? Yes. It's still there."

It never bothered her to travel around Haiti alone, but Gwen and Larry rarely went anywhere just for pleasure:

We liked to have a trip that meant something. We'd go on a Sunday to the mountains or some green valley hoping to find a spring. Larry always had some potential goal, some reason. People would say,

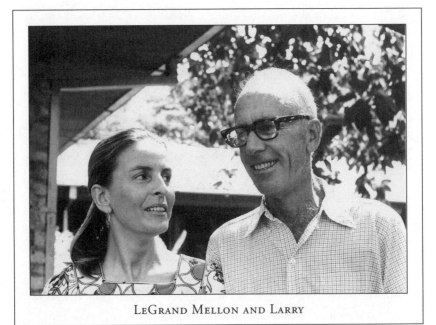

LeGrand Mellon and Larry

"Please come and see—our potatoes have dried up. Can you lift the water up?" So we'd go look and, often as not, Larry would do something about it.

For pleasure, they didn't want or need to travel. Pleasure was at home.

.   .   .

THE GIANT FICUS TREE just outside the Mellons' veranda has lovely green leaves, but its most notable feature is the strange horizontal nature of its branches and strange perpendicular "props" that drop from the lower branches to prop them up. The tree's thick sap knows when to force down a "support" branch, some of which disengage when no longer structurally necessary. The ficus is a bio-architectural wonder with the self-activating instincts of a sophisticated engineer. Its lowest branch is just four feet off the ground but sixty feet long—totally parallel to the ground.

The Mellon home in Deschapelles is surrounded by bougainvillea, flowering ginger, and gorgeous flamboyant trees, cousins to the mimosa, with leaves that hold on to the raindrops and sparkle like a million mirrors in the late afternoon sun. In the distance lie the Cahos mountains. Their river runoffs are the source of an indoor "spring" that pops up and sometimes runs through the middle of Gwen's living room in the rainy season. (She gently steps around it, without comment, and expects visitors to do the same.)

A hundred yards beyond the house are the ruins of a great stone arch and aqueduct from the eighteenth-century French sugar mill whose great wheel, half aboveground and half below, was once occupied with grinding up the raw cane. Those 100-foot-tall remembrances of times past, as eloquent as anything left by the Romans, have become home to a hundred thousand bees swarming around their gigantic hive in its upper reaches. I bid good-evening to some of my favorite zandolites and chameleons.

In Haiti, one soon learns to adjust to the critters that enter daily life. At dinner on the Mellons' veranda, a big frog with huge eyes hops onto a buffet next to the table. With a second hop, he alights perfectly balanced

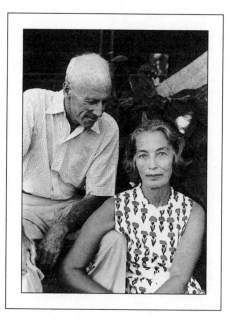

LARRY AND GWEN

on the back of a vacant chair. On his third hop, he lands on the salt cellar. His fourth hop brings him smack into the middle of an empty plate in front of Gwen, who starts a bit in surprise but is otherwise undisturbed. With his fifth hop, he is off the table and gone along his way.

There are no poisonous snakes in Haiti, but one day Gwen was stunned to see an impressive-sized boa in the toilet bowl. Her impulsive reaction was to flush, and the thing disappeared—but of course stopped up the toilet. A Haitian handyman, informed of the problem, said he'd fix it: "She does not like pine oil." He poured some into the bowl, whereupon "she" shot straight up into the air—alive and well—and was removed to the outdoors.[1]

"Snakes here aren't dangerous," says Gwen in the wake of that encounter. "I can move them out of the house without any fear or any squeamishness, and they're big—six feet easily, sometimes as long as a garden hose. We have them living in our attic, but it guarantees we will have no mice or rats, which is a comfort. Right now, it's the season when they're having little ones, and sometimes they come down from the attic. I saw one recently and just picked it up and carried it outdoors."

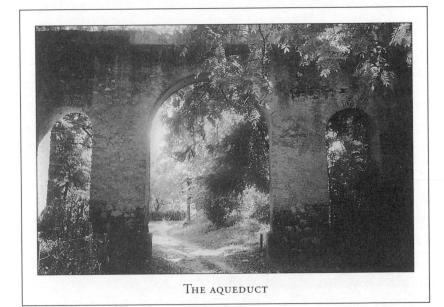

THE AQUEDUCT

Somewhat less charming are the tarantulas that often inhabit the drains of bathtubs and shower stalls. They're fearsome-looking but in fact quite shy. In any encounters with human beings, it's a race to see who can get away faster—and the tarantula always wins.

Jenifer Grant noted that the children of one HAS doctor had a penchant for tarantulas: "They would capture them and pop them into a bottle of formaldehyde. On rainy days they'd take them out with tweezers, line them up and count them. But that hobby came to an end one day when they witnessed their most recent victim just shake himself a bit and walk off."

Albert Schweitzer once told Erica Anderson he found it incomprehensible, as a boy, that "in my evening prayers I should pray for human beings only. So when my mother had prayed with me and kissed me goodnight, I silently added a prayer I composed myself . . . 'Dear God, protect and bless all living things. Keep them from evil, and let them sleep in peace.'"[2]

In Africa, Schweitzer was especially fond of parrots and of their contrariness. "I know a family who tried for months to teach their parrot to say *bon jour*," he told Anderson. "They repeated the phrase over and over, but he would not say it. They got angry and told him how stupid he was: '*Comme vous êtes bête, imbécile!*' [How idiotic you are!] But the parrot stayed silent. One day, a high church dignitary came for dinner. He saw the parrot, went over to the cage, stroked its neck and said, 'What a beautiful bird you are.' The parrot replied, '*Comme vous êtes bête, imbécile!*'"

In Deschapelles, eight beautiful *jako* parrots live close by the Mellons' house, nesting in the old mill ruins and nearby trees. "They feel safe here because the village boys can't shoot them with slingshots. When the light hits them right, you can see their lovely bright green and rose-colored throats. We also have hummingbirds and owls who sit on the wires and a pair of mosquito hawks who roost on the roof and look over the world from there. It's a wonderful sight."

The thriving fields and rice paddies around Deschapelles are graced by handsome green crested herons and snow-white cattle egrets, who serve the symbiotic function of keeping their hosts' ears and flanks free of insect-parasites. "There used to be a lot of flamingos in Haiti, too," says Gwen, "but people in dugout canoes caught them with nets and sent them to the race tracks in Miami." Nowadays, few flamingos are left.

Plants as well as animals came under Schweitzer's protection, and even the sight of cut flowers disturbed him. He asked a visitor who picked a bouquet for a nurse's birthday to do so no more. He would change the location of a building to save a single tree.

Schweitzer's "Reverence for Life" motto, inscribed over the HAS entrance at Deschapelles, was taken to heart by Larry Mellon, who likewise applied it to *all* life. He could no more stand to see an animal than a human being in agony, and would stop his truck to deliver the coup de grace to an injured goat along the roadside. Haitian bystanders, seeing him do so, thought it the height of *blanc* idiosyncrasy.

Former Haitian Congressman Dieutel Toussaint was with Larry one day on an inspection trip in the country, where they saw men with machetes cutting down fruit trees for firewood:

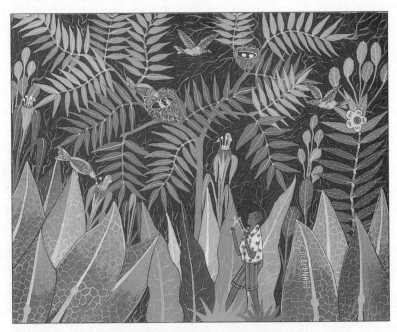

D. Elphabe's *Boy with Slingshot*

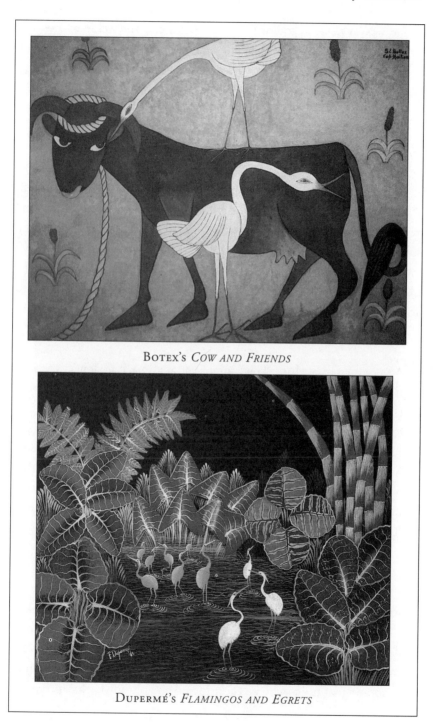

Botex's *Cow and Friends*

Dupermé's *Flamingos and Egrets*

He was so mad he couldn't even drive his car, and he asked me to drive for him. I asked, "Why are you so mad?" He said, "They are devastating nature for no good reason." One day later I was standing around, chopping at a tree with a machete, playing with it like a toy, and he said, "You saw the other day how I was so mad and now you make me mad, too. Why do you ruin the tree?" He was so sorry for it. I never forgot that.

Dutch nurse Udo Hasewinkel, who served at HAS from 1977 to 1985, recalled: "I spent a good deal of time on the HAS soccer field. Two meters within it is a tree. We always wondered why the tree had to be in the middle of the soccer field, but Doc would not let us cut it down. Even today it is still there. However, whenever it rained during a game, all the spectators and players would gather under the tree and get protection from the rain."[3]

Wrote Albert Schweitzer:

A tree grows, bears fruit. Then, after a certain time, it no longer grows. It loses its leaves. Its branches wither. What happens? Why is vital energy checked? Because it did not sink deep enough roots into the earth on which it stands. . . . The same thing has happened with us humans. Humanity has not had deep enough roots [because] the ethical code on which it is based was too narrow. It has concerned itself only with human beings and our relations with human beings. . . . Only if we have an ethical attitude toward all living creatures does our humanity have deep roots and a rich flowering that cannot wither.[4]

.   .   .

A TREAT LIES IN STORE for anyone with taste buds in Haiti, where, for example, even the most delicate Yankee stomachs and palates can savor the *chadeque*, a very tasty kind of grapefruit from which superb marmalade is made. Likewise fabulous is the incredible guava jelly, sweeter than honey. It's a bit harder to acquire a taste for goat steak, the local delicacy, or goat milk, which is considered an aphrodisiac for old men. I wouldn't kid about this. I simply prefer *griyo*—delicious bits of spicy, crisped pork—and other Haitian dishes, many of which are better eaten than seen in the preparation.

Gwen's daughter Jenifer recalls that, during her first summer in St. Marc, "Mother took me, Ian, and his friend Dean (both 15) to the colorful Saturday market. We wound our way through the beautiful vegetables and fruit and into the cooking area, pots bubbling away with soups. Dean looked at a pot and the *marchande* started stirring it, hopeful for a sale. As Dean watched her mix, out of the depths emerged a whole jawbone, teeth attached. Dean fainted on the spot. As we revived him, he murmured under his breath, 'My mother would hate Haiti.'"[5]

Gwen lectures instructively on the subject:

You choose wisely when you eat here. My advice is, eat rice and beans and steer clear of fish. Many people eat seafood from St. Marc, but I've seen fish sitting in a dugout canoe all day there in the sun, then frozen and sold. I'm very careful. There's very little refrigeration, and you can't really trust the iceboxes anywhere. Even here, since the embargo, the electricity turns off every day from 5 A.M. to noon. If you don't think *that* isn't a major problem! We have a deep freeze, which saves my life. A lot of people eat at this house. I have 450 for Christmas—the whole staff, in two sittings.

Christmas here is great. We have griyo, beans, rice, ice cream, cookies, mandarins. Everyone gets the same gift, and I try to think of something that will apply to everybody. They let me know if I haven't chosen well. Last year, it was fanny packs that say "Hôpital Albert Schweitzer." I stood there and put them on everybody. They thought that was great. This year it's going to be baseball hats. But New Year's, and January 2, are bigger celebration days in Haiti, at home with the grandparents, children and all. All families get together, people come back from the States or Port-au-Prince or wherever they live. It's a long weekend, Friday to Tuesday, more important than Christmas. We foreigners are the ones who made Christmas important. They never used to have Christmas trees here when we first came.

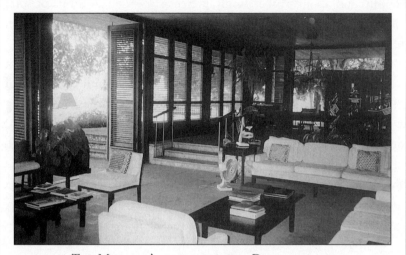

THE MELLONS' LIVING ROOM IN DESCHAPELLES

Gwen and Larry always loved to entertain in their attractive but not extremely spacious stone home. "We really only have one bedroom," she says, "plus a room off the kitchen that I made into living quarters for Frédérique."* Dr. Scalcini describes the house as "not luxurious—which would be offensive because there is so much poverty in Haiti—but just well-introduced into this landscape, and in excellent taste."

Larry only reluctantly agreed to build the house after his hospital architect prevailed upon him. "He said, 'You're going to spend your life here, you need a place of your own,'" Gwen recalls. "It turned out to be a real haven of peace."

It remains so to this day: Birds fly in and out of the open louvre doors, fashioned in pre-Castro Havana. "I saw them there and built the house around them," says Gwen. Those wooden doors are so beautiful, one wonders why they haven't taken hold in the United States. "Because they're not safe," she replies. "You can just put your hand in and turn the doorknob."

Outside, the flamboyant trees "are always doing something different. Right now, the leaves are black, but when it starts to rain, they'll turn a

*Soft-spoken, much-beloved Frédérique Pierre-Jules is the Mellons' longtime friend and trusted assistant, who now serves as unofficial "chief of staff" at the house.

lovely green with beautiful flowers, and the leaves will get very thick and form an umbrella over the house, almost obscuring our front door. I won't cut the branches because they're so beautiful."

Larry's sister Rachel recalls sitting on the porch one day, admiring the mountains but being annoyed by a certain large bush: "I said, 'Larry, cut that thing down. It spoils our view.' He said, 'Those were seeds from Dr. Schweitzer—it's not to be cut down.' So there it is, and there it stays."

In the end, nobody enjoyed the house more than Dr. Mellon.

"After a hard day," says Bill Dunn, his friend, "he'd come home, clean up, have a bite, maybe take a little snooze, and then begin the next part of his day, which was devoted to the things he loved around the house—his music, his languages, good conversation with Mrs. Mellon and their many guests, a relaxed meal in the evening. He was a great conversationalist and liked nothing more than to sit in that living room and turn on the music after dinner with a group of people around."

LeGrand Mellon's second husband, television writer Herb Sargent, recalls one Deschapelles dinner party when Gwen spoke of an amazing attraction she saw years before in New York on Forty-second Street— "Professor Tomlins' Flea Circus":

There was general disbelief by the others. "That's silly . . . no such thing . . . flea circus?"

Gwen did not like being doubted. Or, for that matter, countered, disagreed with, or challenged. And certainly not about a claim to have visited a flea circus. She was trying to organize a defense, but without backup—she had none. Luckily, I was able to save her.

I had seen that flea circus and even booked it on a television program at the time. Now, practically in unison, Gwen and I described the location, the performance, and Professor Tomlins in a small room in the basement of some building on Forty-second Street. Dr. Tomlins, an Englishman, wore a shirt and tie, suspenders, and a pair of wire glasses with very thick lenses. The circus took place under a bright light on a small table. Only five or six people could gather around to watch a performance at the same time. But the fleas were brilliant. They played ball, kicking a tiny pellet around the ring. They danced alone and with each other. They rode tiny tricyles. One flea would pull a tiny cart while another flea rode along in it. They held chariot races. They pushed each other around in little wheelbarrows. From time to time, "The Prof" would stop the show to change their costumes, which were tiny paper tutus applied to their backs. They would spin and pirouette to the tinkling of a music box.

Gwen was delighted with such an immediate confirmation. I was a hero.[6]

There is music, polyglot conversation, and no such thing as a stranger in the Mellon home. "Mrs. Mellon would constantly bring people in and arrange for them to do something productive—not just give them a dole," says Dunn. "Dr. Mellon would say, 'Come and teach me Arabic, or how to play the viola.' With Haitians and everyone else, they were acutely sensitive to what each person needed—always alert to things they could do for people to build their self-respect.

"The Mellons created a certain salon and gracious atmosphere that typified life in Deschapelles—a fulfilling environment for people to step into. The excess and frivolities of life in other cultures were shed and the good feeling that comes with hard, meaningful work was there, as well

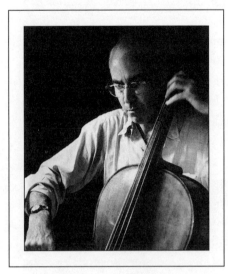

DR. MELLON AS CELLIST

as the enjoyment that came from strong, positive relationships. It's one reason people feel so strongly about their experience at HAS: They find it a formula for a very happy, satisfying life."

Sometimes on Sunday mornings, the Mellons invited Art and Renée Bergner to go swimming with them, as Renée recalls:

> They called it swimming, but it was really just a very modest picnic, something like a cheese sandwich and water in a gin bottle, driving into the countryside and sitting by a stream and playing music. Art was very rusty but that didn't matter to Larry. They'd sit and make these noises and we'd take a dip in the stream. It was never big enough to swim in, but the water was flowing briskly enough so we could get all wet and cool off. Some of these Sunday mornings they'd be skipping church and at some point Larry would say, "I'm going to read my Bible for a bit" and go off under a palm tree to read the Bible in Arabic or Turkish or whatever he happened to be studying at the time.
>
> They came over for Sunday lunch to our house one time when our kids were about four and six. Our daughter Gwen had an interest in horses and the West. Larry went out and lassoed the garbage cans for them. It was still important to him to be able to do it, so he showed them how to lasso all the garbage cans.[7]

Once during a lackluster dinner party at the Mellons, Renée recalls that immediately after the meal Larry said, "Excuse me, I have to go to my office and do some paper work," leaving Gwen stuck with their atypically dull guests. Pretty soon, the telltale sounds of a cello, not paperwork, began wafting in from his study.

.   .   .

The strain and pain of working in Haiti got to some of the doctors at HAS, but it never got to Larry Mellon. His greatest pleasure and the thing that most sustained him after a long work day in the Artibonite was his deep love of music. It had been nurtured early on by his mother, but most of the music and musical abilities he acquired were self-taught.

As a young man in 1920s Paris, he had seen Josephine Baker and thrown flowers to her on the stage. On that occasion, he was transported by a song she sang called "Mon Pays est Paris," which told of her two loves, Africa and Paris.

"My father was of Dr. Mellon's generation, and he too loved Josephine Baker," muses Dr. Scalcini. "She was beautiful and scandalous, but also a great and very intelligent woman. She won the gold medal in France during the World War II for resistance against the Nazis, and after the war, she adopted seven children of all races, as a sign of brotherhood. That song Dr. Mellon loved—I knew it by heart because my father used to sing it."

Larry translated it into Creole and often sang it in Deschapelles as "Mon Pays est Haiti."

Half a century earlier, he had lyrically expressed his profound musical feelings in his little book *Tales, Verses, and Essays*, published at Princeton when he was just 18:

> Next to the human voice, [most] accurate in expressing sentiment comes the violin. The voice and violin constitute in the grand symphony what might correspond in nature to the gentle rain and favorable winds. The stringed instruments might be compared to the music of water—viola, cello and harp representing the rippling lakes and babbling of brooks, while the piano and bass viol take the place of the more profound, slower-moving bodies—the majestic flow of rivers and constant heaving of the ocean. The woodwind instruments are related to terrestrial matter, such as the sound of wind in the treetops and ice-laden branches crackling in a winter forest, whereas the brass seems closely allied to great aerial disturbances such as hurricanes that destroy sturdy ships and whirlwinds that uproot mighty trees.

In Arizona, says Larry's stepdaughter Jenifer, "some of my earliest memories are of Larry playing his accordion or guitar and singing wonderful Western songs—pleasure showing through his wonderful grin: 'I'm going back to Arizona and round 'em up some day, with a whoop and a yell, and a yippie yi yea. . . .'" Larry taught her the basics of accordion at age eight and later encouraged her to pick up the clarinet. As she grew older and traveled to Haiti with her own family, Jenifer never failed to bring along her clarinet and especially cherishes the cello duets Larry played with her son Jeff.

"Larry was a consummate musician," she says. "He could play almost any instrument he set his mind to playing, taking joy in figuring out the fingering of a new concertina or finding the chords that worked well on the bass of an accordion, or finding the balance between breath and notes in wind instruments."[8]

Indeed, Dr. Mellon was proficient in more than half a dozen musical instruments. He played guitar, clarinet, bass, French horn, accordion, cello, and violin (not very well), and he especially loved the oboe, for which he made his own reeds.

"We played together almost every day," says Gwen. "He played the cello, I played the flute. I used to smoke a lot, and I wanted to stop, but I couldn't. One day I said, 'Okay, Larry, you teach me how to read music and how to play the flute, and I'll stop smoking.' He did, and it kept my hands busy. I never played beautifully, but I played."

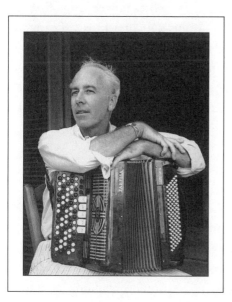

LARRY AND HIS ACCORDION

Larry's encouragement of Gwen to take up the flute opened yet another door for her, says Jenifer, and they would enjoy playing duets together for the rest of his life.

June Sardi, Mrs. Vincent Sardi Jr., a good amateur violinist, played with the Mellons on her trips to Deschapelles and brought extra musical instruments to pass around. But a greater musical pleasure for Larry Mellon was visiting his friend Charlie Ponte's music store on Forty-second Street in New York City.

"Charlie used to save all his broken-down instruments for Larry," says Gwen, "and he'd bring them down and teach someone how to repair them. At one time, we had four marching bands and a music master here. Most of the people couldn't read or write, but they would learn to read music because they couldn't get an instrument unless they could read music. Larry was just crazy about wind instruments. He loved the French horn. When he was so sick, he used to sit on the sofa and put the French horn beside him because he just loved to look at it."

In those declining years of the late 1980s, he could often be found on his living-room couch, feet propped up on the coffee table, scraping an oboe reed. In healthier days, he might serenade the peasants of an evening with "See You in My Dreams." His tastes ranged from classical to cowboy-country. So did the tastes of his daughter-in-law, LeGrand, who shared his love of music and egged him on. When she and Billy first took trips to Haiti together, the three of them would play guitars and perform in public with very little encouragement. LeGrand recounts their repertoire and *tour-de-force* triumphs in the kind of scholarly detail normally reserved for New York Philharmonic program notes:

Without a doubt, our best number was "Wreck of the Sloop John B.," and no one realized we were singing about sailors drinking all night and sheriffs who came to take the drunks away.

Over the years, Larry and I continued to play. Every evening, right after dinner, we would rip out the guitars and go through *The Weavers Songbook*. The first number in the raggedy book was appropriate: "When the Saints Go Marching In." A rousing rendition of this would start us off, and away we would go. Next was "Kisses Sweeter than Wine." We skipped over "Suliram" with its Indonesian words and went straight for "Hard Ain't It Hard"—another rouser.

About the time we were starting into "Follow the Drinking Gourd," Gwen would put away her sewing, mumble some excuse, and scurry out of the room, no doubt to put her head under a pillow. So she missed our best stuff—"This Land Is Your Land," "So Long, It's Been Good to Know Yuh" . . .

Sometimes we took solo turns. Larry would serenade me with "Beside a Western Water Tank a Dying Hobo Lay" or "La Paloma." I had to sing every verse of "Monongahela Sal." Larry said he could see Moat Stanley's steamboat churning through the valley on the Monongahela, then the Ohio, through the Emsworth Dam, past Sewickley, Aliquippa . . . into the Mississippi, ending up at the Gulf of Mexico.

They were looking for new material in 1973 when a friend sent LeGrand a homemade tape of lousy quality, full of people ordering sandwiches and beer in the background. She listened once and forgot about it until a 1976 album appeared with the same names: Willie Nelson's and Waylon Jennings' "The Outlaws." Instantly, "My Heroes Have Always Been Cowboys," "Good-Hearted Woman" and "Heaven or Hell" were added to the rep. Larry ended up owning and loving every Willie Nelson tape ever made, so much so that he asked to be buried with one.*

Though most enthusiastic about folk and country-western, he and LeGrand also spent many hours listening to the classics, agreeing on Bach's Brandenburg Concertos as the best desert-island disk but parting company when it came to Mahler, as LeGrand recalls:

Larry seriously fell in love with Gustav, and I just didn't get it. He did his best to enlighten me—gave me Mahler's complete symphonies on CD. No help. Next he gave me a CD player. He thought I might not be hearing what he was hearing. . . . I tried, but Mahler was still depressing.

*And was.

Finally, Larry gave me a thick book, *Gustav Mahler: The Wunder-horn Years*, and said this analytical study of Mahler's works might open my eyes—or ears. I tried to wade through it, but it was even heavier going than the music. I admired Larry's intellect for conquering it.

I managed to avoid discussion of the Mahler book for a while, but the day finally came when he asked what I had thought of the book. I fudged and said I hadn't had a chance to go through the entire thing, but that I had skimmed and skipped around and found it interesting. His response was, "Really? I couldn't get past page three."[9]

From Mahler to Salvation Army songs—Larry loved them all, though he wasn't quite *au courant*. One day the popular singer Harry Chapin appeared in Deschapelles at the Mellons' door. "Hi, I'm Harry Chapin," he said. "Hi, I'm Larry Mellon," was the reply. "I play the guitar," said Chapin. "So do I," said Larry, who hadn't a clue of Chapin's fame.

Pastor André Sonnal recalls coming to the HAS campus on Sunday evenings as a schoolboy in the 1960s, "just to enjoy a concert. Dr. Mellon's way of playing the guitar was different from anybody else's. He put the head of the guitar up in the air and played it cowboy-style. At Christmas in the chapel, he'd play his guitar and Gwen played her flute. Not only did they care about the people's health, but they gave them music, too."

The way Larry chose from among his various instruments to complement Gwen's flute playing was much the same as the way he interacted with people in general, says Jenifer: "'Come play with me—give it a try, be adventurous, you don't have to be super proficient, just participate with enough seriousness to give yourself confidence. We'll have a fine time.' In reality, it was the way he encouraged us all to participate in life itself."[10]

The love of music permeated Larry's life and fit in perfectly with the philosophy of L'Hôpital Albert Schweitzer and with the Mellons as people: Music was balm for body and soul, his own and the ailing Haitians'. Biographer Peter Michelmore wrote of the day a little girl arrived at the hospital with a cancer that had gnawed her mouth and nose horribly:

> She stood there in distress, looking up at Mellon, her face half pretty and half raw flesh. The doctor picked up the little girl in his arms and carried her to his house. He sat her on a divan on the front porch, and then went to the music stand to play for her. After an hour, Mellon carried the peasant girl back to the hospital and put her in a clean bed. He smoothed the hair back from her forehead and bent close to whisper, "Au revoir, chérie."[11]

In the morning, she was dead.

.   .   .

Music was an integral part of Larry Mellon's life, but art, surprisingly, was not. "I think he was overwhelmed by it," says Gwen. "He didn't have a lot of exposure to the gallery." The Mellons had arrived in Haiti just when the art boom there was first beginning. But it was Gwen, not Larry, who was fascinated by the extraordinary range of Haitian artists and who would later foster the finest ones in Deschapelles herself.

The crisis in late twentieth-century art is that it's neo-everything. There seems no place new to go—no relief from the angst of expressionism, the hi-tech frigidity of photorealism, the ennui of minimalism. One would not expect an impoverished Caribbean island to transcend that crisis, but if there's an antidote to the hopelessness in much of Western painting, it is in the brilliantly imaginative, life-affirming art of Haiti.

How such art emerges from the crushing poverty, illiteracy, and overpopulation of the poorest country in the hemisphere is both a miracle and a woeful mystery, like the social history of Haiti itself. Perhaps because real life is so hard there, Haitian artists have created a fabulous universe of their own. Tourist trash coexists with psycho-expressionist voodoo paintings and the sophisticated poultry satires of Fritzner Lamour, in which chickens watch human cockfights and guinea fowl stand tall and tough, dressed like Tonton Macoutes.

"Haitian artists are fabulists, often conveying their message through animals, like Aesop," says Haitian gallery owner Michel Monnin. "The first time Lamour painted a *macoute* chicken and brought it to me, he was scared to be seen with it on the tap-tap."

Its stunning variety of forms, refinements, and layered subtexts makes Haiti's art arguably the richest and most dynamic in the world. It

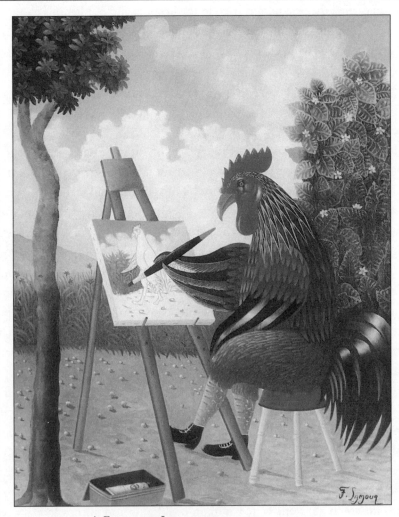

A FRITZNER LAMOUR *MACOUTE* CHICKEN

is, in fact, neither "primitive" nor "naive," except in the sense that it is characterized by spectacular color and a childlike energy and simplicity of design. The "lack" of perspective, for instance, is the deliberate rejection of it. People and animals are the sizes they *should* be, or the sizes you'd *like* them to be, and not the sizes they really are. Jungle scenes with elephants and giraffes abound, though there hasn't been a jungle in Haiti for decades, and there's *never* been a giraffe. The atavisms of Africa are still at work.

In the largely decorative jungle style, there are stunning masters at work—Roland Blain's anteaters, for example, or the paradisaical fantasies of Eric Jean-Louis. Depending on one's view, such canvases are either gorgeous or just imitative of Henri Rousseau. But Haitian painters don't know Rousseau. And jungle painting, in any case, is only the most commercial genre.

Classical precision marks the Botero-like fat ladies and peasant weddings of Saint-Louis Blaise, whose death in 1993 at thirty-six has made him the most expensive Haitian artist of his generation. Brother Serge Moleon Blaise is famous for his epic Napoleonic-revolutionary scenes. Like their late brother Fabulon, all the Blaises are superb artists.

Lush geometric landscapes, on the other hand, are the specialty of Jean-Louis Sénatus, one of the few Haitian artists who is ready, willing, and able to *theorize* about Haitian art. In his Port-au-Prince home on Rue Antoile, he is at his easel in his bare feet, pondering a stylistic change of direction in the painting-within-a-painting on which he's working. Is it finished or not? He doesn't quite know. "It's not voodoo or magic that's at the heart of Haitian painting," Sénatus muses. "It's the *heart* itself."

The Grand Old Man of voodoo artists is André Pierre, a practicing *houngan* in the tradition of Hector Hyppolite, Haiti's first great artist of the 1940s. Pierre is in the picturesque village of Croix-des-Missions outside the capital, working al fresco on a painting of the spirits Damballa and Erzuli. A guinea hen and her train of yellow chicks thread their way around his feet as he paints. When his wife serves demitasses of espresso, he first pours some onto the ground for the *loas*.

"If we don't propitiate, we won't eat," he observes. The ducks and chickens stroll beneath his easel, cocking their heads upward, cooing and mumbling. What *is* voodoo?

"*Un cadeau!*" answers André Pierre. "Unlike Christianity, voodoo is not aggressive. It doesn't make people build churches or tell them what they have to believe or try to convert you." Ah, but the two have a common *modus operandi*, it would seem: Both inculcate fear, be it hell or zombification, and then provide the method of protection from it.

"Voodoo is inside every Catholic church!" he adds with a sly smile, referring to that syncretism of Catholic and voodoo ideas by which the *loas* and the saints have merged. Voodoo believes in just one supreme being, and its *loas* are not gods but spirits, each with its own realm, most importantly:

Erzulie: spirit of love, beauty, femininity, "mistress of all men," symbol of all virtues and vices of women, a combination of Venus and the Virgin Mary, always depicted in a lace dress.

Agoué: spirit of the sea, roughly comparable to St. Peter.

Damballa: spirit of life and wisdom, the serpent-spirit of the sky, corresponding to St. Patrick.

Ogoun: spirit of war and power, always in red, similar to St. George.

Baron Samedi: spirit of death and cemeteries, always in a black or purple suit, top hat, and usually sunglasses (because's he's nocturnal).

The *loas* are found over and over again in Haitian paintings, as are representations of the *vévé*—surely the most ephemeral folk-art form in the world. *Vévés* are complex designs in white flour that are drawn by the priests at the outset of voodoo ceremonies to summon the *loas*, and then obliterated by the feet of the dancers. These and the other magic objects of voodoo are frequently employed in the canvases.

Only *blancs* find that magic threatening. Magic and voodoo are the way things are and have always been in Haiti no less than in Africa. Like "magic realism" in literature, Haitian art and life weave in and out of fantasy and reality, with no clear line between the two. Thus, to treat magic and voodoo as separate or independent phenomena is not only unwise but impossible. Voodoo in Haiti is perhaps not so different from Christianity's permeation of America, the magical elements of which we think quite normal—Christ's miracles and resurrection, for instance—and the tenets of which are applied freely to people's lives. There is no higher compliment than to speak of someone's "Christian" attitude toward the poor. If it's "the Christian thing to do," it automatically receives a positive moral-social judgment.

Compare the Christian idea of eating the body and drinking the blood of Christ with the voodoo practice of requiring chicken and goat blood in its ceremonies. The sacrificial concept is the same; the only difference is the form of the sacrifice. White Westerners are squeamishly averse to the bloodiness of voodoo rites. But Haitians consume the sacrificed animals afterwards, not wasting anything, which is no less civilized than and perhaps superior to Christianity's antiseptic symbolic slaughter. The religious connotations are identical. The bottom line is that Haitian voodoo is a largely positive force with no particular agenda and without the proselytizing (or televangelical abuses) of Christianity.

.   .   .

DR. MELLON WAS neither an aficionado nor a collector of Haitian art. But Mrs. Mellon was both, and HAS campus residents are the beneficiaries. Their homes and the hospital are adorned with hundreds of fine canvasses acquired by Gwen not long after the original collecting boom began, in the late '40s, when the great Dada-surrealist critic André Breton visited Haiti and "discovered" Haitian art for the white West.

Nowadays in Port-au-Prince, collectors go to the beautiful, European-style Galerie Monnin in Pétionville for the most refined "high-style" canvases, and to Issa El-Saieh's sprawling art emporium in Morne l'Hôpital, on a hilltop above the Oloffson Hotel. It is hard to call it a "gallery" because of its staggering volume—thousands of paintings stacked deep against every wall. Just picking a path among them is difficult, but one flips through the paintings with the anticipation of discovery. Oops! There's a 40-year-old Philomé Obin. It's not for sale, but Issa is happy you found it. He's been looking for it.

In the Papa Doc years between 1957 and 1972, Issa almost singlehandedly kept Haitian art alive. Like the Monnins, he has a stable of artists, coddling and cultivating and feuding with them and taking care of their creditors. Issa, whose father was Palestinian and who is also an ethno-musicological authority on voodoo songs, has supported Albert Schweitzer Hospital almost since its inception by donating many of the fine canvases that adorn its walls.

Voodoo, fantasy, landscapes, portraiture—all in striking abundance. One might expect to also find the political and economic conditions of Haiti reflected in its art, but Haitian painting rarely contains beggars, boat people, or other ugly realities. Important political canvases are few: J. E. Gourgue's huge "Papa and Baby Doc," in which the Duvaliers are surrounded by their true emblems, money and cockroaches, and young Frantz Zèphirin's work, full of psychedelic voodoo and biblical symbolism in equal measure. Among Zèphirin's overtly political works are "AIDS Airline" and "Apartheid."

Perhaps the "lack" of politics in most Haitian art is rather a defect in North American perception. Artist Gesner Armand, director of Haiti's Museum of Art, points to a canvas of mother and child solemnly regarding some impossibly huge fruit in a tiny bowl and reminds that in Haiti, "Food is political, too."

If that is the case, which it is, the real political masterpiece of Haitian art is Fritz Saint-Jean's "The Return of the Black Pigs." It is superbly composed and executed and enchanting even on the surface. But to grasp its significance, one must know about a real event: the eradication of the small black pigs, "razorbacks," that were raised by Haitian peasants for generations. Those animals had tufts of stiff hair down their backbone and long legs that made them seem skinny and drawn. But they also had a big lump of fat in the shoulders, which was one of the most valuable things to the Haitians.

In 1984, many black pigs became infected with an African swine-fever virus. At the insistence of the U.S. Department of Agriculture, all 400,000 of them were destroyed by teams of government riflemen, to the enormous trauma of the populace. To replace them, the United States provided thousands of *white* pigs. But while the black pigs foraged for food and ate garbage, the American pigs required a special feed. And Haitians can barely afford to buy food for themselves, let alone livestock.

"That was a real political situation," recalls Gus Ménager. "I was sure, with my competence in livestock, there was no problem that couldn't be solved; that they'd find the white pigs a suitable replacement for the black pigs that had been killed and that we could somehow provide enough feed for them. But now the swine husbandry farmers had to work faster—to produce a 200-pounder in six months. It was a predicament."

Guillaume, the Haitian guide, says with disgust: "Many believe the virus was really a scam. Some of them had it, but there was no need to kill them *all*. The black pigs were the peasants' savings account. When they needed money for a wedding or a funeral, they'd sell one. But the corporations, American and Haitian, had never been able to *organize* the sale of the black pigs, as they could do with the new white ones."

With that tale of woe in mind, regard Saint-Jean's "Return of the

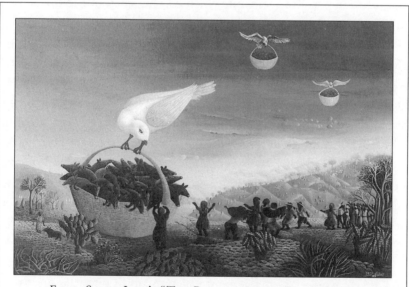

FRITZ SAINT-JEAN'S "THE RETURN OF THE BLACK PIGS"

Black Pigs" again—the wishful resurrection and mythical redepositing of them, from above, to a joyous peasant welcome.

Most Haitian artists, however, eschew such issues. They prefer to celebrate life, or escape from it, rather than lament or reform it. A fine example is Alix Dorleus of Deschapelles, whom Gwen Mellon has cultivated and supported for years and whose exquisite brushwork is much in demand.

Haiti's art is like its people: naïve, brilliantly colorful, full of humor, warmth, and myth. The variety and sheer *density* of the Haitian art scene is unlike any other in the art world today, comparable only to the late Italian Renaissance or Dutch Baroque: Haiti has more per capita artists than any country in the world. For a U.S. parallel in size and population, imagine the state of Maryland with 2,500 full-time working artists, 250 of them world-class in quality. Maryland would be considered the art mecca of the hemisphere.

That such artistic riches come out of such poverty is a great paradox. Voodoo is essential to some Haitian artists and irrelevant to others. But there is no doubt that the earthy mysticism of the art, and of Haiti itself, is tied in part to its religion, which is as impenetrable to the outside world today as it was to the French colonials of Napoleon's time.

The Mellons viewed voodoo ceremonies as private family affairs—often very expensive ones, in fact—and did not disapprove of the ceremonies themselves, only of "their" *blancs* participating in them. In Deschapelles, one often hears the voices chanting all night long, just a few hundred yards away from the hospital. Would the villagers welcome a *blanc* who stumbled in to gawk? Probably not. But the sounds and the excitement are alluring, a unique combination of sexuality and spirituality that characterizes this extraordinary people and their superstitious religion. If a frog urinates in your eye, they say, you'll go blind; if you don't close all your windows tightly at night, evil spirits will get in.

The fascination is not shared by all at HAS.

"I don't have the least curiosity about voodoo," says Dr. Marcella Scalcini. "I worked with a very intelligent Spanish physician here who used to go to voodoo ceremonies. But I didn't want to hear about it, and

Mrs. Mellon is the same. Voodoo is part of the reality, but it's not my field. I remember one doctor saying, 'We are here to fight voodoo.' I said, 'No, to fight malnutrition and illiteracy.' Voodoo is not our enemy. Our enemy is poor health and poor education."

.   .   .

HEALTHY OR SICK, the Haitian people patiently retain their dignity at all times, which is evident in a very moving way on a tour of L'Hôpital Albert Schweitzer. It begins early, of course, in the first light of a gorgeous dawn. Haitian women are already moving briskly up and down the paths, carrying heavy baskets of fruit and vegetables on their heads, often without even one hand to steady the perfectly balanced loads.

One's first full experience of the hospital is almost too much to

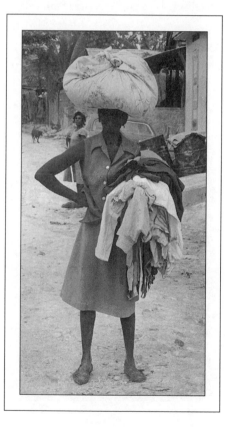

A HAITIAN WOMAN CARRYING A
TYPICALLY HEAVY BUNDLE
TO MARKET

absorb—heart-wrenching and heartening at the same time. Gwen understands this and gently facilitates. It is amazing to see how the patients relate to "Madame Mellon" when she stops by their rooms to say hello: Her presence stirs and brightens them.

At the seven A.M. X-ray diagnostic meeting, seven doctors pool their resources, poring over cloudy film from a faulty developer and comparing notes as to what the pictures reveal. From there, the doctors make surgical rounds, then visit the TB and AIDS patients, among others. Many here are now sick with a mysterious viral flu that bears a similarity to both malaria and hepatitis.

In the car, later, with Mrs. Mellon in the driver's seat in more ways than one, she stops when hailed by a pregnant woman carrying a boy with a large, bloody growth on his head. They exchange a few words to the satisfaction of the woman, who walks on toward the hospital.

"You see a lot of those abscesses on the arms and shoulders, like the one on his head," says Gwen. "Don't ask me how he got it. A lot of times it's because they get a mosquito bite and scratch it and it gets infected."

We're in the car again, a few days later, on our way to the Saturday

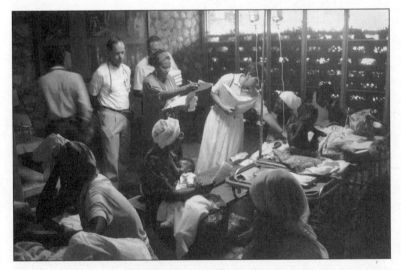

THE DIAGNOSTIC MEETING

market in Verrettes,[12] in search of two crucial but unlikely items, equally difficult to find, onions and cassette tapes. The previous night it had rained heavily—a fabulous long, cool, downpour that reduced the temperature and made sleeping pleasant but also made the roads like rivers.

Haitian highway-building is exactly the opposite of what it should be: the road itself is LOWER than the embankment along the sides, so water runs straight down the highway itself, carving out a deep hollow in the middle. Driving into Verrettes, you could not see the roadbed most of the way, so covered was it with the still-rushing water from the night before. All along the way, women were slowly streaming from the mountain and hinterland paths onto the main road, carrying their well-balanced wares to the market. They are fascinating to watch, as many HAS alumni attest:

My husband, John Roush, who was employed by Lowery Electric Co. in Miami, went down to work on the hospital in 1955," Mary Roush recalled. "One day when he first arrived there he was walking on one of the pathways when he met a Haitian woman with a cow's head upside down on her head. Since the cow's head was still dripping blood, it was a rather startling sight. From a distance he wasn't sure what it was and, of course, having heard the stories about voodoo, he was ready to run the other way. He soon learned that this was not an unusual sight in Haiti.

Haitians start early in life carrying loads on their heads. Little kids four or five years old often carry gallon cans of water on their heads. Some help their mothers by carrying small baskets or wood for the cooking fire. While we were on a walk one day, two boys passed us carrying a bundle of trimmed tree branches about eight feet long. A boy was at each end of the load, supporting it on his head. They were marching, dancing, and singing in a cadence. They would stop, pirouette in unison under the load, all the while carrying on with their dance steps and singing. They went in and out of ditches, around trees. They continued this for half a mile, attracting smiles from passersby and making fun out of work.[13]

On the morning of this particular outing, we were the only *blancs* in the Verettes marketplace. The array of people and goods was stunning. So was Mrs. Mellon's skill in obtaining the avocados, tomatoes, oranges (two for one gourde) and especially those elusive onions she wanted most. It took forever to find them and, once located, the woman vendor was asking an exorbitant price. A fascinating ritual ensued: Gwen kept expressing shock and walking away, only to be called back by the woman's son each time. The irony was lovely: one of the great Mellon family heirs bartering for onions, in Creole, in the proverbial Middle of Nowhere. But Gwen was not about to be taken advantage of, and a fair price was finally settled upon.

Vegetables obtained, everyone piled back into the car and turned to the next challenge: cassette tapes. A small crowd had gathered outside Mrs. Mellon's window, most just curious to get a look at her and the *blanc* visitors but a few still hawking things and asking for handouts. One old man was particularly insistent. Gwen said, in Creole, what she often tells such people: "I don't give out money—but what is it you need?" The man replied that he was hungry, whereupon Gwen dug into her little change purse, pulled out a few gourde notes and handed them out the car window to a boy selling rolls near the old man. The boy gave them to her, and she in turn gave them over to the beggar.

The old man took the rolls and, with something like a curse, crumbled them up in his hands and angrily threw them down on the ground. The crowd laughed. Self-possessed as always, Gwen drew in her hand, raised her chin a bit, and said softly—straight ahead, to no one in particular—"That's too bad. That's sad." She said it with dignity, but was clearly disturbed. The old man was crazy, and Haitians always laugh at craziness. Her distress was for the man, not for his insult.

If the incident upset Mrs. Mellon, it wasn't for long. The story's end is neither happy nor sad but funny: Upon returning home and unpacking the shopping bags, the onions were present and accounted for. The tomatoes were not.

"I forgot to take them," she said, shaking her head with a rueful smile. "I bartered for them, paid for them, counted them—and then left them behind. That woman must have been doubly happy: 'Good price, and she didn't take them!' That isn't cheating on her part. That's my stupidity."

Someone in the marketplace got the best of the *blancs* after all.

．　　．　　．

ONE NIGHT AFTER DINNER in Deschapelles, Gwen tells A Tale of Two Haitians—Pipi and Luquèce.

> Pipi works at the hospital in our generator area and has nine kids but can't send them to school. His oldest boy passed his baccalaureate, which is the last step before you enter the university. Pipi came to see me the other day and said, "I can't afford to send him to medical school." But there's just too much else to be done here, and I told him I couldn't help.
>
> I'd given him a big farm that could have taken care of all the kids, but he never farmed it. It had irrigation and nice rich soil, but the only thing he ever did with it was pick the lemons from the lemon trees. He bought a television set, and you can't even get any television here! He probably could have sent his son to school for a year with what he paid for the TV. He has diabetes and gets a shot every day, free. But he should have done better. Look at Luquèce.

Luquèce Bélizaire was one of Dr. Mellon's most trusted assistants—driver, mechanic, and troubleshooter extraordinaire—and serves the same functions for Mrs. Mellon. He is a powerful, intense man with a commanding, silent presence that speaks volumes in any crisis situation. He is also that rare thing in Haiti: a solvent entrepreneur.

Luquèce owns a car and bought a fair-sized farm with his own money. He also runs Deschapelles' best—actually, its only—restaurant, where delicious *griyo* and fried *akra* are served alfresco by his all-family staff. A measure of Luquèce's sensitivity to the little community is that, during the severe economic crisis and hard times caused by the U.S. embargo of Haiti between 1991 and 1994, he temporarily closed down his restaurant because many villagers were surviving by just selling a bowl of rice or beans to HAS staffers at lunchtime, and he didn't want to compete with them.

"Luquèce is an example of someone who works to his potential," says Gwen. "He's got a lot of vision. [During the military coup period] he used to go to Miami once a month and bring back tapes for people were afraid to write letters. They'd say it on a tape and give it to Luquéce. He'd carry back other things that people needed badly, including money. You have to be a pretty reputable person to do that. Luquèce could do it. For most people, money in the hands is a real problem here."

A related problem is that many of the village children who have grown up around the HAS campus have become very aggressive and "creative" in dunning the staff and visitors. "They're looking for any source of survival," says Dr. Maimon. "They anticipate your comings and goings, they lie in wait for you, they beg quite pathetically or ask to do errands, and when you leave, they want your shoes and clothes and extra gourdes. It's very difficult to say no, but if you say yes—it's like the Pied Piper. You have 100 more."

A personal example: One late afternoon, I walked down to the aqueduct and found a lovely little nook, perfect for reading in the shade and solitude, with no one but a huge tied-up pig for company. Soon enough, a young man on the path spotted me, came up, and explained at length that he wanted to go to the local school but lacked the thirty or forty gourdes for the necessary books—a list of which he produced from his pocket. On the list was a book from the "Ti Malice" Creole-French literacy series that, coincidentally, I had purchased for myself that very morning at the Verettes market place. I considered giving it to him but decided to keep it. I ended up handing him two dollars and making him promise to use it for books. But something in his eyes and suspiciously good English told me, as he took the money and walked away, that wouldn't happen.

Too late, I flashed to the scene of Gwen and the old man with the rolls that morning: I should have risked insult and given him what he said he needed, instead of money. At two dollars, I had suffered no great loss. But the principle—for now and the future in Haiti—is a terribly important one.

.   .   .

As HER REACTION to the forgotten tomatoes suggests, Gwen can laugh at herself, which is necessary for survival anywhere but perhaps especially in Haiti and perhaps even more among people whose life and work involve hospitals.

On the day of my departure, Mrs. Mellon and several HAS staffers accompanied me to Port-au-Prince, where we all had other business and booked into the Hotel Kinam for a day or so. After the jumble of suitcases had been sorted out and sent to their proper rooms, mine turned out to be the only one missing. It contained all of my computer and recording equipment and weeks' worth of interviews. Everyone searched high and low. I knocked on Gwen's door to ask if it had been delivered to her room by mistake. "No," she called out.

Frantically, I went around to the rooms of everyone else in our party. No luck. Stolen, for sure. Hours later, in despair, I decided to make one last desperate check, disturbing everybody a second time and saving Mrs. Mellon's room for last in the hope I might not have to bother her again. This time, instead of calling out, she opened up and there, standing large and square and black beneath her window, was my missing bag.

"Oh!" was the sheepish reaction of Gwen, whose eyesight is notoriously bad. "I thought it was an air conditioner."

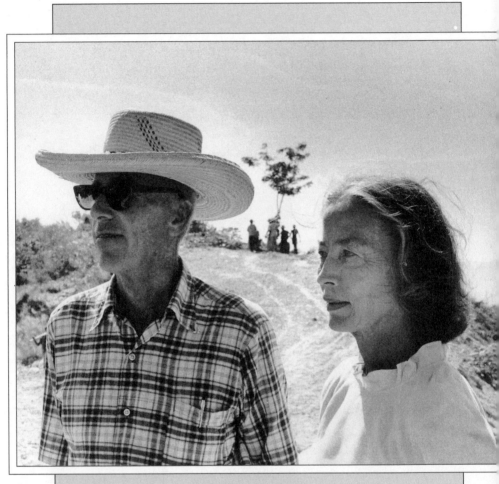

LARRY AND GWEN

CHAPTER 7

ADAGIO
"When the Roll Is Called Up Yonder"

WHAT WOULD Larry do?"

Those who knew Dr. Mellon often asked themselves that question. In important hospital matters, the answer was usually clear-cut. In other cases, especially on his visits to the United States, the answer could be comical.

LeGrand Mellon Sargent remembers Larry calling her from the Westbury Hotel in New York to say, "I'd like you to take me shopping tomorrow. Can you be here at seven A.M.?"

"All right," she replied, "but there's nothing open then."

"Oh, yes, there will be something open," he said. "I'm just looking for the usual things—clothes, music . . ."

LeGrand dutifully showed up at seven and, predictably, they had to stand around outside the shops for two hours, waiting for the store-keepers to open up. ("I couldn't count the number of times I had to do the same thing," adds Gwen.)

Dr. Renée Bergner recalls the time she and her late husband Art, guiding lights of the HAS alumni association, picked Larry up at the Columbia Medical School dormitory where he was staying during a New York visit and took him to the airport for his return flight to Haiti:

As soon as we pulled up, the door of the dorm swung open and Dr. Mellon rushed toward the car. He wore a threadbare winter coat and had a small, battered suitcase held together by cord and a number of heavy cartons with sundry equipment that he was taking back to HAS. He bounced into the car happily and, as we were pulling away, said, "This dorm was a great place to stay. And the best thing about it is it cost only five bucks a night."

When we arrived at Kennedy Airport, Dr. Mellon went to the Pan Am counter to check in with his multiple bundles. Afterwards he walked back toward us in thought. He looked a bit disturbed and finally said, "The young woman forgot to charge me overweight for the cartons. I must go back and tell her." He went back to the counter and paid the extra freight. . . . His ethical behavior became a standard for us to emulate. When faced with ethical decisions, we tended to say, "What would Larry do?" After a while this phrase became such a frequent saying for us, that if we had to decide whether to take the East River Drive or First Avenue, we would joke, "What would Larry do?"[1]

Gwen was wryly amused by the relative treatment she and Larry received on such trips:

Larry and I traveled to the U.S. quite a bit in the last two years, mainly to Presbyterian Hospital in New York for biopsies and for his dentist's appointments, but also for my medical dates. We always had his nurse with us at that time and a car with a driver to pick us up and drop us off and come back.

We'd come out of the Westbury Hotel and Larry would be helped into the car. I was on two crutches, having had my hip operation, but everybody would swarm around Larry to help him and I'd be completely forgotten. Larry would get in the front seat with the chauffeur. I'd walk around on the traffic side and get myself and my two crutches in by myself. The same thing would happen when we got to the destination: The chauffeur would help Larry out with the nurse, and I would be left to get myself out with my crutches. It was so touching!

Renée Bergner, too, has a tale of the absent-minded doctor:

Once Gwen, Larry and [his sister] Peggy Hitchcock were looking for a cab in New York. Gwennie's back hurt and she said, "I must go sit down awhile until we get the cab." Peggy and Larry were laughing and having a great time—remembering songs their mother used to sing, and so forth—and finally they hailed a cab, got in and forgot all about Gwennie sitting and waiting! She had to make her own way home alone.[2]

Usually, the service was more equitable. Once at Kennedy airport, the scenario was highlighted by dueling wheelchairs: Ian and LeGrand met Larry and Gwen and pushed them through the throng, indulging in a kind of chariot race involving the two mobile chairs, two sets of canes and crutches, numerous pieces of luggage, and an entourage of stewards trying to keep pace. Upon their arrival in Port-au-Prince, "There were eleven people there to meet us," remembers Ian, "and we needed every one."

Trips to the United States became more difficult in Dr. Mellon's declining years, but there was always something to laugh or cheer about. In 1984, his whole family, including sisters Rachel and Peggy, joined him at Choate when he was to receive an honorary award.

"Two days before," recalls Gwen, "Larry went to the dentist and had to have a front tooth pulled. The dentist said, 'I'll try and get your teeth replaced for this weekend,' but by Saturday it wasn't ready. Larry said, 'That's all right, nobody will notice.' We have pictures of Larry laughing after his speech, with no front tooth. He truly believed it wouldn't be noticeable."

Linda Gruber, whose husband, Gary, was then chaplain at Choate, described that event:

When Larry received the outstanding alumni prize, he stood on the stage of the Mellon Art Center (a gift of his cousin Paul) and responded with a simple but eloquent speech. Then, in typical Larry

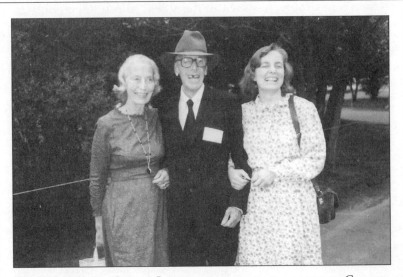

WITH GWEN AND JENNY, LARRY MISSING FRONT TOOTH, AT CHOATE

Mellon fashion, he pulled out his Choate band cap from the days when he was a student there and put it on. At once, I saw both the young boy and giant man all wrapped up in that wonderful person.[*3]

Many years before, when Ian graduated from Trinity College, Larry gave a talk to the parents with these parting words concerning discrimination: "If you have trouble getting into a country club, don't feel badly. Just go out and join a *good* club instead." The remark drew a standing ovation.

Dr. Mellon normally declined honorary degrees because they embarrassed him. But in June of 1989, at the request of his close friend and personal physician, Dr. William Harrington, he agreed to accept one from the University of Miami medical school.

"It was a huge outdoor affair," says Gwen. "Larry was very sick, but they took him around to the back and got him out of the wheelchair

---

*When the Grubers moved to Shipley, they learned that Gwen years earlier had been the first recipient of Shipley's Margaret Speer Award for outstanding humanitarian service. "As in so many things," says Linda, "Gwen was merely leading the way for Larry."

and onto the raised stage. After they read his citation, the whole student body gave him a standing ovation. There was Larry on that stage, so small and frail, and they paid this beautiful homage to him. The president of the University said he'd never seen anything like it before. He left right after to go back to the hospital for his chemotherapy treatment."

As they were leaving, recalled Jenifer, "A man came running up to us and said in excellent French, 'Docteur, excuse me, I am a Haitian. I want to thank you for all that you have done for Haiti.' That touched him even more than the standing ovation."

.   .   .

In *Out of My Life and Thought,* Albert Schweitzer wrote, "To the question whether I am a pessimist or an optimist, I answer that my knowledge is pessimistic, but my willing and hoping are optimistic."

When Norman Cousins visited the doctor in Lambaréné and importuned him to speak out against the nuclear arms race in 1957, Schweitzer rose to the challenge. He wrote and broadcast through Radio Oslo his famous "Declaration of Conscience Against Nuclear Testing," which had an enormous worldwide impact:

> The awareness that we are all human beings has become lost in war and politics. We've reached the point of regarding each other only as members of a people either allied with us or against us and our approach: prejudice, sympathy, or antipathy are all conditioned by that. Now we must rediscover the fact that we—all together—are human beings, and that we must strive to concede to each other what moral capacity we have.

There is a great difference between morality and religion, but Schweitzer, like Mellon, was acutely interested in both. Years earlier, in his first major philosophical publication, *Quest for the Historical Jesus,* Schweitzer outlined an ethical philosophy based on his eschatological interpretations of the life of Christ. But what the hell was eschatology?

Hell, indeed: It's that branch of theology which is concerned with "the end"—death, judgment, heaven, and damnation.

Schweitzer's was a continuation of the nineteenth-century struggle between scientific rationality and faith: the conflict of science versus Christianity. If the true historical Jesus were brought to light, Schweitzer hoped, it would help liberal theologians defeat dogmatism. But the real figure of Christ evaded his, as everyone else's, grasp. Early Christians failed to explore the factual life of Jesus, and the gospels shed little light on it or on the "Messianic secret" that Christ kept until the end. All other biographical accounts were hypothetical constructions.

To Schweitzer, the key to the historical Jesus was simply his "overwhelming heroic greatness" for posterity. Whether Christ appeared as the Messiah all along or revealed that only to his closest confidants at the end does not help understand him: It is pointless to try to explain psychologically a person who "knows that with his actions and his death, he is creating a moral world which will bear his name." The supernatural sphere was beyond the thinker. To Schweitzer, the incomprehensibility of Christ's dual nature is in itself the answer. *Quest for the Historical Jesus* was unusual in scholarly theological literature, a combination of missionary ardor and strict objectivity.

Larimer Mellon was as objective as his mentor but his own theological beliefs, by contrast, lacked any such polemics.

"This will make you laugh," he apologized by way of preface in a letter to Dr. Schweitzer, "[but] you must realize that Presbyterians, more than other Christians, carry painful duties and heavy responsibilities. Not necessarily, alas, bringing more spiritual satisfaction. . . . Excuse me, my dear respected friend, for inferring that these remarks contribute to your understanding of religion. These ideas are due to Presbyterianism which I absorbed in my upbringing surrounded by my Scottish family."[4]

Bill Dunn said that "one of the most interesting things about Dr. Mellon, was his deep respect for the beliefs of other people. He disliked evangelism and, among his own staff, did not tolerate people trying to sell their religion to others. Rather, he wanted to make sure we encouraged everyone who came to HAS to bring their faith with them and mesh with the others on the team. He had confidence that when people of good will put their beliefs to work, good things would come of it. And he was right."

Though many religious groups sent valuable aid and personnel to HAS, Mellon often declared: "This is not a missionary hospital. Religion is a means of sustaining oneself and is not to be disseminated." One day he walked into the hospital and noticed a crucifix on the wall, placed there by his beloved Catholic sister-nurses. He politely asked them to remove it.

How did the nuns react? "They accepted it," Gwen recalls. "It was just the rule, and it was applied uniformly. The sisters were so marvelous. In the days when they had to wear full habits, I always thought they looked so glamorous. I rather envied them—all the imperfections of middle age covered up! We did all their laundry, and, God, you couldn't believe it. All those layers, and in such heat. But if it bothered them, they never talked about it."

Larry was upset once when his friend Emory Ross gave a sermon in Deschapelles referring to Christianity as "the greatest religion." Some of those in attendance got up and left.

No one ever heard Dr. Mellon raise his voice. He was a very quiet, private man, and he thought religion a very quiet, private matter. The HAS campus chapel, which he authorized and brought into being in 1956, was for any Protestant pastor, Catholic priest, or Jewish rabbi who wished to preach in it. In the years since, every variety of religious service has been held there. At the time, says Dr. Scalcini, "Many people didn't like it. It was too ecumenical. He was ahead of his time."

HAS's former Pastor André Sonnal first came to that chapel as a small boy in 1965. He befriended some of the Mennonites there and later attended Bible College in Indiana. After graduation, he returned to Haiti and became pastor in 1989, shortly before Dr. Mellon died. The hospital chaplain's post is a prestigious one. Sonnal was highly respected as a counselor and minister to the sick, and much valued by Gwen Mellon as a good friend and skillful arbiter.

"One of the sermons I preached was called 'The Value of Christmas,'" Pastor Sonnal recalls. "I said there was no bank in this world that could contain an amount of money as valuable as Christmas. Dr. Mellon liked that. He came to me afterward and said, 'That was the first Christmas message I enjoyed so much.'"

Albert Schweitzer liked to preside over the Sunday services at his own hospital, preaching to the natives in French while two interpreters translated his words into the Pahouin and Gaban dialects. Larry Mellon seldom conducted a religious service at the HAS chapel. On one of those rare occasions, he cited a biblical quotation concerning brevity and said, "In keeping with that, my sermon will be brief. In fact, it's over now."

His Mennonite friend, Edgar Stoesz, says people are handicapped in attempts to understand Larry's spirituality by the fact that he chose not to say or write much on the subject, unlike his mentor Schweitzer:

> Dr. Mellon changed in the course of his lifetime, as we all do. [But] through thirty-four tumultuous years in Haiti, his faith did for him what faith is supposed to do: It sustained him. In the end, he was able to leave with no regrets. It was a faith that generously and genuinely made room for people of other persuasions. It was, in a sense, the application of Reverence for Life to the spirit world. Just as all creatures were to be reverenced, so he reverenced the spirituality of others.[5]

That practice of reverence for life rubbed off on the other HAS physicians.

"I have no religious feelings about abortion, for example," said Dr. Art Maimon, "but in view of Larry's attitude, I never could feel that doctors should be associated with it. It's troubling, and I'll never resolve it. It goes back to basic concern for life and the old Hippocratic concept *no le nocere*—'if you can't help them, don't hurt them.' Larry put this to work, and his life was a testament to it."

Dr. Scalcini, who knew Larry's family history, once asked, "Dr. Mellon, did you do this because you are a philanthropist?" His reply was, "No, Marcella, to follow Christ."

"If you didn't ask," she says, "he never talked about God. But I always remembered those words, 'to follow Christ.' Another time we were talking about new physicians applying here. They had to fill out a form asking what religion they were, and I said, 'Dr. Mellon, I don't like this. I don't care if the doctors I work with are Catholic, Protestant, or atheists.' He said 'Yes,' like he agreed with me, but then he said, 'Only religious people last long in a place like this.' Those were the only two times I ever heard him say anything about religion."

Pastor Sonnal, too, often wondered "why a person from such a rich family, instead of staying in the U.S.A. and enjoying his money, buying yachts and mansions, would come with his wife to this poor country to help people and live a poor life this way." But they never discussed it in religious terms.

"Dr. Mellon didn't give you a chance to do that," he says. "It wasn't religion that mattered to him, it was the health of the people. He wasn't perfect, but he lived his religion. You could see Christ within him by the way he lived—so mild and simple and kind. When he was out working all day on the pipelines, Gwen would want to give him a sandwich and he would say, 'No, the workers have no sandwich, so I won't either.' He didn't think he should have better food. He had a right to, but he didn't. He was very sensitive to the people."

Larimer Mellon, the pastor concludes, "did not belong to Haiti or to the United States. He was a citizen of the world. He didn't act like an American. It was hard to know what nationality he and Mrs. Mellon were. The Haitians never asked where he was from. The Mellons lived here, so they were Haitians. People didn't call them *blancs*. At the end of his life, he didn't want to leave Haiti. He wanted to die here."

He was, in fact, suffering from Parkinson's Disease and skin cancer. It was a time of completion, not only for Dr. Mellon. In 1987, the school over which he and Hal May had struggled so mightily was celebrating its 25th anniversary. Dr. May was invited to speak at the ceremony and accepted: "I wanted to make sure to stay with Larry and Gwen, and they felt the same. There had been that rupture, that one big difference of opinion. But we wanted everybody to know we loved each other very

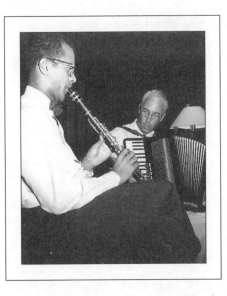

DR. HAL MAY AND LARRY

much. I felt close to Larry until his last breath, and I've always felt very close to Gwen."

It was Hal's first return to Deschapelles in two decades, since leaving so unhappily in 1970, bringing the school rift to bittersweet closure. There would be no final grudge between two gentle, stubborn men who practiced what they preached.

.   .   .

LATE IN ALBERT SCHWEITZER'S LIFE, Larry offered to send him an upholstered arm chair for his spartan quarters in Lambaréné. "No, thank you," said Dr. Schweitzer, "I'm not ready to go to sleep yet." Dr. Mellon's own health was now failing. He was getting ready.

Marcella Scalcini, among other HAS doctors, attended him at the house during the last years:*

He never complained. He was very compliant with whatever the phy- sicians told him and entrusted himself to them. He was very patient

*She also became Mrs. Mellon's personal physician, by referral from Dr. Mellon. "Marcella gave me a good physical," he told Gwen after Dr. Scalcini first examined him. "You should see her, too."

in those last years, which were quite painful—not physically, but mentally for him, and also for Mrs. Mellon.

One day, he had shaking and chills, and I thought he had malaria. So I gave him the malaria protocol (chloroquine). The next time I saw him, he had cellulitis and an infection of the skin, which can spread very quickly. I was a little scared because he had a prosthetic shoulder and that kind of infection can go into the shoulder. We didn't have many antibiotics at the time, but I found a few vials of cephalosporin. I sent a nurse to Port-au-Prince to buy more, and she couldn't find any. But I was lucky because he responded well.

After he recovered, he went to New York and when he came back, he brought me a beautiful sweater. I still have it. It is so dear to my heart. People say he was like a cowboy. I don't know this type of American, but I think his life here was not too different from the life he had on his ranch in the United States, only this one was more altruistic. He didn't spare himself.[6]

Albert Schweitzer once said:

You know what I would really like to do? Just once or twice, to get up without feeling tired and to go to bed without knowing how many things are still left undone. What a luxury that would be. [But] basically, I am very lazy. That is why I must work so hard . . . The only remedy against old age is to work harder than ever before.[7]

The last HAS staff meeting Dr. Mellon attended left a profound impact on those present. Upon learning of serious friction in the staff, he summoned everyone to the hospital library. He sat and listened as the various factions voiced their gripes and recriminations. When they were done, he sat silently for quite a while. Everyone waited for his response. What position and whose side would he take? Finally, he said, "We should never hurt each other's feelings in dealing with each other— that's no way to run a good hospital." With that, he stood up and left.

In late July 1989, Gwen recalls, "he said, 'I have nothing for your birthday.' I said, 'Don't worry, I don't need anything.' But he was sad about it, and I wanted to cheer him up. So I cut a picture of an Alfa Romeo out of a newspaper and said, 'I'll put this on your lampshade, and on July 22 you hand it to me, and that'll be my present.' He knew I always loved cars and he said, 'I'll order it for you.' I said, 'No, just the picture—just symbolic.' He said, 'I'll be waiting for you in the Alfa Romeo, and don't worry about what you're going to wear because we'll both be wearing feathers of angels.' Imagine, an Alfa Romeo up in the sky! It makes me weep, but it was lovely. Living here forty years teaches you a lot about what really counts."

Larry had just two weeks to live.

.   .   .

A HAITIAN MAN once sent word to Mrs. Mellon that he was dying and asked her to come and see him. She went, found him lying in bed. According to Haitian custom, his shoes lay by his head; his coffin was stowed directly above him in the rafters. He wanted to thank her, one last time, for a single life-saving treatment he had received at HAS many years before.

Around New Year's of 1989, Dr. Mellon had Luquèce drive him and Gwen to Petite Rivière to order two coffins—extremely simple ones, costing about thirty-five dollars apiece, in the hope that their frugality might serve as an example.

His belief was, "*Pas mette l'argent en bas terre* (Don't throw money away)," says Maître Delenois, a longtime friend of the Mellons. "He saw too much need for it elsewhere. I made the coffin myself, half wood and half carton—an ordinary one, the same as I make for people in my *asile* (old folks home)."[8] It consisted of a crude wood frame, the top and sides fashioned out of brown cardboard from a refrigerator box.

A few weeks later on a Sunday night, Larry called Bill Dunn and said, "I think it's time to go over and get those coffins." Dunn said he would attend to it the next day. Mellon replied, "Bill, when I call you on a Sunday evening, I don't intend to have it done on Monday morning. I think we should get them now."

Dunn got the message and located Luquèce, who drove to 'Ti Rivière that night. Upon his return, the two men unloaded the coffins and put them in a storage room, available when needed.

When he himself was hospitalized at HAS, Larry insisted on the standard room, bed, and food. "Everyone scurried around and worked hard to choose the best room," recalled Raphael Valery, a former HAS agronomist. "They found some pj's for him. Doc said, '*Merci beaucoup*, but just bring me the regular johnny coat. We don't have two types of sick people . . . Give me the same arrangement as everyone else.'"[9]

Back at home for his last days, he was attended by faithful Frédérique Pierre-Jules, who provides a sweetly comical example of Dr. Mellon's unfailing concern for others to the very end:

I had been up many nights with him and was becoming tired. Mme. Mellon asked [Belgian nurse] Paul Vissers to do the night shift, and he covered for me that night. He slept where I usually slept, in the study. During the night, Doc got up on his own, walked by Paul's room and came to my room and knocked. "What do you want?" I asked. "A little something to eat," Doc said. I got up, went with him and prepared the food, and when he was finished, I escorted him back to bed. Doc looked in at Paul and said, "Maybe he is hungry." I said, "No, I don't think he is hungry." Doc insisted, and woke him up. Paul, thinking that Dr. Mellon wanted to eat, unaware he already had his little meal, said, "Yes, I'm hungry." Doc said, "Go ahead, prepare something for yourself, I've already eaten."[10]

Annie Williams, who served at HAS with her husband, Roger, in the late 1980s, later wrote Gwen: "It's easy—easier—to live your philosophy when you're feeling well, young, and energetic. The way he continued when his body was nearly gone was amazing to me . . . how unselfconsciously [he] struggled to get his guitar strap over his shoulder and play an occasional chord while he entertained us with one of his favorite cowboy songs. You started to help him, but then you realized that you didn't need to . . . He was showing us that you must always try to do what you can with whatever strength you've got."

Dr. Maimon says Dr. Mellon lived "about three years longer than expected. About one-third of Parkinson's disease patients have senile dementia, but Larry never did." Dr. Jaime Ollé, one of Larry's favorites, had returned to Deschapelles that May and visited him frequently:

> He wasn't talking much at the end. But with some people you establish a link without talking, with some part of their souls, and I always felt this with him. We didn't talk about the hospital. We talked about literature. He was so well-read. He spoke Spanish and Portuguese and even a little Catalan. He gave me a leather-bound book by Valle-Inclán, the great author of Galicia. I would tease him and say, "I know you were a spy in Barcelona," because he knew the hot spots there—the bars and nightclubs. He liked to talk about Barcelona with me.
>
> A few weeks before he died, I was at his bedside and he said, "Jaime, why aren't we in Barcelona?" I thought, that sums it up—he has seen the other side. Barcelona was a symbol: "I am dying here, but I know there's still a Barcelona." He was getting weaker and weaker, but his mind was sharp to the end.

Albert Schweitzer, watching the autumn leaves drift slowly to earth in Günsbach, once mused that people should be allowed to die the same way—naturally, gracefully, without pain:

> The main question in life is, how do you feel about death? Everything that captivates and engages us is only of relative and temporary worth. In an instant, in the very next hour, it may become utterly valueless.
>
> For centuries, sermons have been preached on the terror of death in order to frighten men into believing in eternal life . . . All we ask is that death not be mentioned, and thus a conspiracy of silence has descended. We all pretend to our neighbor that the possibility of his death could never happen. No other rule of behavior is so scrupulously observed as this.
>
> [But] we must all become familiar with the thought of death if we want to grow into really good people. When we are familiar with

death, we accept each week, each day as a gift. Only if we are able thus to accept life bit by bit does it become precious. Only familiarity with the thought of death creates true inward freedom from material things. The ambition, greed, and love of power that shackle us to this life . . . cannot in the long run deceive the man who looks death in the face. . . .

What holds the deepest meaning in life is not what we hope for, not what we wish from life, but the near and far people who are in need of us. Fear overcomes us when we look at those who mean something to us and ask ourselves in horror, what would our life be without them? Face up to this fear, too. Don't push it into the farthest corner of your thoughts. Have the courage to put it into words at the proper time. There's something deep and sanctifying that takes place when people who belong to each other share the thought that every hour, each coming hour may separate them.

In this awareness, we always find that the initial anxiety about those who are left behind gives way to a deeper question: What will happen to that which was between us? Have we given each other everything we could? Have we been everything we might have been to one another?[11]

·   ·   ·

DR. WILLIAM LARIMER MELLON's thirty-five-year labors in Haiti ended on Thursday August 3, 1989, at 6:18 P.M., when he lost his long battle against Parkinson's and cancer at the age of seventy-nine. Death came peacefully at home, with Gwen by his side. His bedroom doors were open as usual to the view of the Artibonite Valley.

"Mother and I," says Jenifer, "gave him a few things to take along: a handkerchief (he was never without one), his knife, the Parker pen his mother had given him, a gnarled wooden cane he'd recently made himself with a string looped through the top so it would be easy to hang on doorknobs or chairs, his slippers . . . and of course some music—a Haydn Horn Concerto and Willie Nelson."

Early the next morning, he was taken in his simple coffin to the hospital, where hundreds of friends awaited, and carried from there by Frédérique, Bos André, Sabiel Paul, Antoine Cenon-Dieu, Ti Blanc, and Andrew Rawson down to the HAS cemetery. The cortege was "Haitian in every way," says Jenifer, "except for the silence, as requested by Pastor André Sonnal in deference to our traditions." The graveside service began with "When the Roll Is Called up Yonder," sung in Creole, and ended with "Amazing Grace." Pastor Sonnal, chairman of the funeral committee, presided. Dr. Mellon, he said, had left a monument:

> We pay our taxes, and the government should provide us with a hospital, but they don't. This man, instead of helping people from his own country, came here and helped us. What he did here will never die. Why were we the ones who benefitted? He and Mme. Mellon traveled to South America, Mexico, Africa. Finally, after visiting all the other places in Haiti, they came here and saw that if the people of the Artibonite Valley could be healthy and produce food, it would help the rest of the country because we are in the center. Everybody would walk the same distance, no one much more than another. I think God brought them here.

Dr. Mellon's simple burial provided an example, as intended, to people who often spent a year's income on the funerals of their loved ones. Guards were posted for weeks in the little tree-shaded cemetery just beyond his home because, in Haiti, the bodies of people considered saints are often stolen.

"The Haitians have an interesting theory about Dr. Mellon's death," says former HAS medical director Michel Jean-Baptiste. "They don't know anything of Parkinson's. They think what happened to Dr. Mellon was that he was too active when he was young and that he used himself up. In a sense, they are right."

On Monday, forty-eight hours after his burial, Gwen and Bill Dunn met with the staff, reassuring all that the hospital and its work would continue, as Larry directed, in the capable hands of his best friend, Gwen, as president of the Grant Foundation.

"Larry truly loved me but seldom said so," she reflects. "We never argued, luckily, because our decisions were almost always the same. Once I mentioned that over the years we got on pretty well and did not have arguments. He said, 'Yes, but I was mad at you once.' I asked what I had done. He replied that he couldn't remember."[12]

Gwen Grant Mellon, the dynamic woman behind the dynamic man, eulogized her husband's spirit as "like a crystal with many facets, found on the handle of a door, on the end of a stethoscope, on the edge of a scalpel, under the saddle of a horse. It is a letter of love written by illiterates on the rocks, the hills, and within the homes of thousands in Haiti. Having seen it is a legacy to teach by. It cannot be stifled. It is a real and living thing."

.   .   .

HIS HAITIAN FRIEND Amino Noel said Dr. Mellon "had a head that nobody else can have in the world again. He was so many things and he had so many things in his head—if I could take his head and put it on one of my sons, I would be a rich man."

On a hot afternoon in the nearby village of Estrale, another old friend reminisces about the wells he and Larry installed together and concludes, "We can't find anybody else like him."

Haiti's social and economic problems are magnified by the symbiotic complications of its poverty. A program to plant coconut seedlings, for example, was aborted when all the young trees were dug up and eaten by hungry villagers.

"Larry told me of the time he stopped by to visit a Haitian friend, who was eating an enormous bowl of rice," LeGrand Mellon Sargent recalls. "There was way too much food for one meal, but the man seemed determined to finish it all. He was saving none for the next day when he'd be hungry again. It wasn't greed, it was that he couldn't plan for tomorrow. He had to take advantage of what was before him before it disappeared or was taken away. He had no concept of 'future' because his country had never had one. The hospital's value was not only as a medical center but as something that had a future—something that would last."[13]

The socioeconomic predicament is inseparable from politics, but the Mellons always understood that they were guests in Haiti and, in four decades, never uttered a word against any of its leaders or ruling cliques. "I'm only a visitor here," said Larry, "and have no right to criticize long-established customs and traditions," including the tradition of corruption. A USAID official estimated that $11 million out of $24 million sent to Haiti from Washington for a certain farm program was stolen by grafters.

Larry was constantly on guard, against the Americans as well as the Haitians. "I feel strongly opposed to accepting funds from any government," he wrote his friend Addison Vestal in 1978. When a USAID official advised Vestal, "Sup with the devil but use long spoons," Mellon's response was, "The hell with the devil, if we have to eat with our fingers."[14] Once one got involved with government agencies, he felt, they made demands. He was especially careful to steer clear of the quagmire of internal Haitian politics—quite successfully so.

"The Duvaliers never interfered with us ever," says Gwen. "In all those years, Dr. Duvalier only sent us two referrals. He could have done thousands because he was a doctor; it would have been legitimate. I think he later told his son, 'Just leave them alone.' Neither of them ever came out to see what was going on, though of course they had all kinds of other ways to find out."

After Jean-Claude "Baby Doc" Duvalier succeeded his father in 1971, USAID undertook to make Haiti the "Taiwan of the Caribbean" with deeper market dependence on the United States. American plants greatly benefited from the huge unemployment, lack of unions, and fourteen-cents-an-hour wages. A new law required all political parties to recognize President-for-Life Duvalier. The Reagan Administration, meanwhile, certified to Congress that "democratic development" was progressing sufficiently for U.S. military and economic aid to keep flowing—mainly into the pockets of Baby Doc and his friends.[15]

Increased terrorism by the Tonton Macoutes produced pressure from U.S. President Jimmy Carter and, most significant, an emotional visit to Haiti by Pope John Paul II ("Things must change," he declared) that caused the Duvaliers to lose control. Everyone was thrilled when the regime finally collapsed in 1986.

But Haitians, by and large, are apolitical; revolutions always seem to leave them worse off. In the post-Duvalier instability, Haiti became even more isolated. Tourism, once the main industry, evaporated for fear of violence and AIDS. Haiti's Club Med, once the Caribbean's best, shut down. Such was the country's "bad rep" that the sole remaining cruise line servicing it listed the coastal town of Labadie as a port of call but discreetly omitted the word Haiti after it.

The election of populist Jean-Bertrand Aristide, a Roman Catholic priest, as Haiti's first democratically chosen president produced short-lived elation among the populace. Swept into office by a grass-roots tidal wave, Aristide was sworn in on February 7, 1991. But his anticorruption campaign, attempted streamlining of the bloated government bureaucracy, and efforts to end the contraband trade enraged the "kleptocracy"—Haiti's unscrupulously wealthy elite.[16] Seven months after Aristide took office, dissident generals seized control and replaced him with a military junta. In 1992, after the army broke an accord to restore the exiled Aristide to power, a U.S.-led international economic blockade was reimposed on Haiti.

That cruel embargo brought even worse hardships and more malnutrition to an already devastated people. In rural areas, the disruptions and the 50 percent annual inflation caused by the embargo made it impossible for many to carry on farming. More peasants sold their land than ever before, to rich people or businesses. With larger, fewer farms and hired labor came such compounded social ills as the growth of a new ruthless class of money lenders. Some farmers, desperate to avoid selling, borrowed cash at terms of 100 to 200 percent interest—only to end up selling anyway.

Agriculture was only one facet of Haiti's economy to be ravaged by the embargo. The little workshop industries at HAS provide a microcosmic example of what happened everywhere:

"We made good furniture, good ceramics, good rugs, and so forth, and we had a big inventory stored to fill orders from the States," says

Gwen. "But we couldn't ship it out. We had to close down the carpentry shop, even though it was the only means of survival for the people who worked there. Ceramics was closed because there was no electricity for the kilns. In weaving, we had to let everybody go except the head of the shop, and we didn't really even need her. Somebody said, 'Put her in another department—she's an honest girl who weaves very nicely.' But nobody needs another person who can't read or write."

The nonprofit hospital's cottage industries fell victim to a Catch-22 bind:

> Before the embargo, we were holding on. We didn't make money, but at least we didn't lose much. After the embargo, the accountants said, "Mrs. Mellon, we have to close the boutique. We can't continue to lose money." I said, "Give me a chance." Pretty soon, we were making a little. Then they said, "We can't make money—we're a charitable institution." The object is to break even. Before the embargo, it pretty much ran that way. After, it all fell apart—the weaving operation, for example, involved thirty-two people who got five dollars a week to clean cotton. A hundred families were solvent because of that income, maybe 200 when you counted people spinning thread up in the mountains. All those petty but life-saving little amounts.

When the 1991 military coup occurred and the U.S. embassy advised all Americans to leave the country, twenty-five or thirty of those at HAS did so. The ten who did not included Gwen Mellon.

"My mother and the critical American members of the staff decided to stay," says Jenifer Grant. "She has received many letters from Haitians thanking her for staying in those difficult times. She is admired for her courage."

One of the others who stayed through that chaotic time was Dr. Steve Williams, a recently arrived internist. The embargo and resulting lack of supplies "put a lot of restrictions and stress on the hospital," he says, "but HAS was one of the few hospitals in the country that continued to function and provide medical care as it had prior to the coup."

The name l'Hôpital Albert Schweitzer means something, says Gwen: "In all the tempestuous times in Haiti, we've never felt truly frightened, except momentarily once or twice. I don't know about Port-au-Prince, but it's calm in Deschapelles."

In September 1994, a peace mission led by Jimmy Carter reached a compromise with the coup leaders and, the following month, a multinational (mostly American) force of 20,000 landed in Haiti. Restored to office, Aristide moved quickly to replace the police force and downsize the military—there being no sane reason for a large army in Haiti, its only potential "enemy" is the neighboring Dominican Republic, which has no conceivable geopolitical reason to invade.

A corrupt infrastructure was supplanted with a weak one, but it was a crucial step in the fledgling democratic direction. Another significant step, belying the cynics' predictions, was Aristide's fulfillment of his pledge to leave office on schedule.

The winner of the second free presidential race in Haiti's history was René Préval, a U.S.-educated Aristide protegé, elected in December

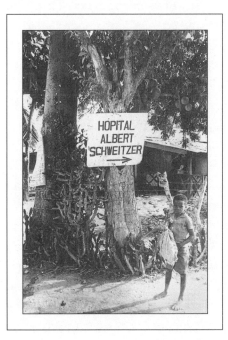

"WE HAVE A LITTLE HOSPITAL AND WE WANT A LITTLE SIGN."

1995 and inaugurated in February 1996. The new leader was friendly toward HAS in general and Mrs. Mellon in particular. She is convinced—
and states in her politically muted way—that "he has the interests of the
country at heart," and most international observers agreed.

But the subsequent parliamentary elections were not so certifiably
democratic as Préval's, resulting in governmental paralysis over cabinet
appointments and a two-year, ruling-class power struggle in which the
president's and the parliament's efforts to bypass each other delayed des-
perately needed foreign aid and investment.

For decades, Haiti's most urgent issue was human rights and political
freedom. Now, it is the economic deterioration that is jeopardizing the
nation's recent political gains. The government is being reduced by massive downsizing and is further abdicating its economic role to privatiza-
tion. That, according to Haiti-watcher Jonathan Pitts, has ominous
implications for a country with a history of unregulated monopoly
abuses. Public utilities such as the phone, water, and electric companies
are headed toward multinational corporate takeovers. Of 7 million
Haitians, about 140,000 have electricity. Private monopolies have even
less incentive than public ones to expand services to the poor. Privatiza-
tion means casting adrift the hemisphere's weakest, most uncompetitive
economy in the global one, a defenseless sacrifice on the altar of free
trade. One example:

Imports of heavily subsidized American rice have shot up astronomi-
cally, from 7,000 metric tons in 1985 to 140,000 tons in 1995. Haiti's
peasant economy lacks most crucial agricultural infrastructure (irrigation, telecommunications, electricity, roads) and access to formal cir-
cuits of credit; informal loans cost 20 to 100 percent a month. Haitian
peasant rice producers are thus expected to compete with North American agribusiness, which enjoys all manner of high-tech advantages and
subsidies. As more and more rural families find it impossible to make a
living on the land, they join the exodus to the chronically overpopu-
lated slums of Port-au-Prince, complicating the already massive social
and health problems there. It is, all in all, a cruel paradigm of what crit-
ics call "sado-monetarism." The challenge for Préval and his successors

is to substitute a gradual for a brutal integration of Haiti's economy with the world's.[17]

It is a Yankee myth that democratic elections lead automatically to economic democracy, the sharing of a country's wealth in equitable ways that narrow the gap between millionaires and paupers. Haiti's once-rich coffee business is gone, and its agriculture is so undeveloped that most peasants do not even use wheelbarrows. Thanks to the embargo, unemployment in Port-au-Prince is an unfathomable 75 percent, half the population survives on an income of under $60 per year, and the sole steady source of foreign income is the $300 million lifeline that Haitian emigrés working abroad send home.

Haiti, still groping for its own form of social and economic glasnost, needs more time to surmount the imperialist handicaps left over from 200 years. But enormously important accomplishments have taken place: not least, the peaceful transition of power and the end of secret-police terrorism.

"Many thinking people in Haiti today are optimistic about the country's future since the Préval government came to power," says Mrs. Mellon, who in 1997 was awarded a presidential citation of merit by the new leader personally. L'Hôpital Albert Schweitzer is seeking to extend its collaboration with the ministry of health and to create a more synergistic partnership to meet the health needs of the Artibonite. Though poverty and overpopulation still prevail, deprivation has not killed the spirit of the people or of the hospital trying to serve them.

Haitian resilience has surprised the world before. Or, as HAS alumna, Anne-Marie Judson, put it: "Things don't work in Haiti, but things work *out*."

Dr. Ollé elaborated: "If you are surrounded by a nonfunctioning society, to keep something like HAS functioning is a very difficult show. When the Duvaliers were here, it was bad, but at least you knew who was the boss. Now things change every six months. I'm not defending Baby Doc. But each time the people are squashed down, there's more cynicism."

Ollé, who has spent much of his professional life practicing medicine on third-world assignments in Africa, Latin America, and the Caribbean, thinks the general state of public health in Haiti is worse now than it was fifteen years ago—worse, even, than in Burundi or Mali, for complex reasons:

> Sociologically, Haiti is a dramatic country from its very origins. People were brought here from totally destroyed societies in different parts of Africa. Then the white bosses ran out and left a void, leaving all those people from different places with different languages by themselves. Hierarchically, it was totally broken up here, unlike in Africa.
>
> Africa has some terrible diseases like schistosomiasis or sleeping sickness that do not exist here. People there live on a very low level of subsistence, and now and then they have a big disaster like droughts or war. But when things are normal and they're not killing each other, you don't see the malnutrition you see here. The villages are poor, but when problems come up there is a clear line of authority. Society is pretty well structured.
>
> The reason why sanitation and the health structure don't function in Haiti is because the government doesn't function. The other factor is pacificity. People here, to survive, must be ready to accept everything. So many politicians come and go that the people don't believe in anybody or anything. That makes it very hard to mobilize them. There is no political structure except maybe in Port-au-Prince and a few big cities. Last year's leaders are in hiding. That makes people reluctant; they don't feel they have a *right* to anything. They just try to survive day to day. In other Caribbean countries, the Spanish and British left something. Here, the French were kicked out sooner and left total chaos.

Haiti's existential dilemma, says Dr. Ollé, manifests itself in various ways at HAS, such as the complaint by some staff members that the hospital should be run by Haitians. That was, in fact, the original idea.

"One of the aims of Dr. Mellon was to totally Haitianize the hospital," says Dr. Ollé. "A Haitian doctor in Port-au-Prince once said to me, 'You're all a bunch of spies.' I said, 'Why don't you come here and see for yourself? First, there's nothing to spy on. Second, they would love to have more Haitian doctors. If they could find more Haitians, they wouldn't need me. So just apply and come and then you can spy for yourself.' This anti-American feeling is very deeply rooted.

"HAS has survived because it has Haitianized up to a point, but if it were run totally by Haitians, it would last forty-eight hours. There would immediately be a power struggle. This is the biggest hospital in Haiti, so it would be a means of obtaining power."

HAS is not just a hospital. It is also an employer that provides a livelihood for hundreds of local families and, as such, is subject to constant pressure from workers who want higher pay. It thus has the typical problems of any big business, including theft. Dr. Ollé provides a humorous, firsthand illustration:

Here, like everywhere else, people steal. But it's more dramatic because if you steal food here, you are probably letting somebody else starve. When we catch someone stealing, should we punish him? Kick him out? To what point do we pursue him? Do you turn petty theft over to the law? There's only one gendarme in the village. Dr. Mellon did not like to make waves. He tried to correct things without making a big deal about it, but that's a policy that has been argued against. Our medical director, for instance, has had death threats. What do you do about that?

To give you a simple example, once somebody broke into my house. I had nothing valuable. They took a little radio—I didn't really care about it, but I thought, "If it's an insider here, I'm going to find out." I have my network of children, and I put them on the case—"Find out where the radio is!" Sure enough, a few weeks later, I found out. I thought, how do I handle this? Some people told me, don't say anything because you'll get killed if you try to recover it. But I said, I'm going to get this radio. There is a point where you draw a line. I knew who the bastard was, and I was going to get him.

It was an employee, who didn't take it herself but had somebody else take it for her. So one morning, I took a bicycle and went up when I knew she was working. I went into the house, and there was the radio. I didn't take it. What to do? I went to the kid who stole it and said very diplomatically, "I'm looking for this radio." But the radio didn't come back. So then I went to the local gendarme and said, "Look, I know where the radio is and I want to get it back without accusing anybody." He said, "This is impossible. You need a legal order." So I invited him home and we had a little rum. Two days later, he says, "I have your radio." But he didn't bring it. We had a little rum again, and I gave him twenty dollars for his expenses. I said, "I know you've been through a lot and it took you a lot of work." The matter was solved. I got it back. Later, when I saw the thief, I said, "I got my radio back and you'd better watch out." So I had recovered the radio without getting killed.

And without getting the thief killed. Sometimes, says Dr. Skeets Marshall, "You'd even catch the person walking down the street wearing an article of yours. But you didn't report them, unless it was a big item or a whole lot of money, and nobody kept a lot of money around. Awful things happened if they were taken to the justice of peace in Verrettes or St. Marc. Prisoners were so badly beaten, they were almost killed. This happened to a man who was caught and later appeared at the hospital, dying, in such a horrible state that it made you think twice before reporting anybody to the authorities. Especially in rural Haiti, it is very serious to steal even a couple ears of corn."[18]

Such stories illustrate Dr. Mellon's philosophy that "you can't come here and think you're going to correct everything," says Dr. Ollé. "People are the same everywhere, but here conditions are worse and surviving is harder. Temptation is stronger. We had a big hospital kitchen here that served food to all the employees up to a few years ago. They had to stop because it was one of the biggest outlets of disappearing supplies. That turned out to be a good move: Now the employees have to eat outside, and it created little businesses for the local people, little lunch stands. Sometimes in Haiti things work out for the best, but not the way you thought or planned them to work out."

.   .   .

THE SCOPE OF Haiti's coexistence with misery, and of how the Mellons submerged and enriched their own lives in the Haitians', is suggested by a typical clinic day at HAS. Some 300 patients show up at the regular Monday, Wednesday, and Friday clinics. Doctors first screen out the emergency cases for immediate attention. An outdoor inoculation station in the courtyard is kept constantly busy. The care is efficient and in keeping with Dr. Mellon's motto, "Keep it simple"—for reasons of economy as well as efficiency. HAS collects only about $100 a day in fees, far less than one-tenth the cost of its operation.

On one bright clinic morning, Dr. Maimon provides a running commentary during his examinations: "You can't prescribe the optimal, *au courant* drugs in Deschapelles. I am appalled at the cost of drugs. As a kid, I raised cattle and sheep and wormed them with a preparation the vet gave me called Lovamisole. It cost $14 to worm a couple of sheep. That same drug is now being put out by a major U.S. pharmaceutical company to treat patients who've had a resection for carcinoma of the colon, and it costs $2,000 a year. There's an obscenity there."

With a Creole translator standing by, Dr. Maimon turns his attention to a stomach-ulcer patient:

"It's amazing that they stay as healthy as they do here. . . . We'll give him two antacids. You can't recommend a specific diet, because they can only eat what they have. What does he usually have for breakfast? Rice and beans? Does he put Tabasco on it? No. That's good. Most Haitians put cloves and Tabasco on their food, which doesn't do them much good."

Next case is a man from whom Dr. Maimon has difficulty eliciting information.

"If you ask a specific question, it's like leading the witness, you get a yes or no—either 100 percent right or 100 percent wrong. If it's 100 percent wrong, you've been thrown a curve and you'll never get anywhere.

So you start out with a general history, and you try to condense it and lead them into something specific about the complaint in their own words."

He studies the man's chart for a while: "Somebody was under the impression that he had diabetes at one time. He just says *suc* [sweet]. The first patient I saw here years ago told me he had diabetes. I said, 'How do you know?' He said, 'Because where I pee, the ants congregate. I tasted my urine, and it was sweet.' It was a good pickup, and he was right. I gave him the proper medication, and he came back a week later and gave me a sack of grapefruit! These patients are eternally grateful."

His interpreter says the patient at hand is also complaining of blurred vision.

"The greatest cause of blindness in the United States is diabetes," Dr. Maimon observes. "He probably has either retinal degeneration or cataracts. But we don't have an ophthalmologist here anymore."

With his pen light, he looks in the man's eyes.

"He has cataracts. See how opaque his lenses are? The light is not getting through. He'd need two operations . . . The diagnosis is probably diabetes mellitus, maturity-onset type. We'll get a blood sugar on him and a urinalysis. These are cursory exams. You can't spend the day micromanaging a case. You try to cover the bases with a systemic review. So we'll get these two lab tests, and I'll see him again."

Next case: an enormously overweight woman complaining of neck, back, and stomach pain.

"How can anybody be this obese in Haiti?" says the doctor in a rhetorical mumble. "It defies probability. Where does she work? What does she do?"

The interpreter and the woman converse.

She sells in the marketplace. She has access to food, that's why she has this problem—the same problem I have, but to a lesser extent. Looking quickly back at her recent visits . . . No previous history of stomach disorder. Haitians, to survive, have a stomach like a billygoat. They can eat very little or very badly and get along, but they almost all have epigastric distress. But at least the hyperacidity prevents parasitism of the lower gut. The bugs can't live in that hyperacid condition. It's sort of a blessing in disguise . . .

She was here in April, complaining of backache. Some American doctor wrote she had "lumbalgia." That's a twenty-five-dollar term. That means you have pain in your lumbar area. I've never seen that word in my life. . . . She also has hypertension, which you'd expect in somebody so obese, and she has back and neck pain. . . . What else is she complaining of?

The interpreter asks and relays the answer.

Headaches, earache, and a rash. . . . We'll write a note for cortisone cream. I'd like to do a pelvic exam for fibroids, but I don't have a place to do that today. . . . She goes back to 1959 here. Here's Larry Mellon's signature on the chart! July 6, 1959: "Gas in abdomen, rash on both arms. Eczematory serous lesion. Feels hot, no diarrhea." He treated her for worms, and she had a positive serology for syphilis. He practiced total medicine. He would always treat *something*—you can't treat everything today. You could spend a week or a lifetime trying to treat this lady. She can't afford it, and we can't afford the time. You do what you can. You pick your disease of the day.

Larry did such great work. He always was interested and heard them out, made them feel he cared, and did something. . . . Here's me in her chart from 1968: "Headache, fever, constipation." I gave her aspirin, vitamins, and food. She was hungry. So we're old friends.

Maimon frowns and reflects for a moment.

You know, no matter how much time Larry Mellon or I or any other physician spends treating this woman, the health of the nation has less to do with medical care than with genetics, with what you eat, where you live, what kind of bugs you're breathing, whether your sewers are good. The Swedes, for example, won't go into any third-world country to do any health care unless the infrastructure is in place. If you treat this woman for typhoid and she comes back in three months with more typhoid, you're just spinning your wheels. She's going back to the same environment. If she keeps being eaten alive by malarial mosquitos, you'll be treating her for malaria from now till Doomsday.

Dr. Maimon's last patient of a long morning is an elderly woman with bloody diarrhea:

Looking quickly through her chart . . . this lady's diarrhea was treated eight times here. She is a good candidate for a diagnosis of tropical sprue—chronic diarrhea, unresponsive to the usual things. What are we going to do for her? We treat her with folic acid, which helps heal some of this. She could be on Kaopectate the rest of her life, but that wouldn't help her nutrition. She's got a lousy gut but good arteries. She's eighty years old—and somehow she's survived it all.

.   .   .

Expatriate doctors at HAS—as anywhere else—include realists, idealists, and cynics. If Dr. Maimon exemplifies the first type, Dr. Richard Pantalone represents the second and provides insight into the third. Haiti's vast, unquenchable needs attract some well-intentioned people who fail to influence let alone correct its conditions, he says. As a young surgeon in 1986, fresh out of a University of Pittsburgh residency, Dr. Pantalone's experience was a parable:

With more naivete than knowledge and more enthusiasm than experience, I wanted to accomplish my childhood dream of running an efficient, comprehensive surgery department in a "mission" hospital. But from the night of our arrival in Deschapelles—when Bill Dunn told my wife and me there was a "strike in the OR"—until we left eighteen months later, it was a constant psychological struggle to rationalize the circumstances of life in Haiti such that my daily work was tolerable, without continually conceding the basic surgical principles I had struggled so hard to learn.

Each day brought a parade of surgical pathologies which would have been better understood and more practically treated by reading 1939 instead of 1999 texts. Many of the problems had no meaningful solutions, as the disease process had been neglected for far too long. Explaining in broken Creole, trying to find words which made sense, that a huge malodorous tumor exiting from some orifice or limb was incurable, was alien to my "cut and cure" tradition and insulted my professional ego. But with the fatalistic thinking of their society and lack of other options, most patients understood the hopelessness on their own terms. It was just one more desperate fact of their lives.

Many who work in such circumstances suffer "compassion fatigue" quickly. They either lack the religious faith which pulls one along with promises of salvation or they are unable to adapt to the society. It is difficult to balance the reality of daily existence with the compromises one must make. Finally, you either transform in some way and stay—perhaps the ultimate compromise—or you repatriate.

I, too, left eventually, but not without undergoing my own transformation. Late one winter afternoon, the last patient examined, the last emergency operation performed (hopefully), I left through the front entrance of the hospital for the short walk home. The low-lying sun was casting a golden patina on the scene. I was trying to reconcile the day's surgical calamities (bulging abscesses, inoperable cancers, ugly traumas) with the belief in a benevolent God: it was incomprehensible to me how the two could be compatible. I casually glanced up at the Schweitzer motto "Reverence for Life" carved above the entrance of the hospital, which I'd read many times and thought I understood. But only then did I fully internalize the words and get an antidote to my disquietude.

Rather than be overwhelmed by the countless unsolvable problems I felt responsible for, I should and could only focus on each individual "Child of God" who came randomly to me as a patient. Though a product of twelve years of Catholic education, I had never been reli-

giously motivated, yet this quiet, simple credo suddenly made infinitely deeper sense to me: not "Reverence for Life" in theory for the
world, but in practice with the single man, woman, or child lying
helpless in front of me. Only then did I begin to understand what it
really meant, and how a Mellon or a Schweitzer could sustain themselves through the years.[19]

.   .   .

L'ESCALE, the HAS tuberculosis village, is sadly busier than ever these
days, treating well over 1,000 cases a year. The prevalence of TB in Haiti
has always been extraordinary, but is getting much worse.

"We have a three-month treatment for TB," says Gwen. "It's a new,
expensive drug that's tough to afford—but we can treat it. The problem
is, TB is complicated now by AIDS. If you have AIDS, you're much
more highly susceptible to TB. And if you have TB, you are more susceptible to AIDS. When people come in with pulmonary difficulties,
we're not sure which disease it really is. AIDS is so devastating."

The number of AIDS cases and the load on HAS physicians have increased dramatically. The patients are more desperate, since any prior af-
flictions—especially tuberculosis and infectious diseases such as malaria,
typhoid, sepsis of all kinds—are heavily compounded by AIDS. More
TB cases are failing to respond to first-line TB therapy and medication,
and some are totally resistant to *any* therapy. Nowadays in Haiti, many
if not most adult TB patients are essentially AIDS patients, or vice versa,
due to their immuno-compromised state. Demographic studies by Dr.
Jean Pape, Haiti's great AIDS expert, show a 5 to 7 percent HIV positiv-
ity in childbearing women in the Artibonite Valley, suggesting a forthcoming tremendous increase in vertically transmitted AIDS. As it is,
AIDS is the leading cause of death between ages fifteen to thirty-five in
Haiti.

In the early 1980s when AIDS was first identified, it was said to afflict
only "the four H's"—homosexuals, hemophiliacs, heroin addicts, and
Haitians. That myth has since been corrected. But even so, why did
Haiti become such a hotbed for AIDS?

One theory is that, in the late Duvalier years, there was great movement by the emerging Haitian middle class, who traveled to other French-speaking countries, particularly in Africa, where the disease may have originated. Medical anthropologists say, as early as 1956, AIDS was endemic in monkeys and other simian forms in the Belgian Congo, where natives smeared monkey blood on their genitalia as an enhancement to intercourse. A corollary is that, with the "shrinking" of the world through international travel in the '60s and '70s before AIDS was identified, more tourists came to Haiti, including many homosexual North Americans attracted by the country's fabulous art, its gay-oriented resorts, and its relatively liberal sexual mores.

Both theories are supported in some quarters and vehemently contradicted in others as racist, sexist, or both.

Other than those infected from mother to child, most AIDS cases come from sexual contact; in richer countries, drugs and dirty needles are also a cause. In Haiti, a patient with congenital AIDS will probably be dead by age seven. Sexual activity begins at about twelve. So the only category not likely to be HIV-infected is between ages seven to twelve. That is the only real window for non-AIDS patients who are likely to be seen at HAS.

.   .   .

AIDS AND MALNUTRITION are the greatest of the challenges, yet only two of many facing HAS. Now as in the past, its success depends largely on focus. Dr. Mellon's ability to reject, limit, and terminate projects, however painful, has crucial implications in his absence for the hospital's future.

In shutting down the school and Hal May's dreams for it, he lost the services, and for many years the friendship, of one of his most talented physicians and devoted administrators. In Larry's opinion, the school wasn't working economically. It was a different business. Right or wrong, Larry killed it. For similar reasons, he nipped the proposals to establish a tropical disease center at Deschapelles in the bud. Why should such a marvelous institution as HAS not embrace a larger sphere of closely related activity?

"He said, 'These are our patients, not guinea pigs,'" Gwen answers.

"We did surgery, vaccinations, child care. We just wanted to be a good general hospital. Keep it simple. Take care of the people in your area. It was defined very early in the game. If you go to something bigger, the focus would change. You'd have people coming here because of that school for tropical medicine. You wouldn't get regular interns interested in all aspects of illness. Tropical medicine is in with all the other work here. Why pull it out? Every doctor on the staff takes care of TB patients, for instance—it involves surgery, medicine, pediatrics—yet it's not 'a TB hospital.' If we have a lot of TB, we'll take care of it. If there's another community problem, we'll try to take care of that, too. But we're primarily here to take care of people and their medical ills."

Dr. Lepreau says Mellon flatly "didn't want students around," following the example of his guiding light, Schweitzer, who wanted the patients to be treated and none of the academic business. "But I was interested in teaching somebody, so he went along and allowed me to have residents from major teaching institutions such as Yale, which regularly sent opthalmologists. They came and spent three or four months as senior-type assistant residents in surgery. Same in pediatrics from Cincinnati and Philadelphia, and in medicine from the University of Vermont—a tremendous impetus to the elevation of medical care." Over the years, hundreds of specialists contributed their services.[20]

Lepreau coordinated it all. But the programs declined after he left. Gwen cites Larry's cornerstone speech for the reasons:

"He said the hospital was a center for learning, not teaching: Learn what the people need. Before you start to work, find out what the illnesses are and where to put your effort and resources. You're ignorant when you begin. It was a learning process to understand the Haitian people, what they value—and there's nothing more important in dealing with the people you're trying to help. The docket was full without a school. We already had too much to do. Certain kinds of statistical studies or clinical research we've approved, but when people ask if they can use us to find out the value of a drug, the answer is no."

That relates to the HAS aversion toward "state-of-the-art" medical equipment, much of it computerized and all of it hard to repair. A rare exception was Gwen's acceptance of the gift of a new ultrasound diagnostic instrument.

"It's tricky to use, but you can look at all the organs like an X ray. By telling you where the trouble is and evaluating it, it has helped to avoid surgery in a lot of instances. A Swiss man came and demonstrated it, and we hoped he'd leave it. He didn't, but he helped us get one at a good price—a little under $50,000. It's very valuable. Even that, we debated and thought about for quite a while."

Young residents who come to Deschapelles learn that if they do a good history and physical and minimal lab work and an X ray if indicated, they can make most of their diagnoses without any fabulous American high-tech equipment. Paul Vissers illustrated the wisdom of "Keep it simple" in his own department:

> We received a gift of some wonderful new hospital beds. The other nurses and I were overjoyed because they had little motors which would adjust the beds mechanically. No more bad backs for us! However, after a few days off, I returned to the ward to discover that the beds were all gone. [Maintenance] had decided to remove the motors, as they were really too complicated to operate on the wards; they were afraid they would start breaking down, and they believed they could be more useful in other areas of the hospital. I asked why they had also removed the beds. The answer was, "How many people can sleep under one of these beds?" Many of the sickest patients have a relative stay with them who often use the space under the bed to sleep. The new wonderful hospital beds with their thick mattresses were too low to the ground and lacked the airy space provided by the older beds.[21]

Gwen has no apologies for the back-to-basics rule of thumb:

> We just had a U.S.-trained pediatric psychiatrist here whose specialty was parent-child relationships. She worked on the wards and we listened carefully to what she had to say, which in essence was, "These mothers don't relate to their children very well. They don't sing or

play games with them." It was true. They hold the kid if he's crying or feed him if he's hungry, but that's about it. Then they go and do all the other things they have to do. So this woman went on: "It's been shown that if the parent goes in with some nice toys and spends time with the kids, they pick up faster." She said she'd be sending us some toys, and later she did send a few.

My reaction was, it's great to teach a mother how to relate to kids, but why bring in trucks and all these things you get in the States? When the Haitian kids go home, they're not going to have them. Why not use things they have at home, instead of a truck that'll be broken in a week? Skip-rope, or something they can make themselves. Nobody paid any attention to me. It's fine for pediatric wards in the States to be full of wonderful toys—but kids there have them at home, too. If they have wonderful things in the hospital, they'll have a deprivation syndrome when they go home without them. I used to give out toys to kids here at Christmas, until I figured out they were gone by December 26.

.   .   .

THE MIXTURE OF compassion and no-nonsense pragmatism that characterizes Gwen is why her husband's last pivotal decision did not come as a surprise: A few days before he died, Dr. Mellon named Gwen Mellon his successor as president of the Grant Foundation and effective head of l'Hôpital Schweitzer.

On her first visit to New York after Larry's death, she stayed with LeGrand and Herb Sargent. His account:

I had never been alone with Gwen and decided to invite her to lunch. It was a mild, late fall day, and the two of us walked over to a neighborhood Madison Avenue restaurant. She hadn't done any recent shopping but her stylish look was both current and timeless. When we entered the restaurant, I was strongly aware of the attention she drew from diners along the way from the door to our table. She had the carriage and face of a mature aristocratic fashion model.

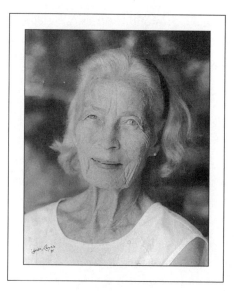

GWEN GRANT MELLON,
HER HUSBAND'S SUCCESSOR
AS HEAD OF
L'HÔPITAL ALBERT SCHWEITZER

I think going out to lunch was the first thing she had done on her own since being alone. We talked about Haiti, the hospital, New York food, and Larry. She told me how much she missed him and admitted to the extent of her loneliness. However, something told me that Gwen, at that moment, subconsciously had started to become aware of herself as a singular forceful entity. She described Larry as her "lodestar for over half a century," but she soon became the guiding light for many others.[22]

Dr. Lucien Rousseau feels Mrs. Mellon has carried on precisely as her husband would have done: "She is not a very extroverted person. She is rather discreet. You have to find the gold inside of her by watching her and understanding what she is doing. There may be problems and changes in the hospital policy. She cannot keep everything as it was in 1956. But she keeps the ship in the right direction, taking advantage of certain new ideas and rejecting others. She will not accept attractive propositions if she thinks they are not compatible with the philosophy of Dr. Mellon."

I witness a demonstration: We are chatting on the veranda when a staff doctor arrives to inform Gwen that a prestigious American medical school is offering HAS a new meningitis vaccine on an experimental basis. She politely and predictably declines. Surprised and disappointed, the doctor asks why.

"First of all," she replies, "Dr. Mellon never wanted anyone to experiment on the patients. And secondly, monitoring the thing would take up too much of our resources."

There are more dramatic instances of the toughness Gwen can summon on demand. Her husband's sister Rachel recalled, "She was wonderful the day the mob came out." Rachel Mellon Walton was in Deschapelles shortly after Baby Doc was deposed in February 1986, when vigilantes went looking for Macoutes and others who had taken jobs or profited from the Duvaliers.

"Bill Dunn had just arrived and a mob of unhappy people appeared in front of the garage," Gwen recalls. "Larry was sick, so I ran out. They were all standing outside looking tough, most of them poor people with no shirts, but people I know—I had friends among them—so I said, 'What do you want?' They talked together and then they said, 'We want air.' I said, 'Air? What do you mean?' For electricity conservation, someone had cut off the hose they used to inflate tires. I said, 'Sure. We can give it to you.' So we gave it to them. I went home. They dispersed but, an hour later, they were back again by the business office.

"I ran up from the house again, with Bill beside me. They said, 'We want de Vastey [HAS' longtime chief financial officer]. I said, 'You can't have him.' They started to come over the fence and I said, 'Don't come over, please.' One shouted, 'Mrs. Mellon, don't get into this. This is not your problem.' I said, 'It *is* my problem. He's not yours, he's mine.'"

"No one from the business office came and stood beside me. Everybody disappeared except for Ti Blanc. I said, 'Ti Blanc, go away, this will do you no good.' But he wouldn't. He and Bill stood beside me. They wanted to *dechouké* the man—burn down his house and everything—because they felt he only hired people from St. Marc, his hometown. Eventually, we dressed him and his wife up in green operating gowns and smuggled them out on stretchers in a pickup truck to St. Marc, where they were safe. But it was a humiliating, terrible thing.

"Larry was so sensitive, it would have made him more ill—this was just a year or so before he died. But he never knew what was going on, and finally the people left. It didn't get violent, but it could have. When I went back into the hospital, the medical director at the time—who didn't come down and help me—said, 'Mrs. Mellon, you're a very foolish woman. You could have been killed.' I just looked at him."

.   .   .

FOR YEARS, donations to HAS were unsolicited, as the founder wanted it. Whenever Bill Dunn raised the "f" word—fund-raising—Dr. Mellon would respond, "You're not going to write one of those begging letters, are you?"

With a name like Mellon, Larry didn't feel comfortable asking for money. But in 1959, he authorized his son, Bill, to produce a brochure (with Billy's own text and photos), telling about the hospital with only a gentle suggestion that support would be appreciated. It became an annual project, handled by daughter-in-law LeGrand for years.* Since the brochure was sent out in the fall, she visited HAS for ten days at the end of each summer to get the latest Deschapelles scoops.

"For the first two or three days," says LeGrand, "I would ride around with Larry or hang out around the hospital with Gwen while they brought me up to date. Then I would go off and write a little, then check the text with them. Then I'd ride around a little more, write a little more. . . . The day before my departure, we'd finally have the full, accepted version. All that would be left was to come up with items for our "$25 Will Provide . . ." section at the end. By then, we would be in that loony state one reaches after final exams, and it turned into a competition to see who could come up with the most unlikely items. Some of the winners were: '$25 will provide 1 pair ladies' snowshoes, 4 boxes of "After Dinner" mints, 3 feather boas, 1 dozen monogrammed golf balls, 5 eyelash curlers. . . .'"[23]

HAS' annual budget today ($4 million in 1999) derives about 18 percent from investment income on Grant Foundation funds, 9 percent

---

*Ian Rawson took over the brochure job in 1977 and did it for eleven years, when it was turned over to his son, Andrew, and Jenifer Grant's daughter, Susannah.

from Haiti (patients' fees, the HAS farm operations, boutique, etc.), and the 73 percent balance from individual contributions and expatriate foundation-program grants.

The Grant Foundation's initial (and ongoing partial) provision for operating expenses was a gift of almost all of Larry's personal fortune. "The only real property I have left in the world is a trunk in somebody's basement in New York; it contains a full-dress suit," he once said, only half-kidding.[24]

Even during his lifetime, Larimer Mellon's own money accounted for about half of his Haitian hospital's annual expenses. He always opposed outside grant-seeking "for sound economic reasons," says his wife, "but also for certain personal and family reasons, because he was who he was."

Following Schweitzer's advice, Larry structured his hospital in Haiti for independence. That structure has moved into a different mode under Gwen, as she ponders the financial future and her own succession at the hospital. Hers was an intensely poignant version of the ethical-philosophical question facing everyone who came to Deschapelles, a question similar to Christ's first words in the Gospel of St. Luke: "What do you seek?"

After Larry Mellon's death in 1989, said Bill Dunn, "The first thing we had to do was tighten the belt: a 13 percent reduction in operating expenses to pare down to the bare minimum and develop a plan for a stronger financial base. This hospital during Dr. Mellon's life was heavily dependent upon funds he personally contributed to it. But most Mellon family trust funds are discontinued at the time of death.

"One of the things he and I had great discussions about, because we were on opposite sides, was endowments. He felt they created weak institutions; that institutions should live or die based on the work they were doing. If they were worth having, people would support them. His philosophy was not to become beholden to any government. Dr. Schweitzer had advised him so, and Dr. Mellon adhered to that to his dying day. In 36 years, with all the come-and-go governments and problems in Haiti, his dedication to remain apolitical served the hospital very well."

After Larry's death, it was reluctantly decided that HAS had to apply for outside grants—one of very few of her husband's policies Mrs. Mellon reversed. "It was hard," she says, "but we had to do it if we were to continue to have community health. Grants are hard to handle and involve a lot of paperwork and a big time lag. You have to adhere to statements you've made much earlier—asking for money to fix the drains on the road to Verrettes, for example, then finding out it's impossible on that amount but also impossible to change because of the wording of the grant."

It was only very late in his life that Larry Mellon even permitted the formation of HAS alumni groups. "We don't lean on them much," says Dunn. "Larry was very sensitive about it. When the Alumni Association was formed in the U.S. and Canada in 1981, he wasn't sure it was a good idea. He wanted it done for the right reasons, and the right reasons, as far as he was concerned, did not include fund-raising. His philosophy was that these people had already contributed to Albert Schweitzer Hospital with their time and energy, and he did not want them badgered for money. So from the outset, an astute effort was made to keep fund-raising out of the Alumni Association portfolio but, in recent years, certain individual alumni have become very active fund-raisers on their own."

One main function of the alumni groups is recruitment, helping to overcome reluctance due to Haiti's "bad press" and living conditions. Over the years, a few HAS doctors and nurses contracted typhoid (easily curable if treated quickly), and some, inevitably, suffered from amoeba-related intestinal problems. But by and large, few have been harmed by coming to HAS. On the contrary, many say the greatest experiences of their lives and the lives of their children took place there.

Dunn attributes that to the expatriates' compliance with Larry Mellon's philosophy of being a guest in Haiti, and to the basic humility that attitude implies:

"I was coming back from Port-au-Prince once, and as I turned the corner from the main road up to the hospital, I noticed that the one and only 'Hôpital Albert Schweitzer' sign with the arrow was missing. I stopped and found it on the ground, all messed up and dirty, and I took it in and gave it to Mr. Angus, the chief of housekeeping, and asked him to wash it off. The next day he said, 'You know, there really should be a bigger sign out there,' but I said, 'No, I think that old sign will do just fine.'

"When I told Dr. Mellon about that later, he said, 'Bravo! That's just what we want. We have a little hospital and we want a little sign!' His concept was, this is a simple, rural hospital that would best serve the people if seen in those terms."

As of 1999, there were forty nurses and fourteen doctors at HAS, serving some 185,000 people in the Artibonite Valley. The hospital's 116 beds hold 2,500 patients a year, and an additional 50,000 are served as outpatients. HAS employed 400 in its nursing, pharmacy, laboratory, records, and X ray departments, and in its kitchen, laundry, and farm. There is a basic, inviolable rule of "containment" to which Dunn and Gwen Mellon remain committed.

"The first day I came to work as hospital administrator, September 5, 1985, Dr. Mellon came to my office and gave me a three-by-five index card," Dunn recalls. "On it were the number of beds in each department—pediatrics, so many beds, surgery, so many, and so on—totaling 116 beds. He handed that to me and said, 'Bill, you have a bulletin board here? I'd like you to put this up and understand it's the framework in which this hospital has to function. If we'd wanted more beds, we could have done it over the years, and we'd be a 300- or 400- bed hospital. There's no limit to where it could stop. So *we* have to do the limiting. As long as you're here, I expect you to control that, and I'd anticipate never finding more than 116 beds in this hospital.'

"And we listened to him. That card is still on the bulletin board of the administrator's office."

CHAPTER 8

FINALE
Reverence for Life

A DEBT WEIGHS ON US and our civilization," wrote Albert Schweitzer. "We are not free to choose whether we will or will not do good to the colored people; we owe it to them. The good which we do them is an act not of charity, but of reparations. . . . After we've done everything there is in our power to do, we shall have repaired only a small part of the mistakes committed against them."[1]

Larry Mellon would never have written that, or at least not with such political bluntness from the pulpit. He and his mentor were "two kindred spirits who had found common goals and shared their experiences, the failures as well as the successes," says his stepson, Michael Rawson. But their basic attitudes—Mellon's modern American pragmatism versus Schweitzer's turn-of-the-century European paternalism—were profoundly dissimilar in many ways. Dr. Michel Jean-Baptiste, longtime medical director of L'Hôpital Albert Schweitzer, warned against facile comparisons between its founder and its namesake:

> One of the main differences between them is that Dr. Mellon came to a country that had been independent for many, many years and had its own culture and government. Haitians are proud people, very proud of their culture and language. It was different from Dr. Schweitzer's situation in Gabon, which was still a colony where the white man was seen as superior and blacks were very deferential.

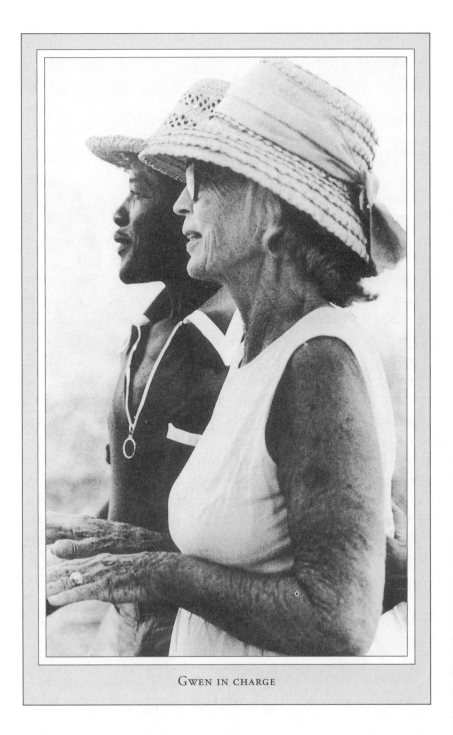

GWEN IN CHARGE

Haitians are also xenophobic. Their first reaction to a foreigner is to keep their distance. Haiti was discovered by Columbus and the Spaniards, who killed off all the Indians or made them slaves, and then came the French and English and American occupations. So Haitians as a rule are not going to open up to foreigners right away. They are suspicious at first.

The first thing Dr. Mellon had to do when he came here was to gain their trust, and it didn't take him long because they realized that this guy was serious. He meant business. He set the example right away. The first day he opened up the clinic, he didn't stay down at his house while the other doctors worked. He and his wife worked here till eleven o'clock at night. To this day, I've never heard anybody say anything bad or irreverent about Dr. Mellon, which is remarkable in itself. And why?

Because he made the people feel that he appreciated their culture, not that he was the great American who came to save them. He genuinely loved the Haitians. I don't know why. I'm Haitian, so personally, I like Haitians. Once in a while, you meet someone from another country, like Dr. Mellon, who just falls in love with the Haitian people. He respected them. He didn't think, "Look at these stupid people and their backward culture." He tried to understand them, even if he didn't believe what they believed, and people really appreciated that.[2]

What he enjoyed most was working out problems, whether it was the best sequence of breaths to play an oboe piece or the exact amount of flour a baker needed for the week, says stepson Ian Rawson. But he always remained something of an enigma:

Larry wasn't comfortable expressing his deep thoughts or motivations. People were frustrated if they wanted him to explain why he had sacrificed a life of comfort to serve the poor farmers of the Artibonite Valley. His answers were rarely expressed as abstract truths or quotable sound bites. Instead, he would invite them to go out with him on his regular rounds to visit the bakery or the cotton cleaners. What people would get out of several hours in the Land Rover with him was not a philosophical discussion but something much deeper, if they were observant. They would see him show the deepest respect for an old gentleman in tattered pants who cleaned cotton balls for the weavers and depended on the payments Larry gave him. They would see Larry stop the car in the middle of a road, get out, lift a heavy basket into the back, and open the front door for the basket's owner with as much grace as if she were the Duchess of Kent, then drive her to her courtyard, even if it was miles out of his way. They would see in his smallest actions the deep love he had for the people of Haiti.[3]

Larry's niece, Farley Whetzel, and her husband, Josh, got firsthand proof of that on their initial visit to Deschapelles in 1962. The big event that week was the christening of a baby whose ancient grandmother Larry knew and liked. The Mellons would all go, he announced—on foot, up a steep mountain near the hospital. Matter of factly, he mentioned that grandma couldn't walk and that he and Josh would carry her up on a stretcher. It was a strenuous climb on a rocky path, but they did it. Once there, they found some musicians assembled, Dr. Mellon joined them on his accordion, and a good time was had by all.

"Larry didn't make a big deal of it or play the hero," says Farley, daughter of Rachel Walton. "It seemed perfectly natural for him to do this."[4] From Uncle Larry in Haiti, the Whetzels went to visit Uncle Matthew in Jamaica. The big event *there* was a lavish party on his grand estate, with celebrities strolling through the exquisite gardens. The contrast was striking, they thought, like the brothers—the yin and yang of Mellons.

"Dr. Mellon was such a great man that it's difficult for us to understand him and even more difficult to try to emulate him," says the Harvard-trained Dr. Jean-Baptiste. "As medical director, I've tried to deal with the patients in a way that I think he would do or would like me to do."

"The other night they called me at home and said there's a guy out here who was cut up badly by a machete a week ago. He's been to two other hospitals, one in Port-au-Prince, and now he's here—he's not from our district. We have to be strict about that or the whole country would come here. What would Dr. Mellon do in my place? The nurses wanted to get rid of him, but once I asked myself that question, I had no choice: Bring him in. It was the right decision, of course. To come that distance, you knew the guy was desperate. I have to do that—and go through that intellectual exercise—all the time."[5]

Indeed, the hospital is constantly wrestling with how to screen and limit its patients to the Artibonite. Color-coded cards? Baptismal records? Picture ID's? "It's very tricky," says Gwen. "We have to be careful not to do anything shocking that might produce a bad reaction or public indignation. I've suggested telling people, 'Today we will see you, but you must not return.' A lot of people who live in Port-au-Prince come out here for surgery because we do it for $10 instead of $150 there."

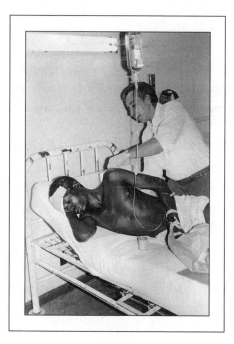

HAS MEDICAL DIRECTOR
MICHEL JEAN-BAPTISTE
AT WORK

The choice is painfully difficult: Those most likely to be turned away are the ones who have traveled the farthest. What to do with a peasant—as opposed to someone coming from Port-au-Prince to take advantage—who has made a long trek on foot? "The nurse will decide if it's an emergency or call in a doctor to decide," says Gwen. "If there's any doubt, they usually say yes."

Dr. Mellon was an administrator and philanthropist but, above all, a physician, and it was the last of those three roles that determined most of his judgments. "He was the guru," says Dr. Jean-Baptiste. "That's what he represented for us." Former HAS veterinarian, Julian Strauss, speaks in the same terms:

"I thought of him as a holy man in a sense. He had weaknesses, but that only made him more human and wonderful. I knew he was wise, so one day on the way to Drouin I decided to ask him what I should be doing with my life and where I should be heading from here. It only took four or five bumps on the road to get it all. 'When I was your age,' he said, 'I'd just gotten a divorce and was working in my daddy's bank.' That was it. So humble. It was life-changing. Not a day goes by I don't think of the hospital and Dr. Mellon. I miss him."[6]

When Larry died, says Michel Jean-Baptiste, "we lost our spiritual leader. But Mrs. Mellon has matured. You say, 'What? This woman is eighty-five years old and you're telling me in the past three years she has matured?' Yes. I've seen a major change in her. Now *she* is the respected authority figure.

"The task is to make it continue to work—to keep the hospital functioning using his principles. It's not easy. It's one thing for me to say I understand Dr. Mellon's philosophy, but I have to translate that into action and pass it on to the Haitian staff. We have to have Haitians who believe in what Dr. Mellon and Mrs. Mellon were doing, and we do. Only, we need *more* of them. If a staff member believes in Mrs. Mellon, he's going to take care of the patients properly because that's what Mrs. Mellon does—she comes every Sunday and visits *every single patient* in the hospital. I am here then and I see it. You have no idea how good that makes the patients feel. It's very important. They love it."

Dr. Jaime Ollé, the visiting doctor from Barcelona, agrees. "She's like the Holy Spirit," he says. "She's everywhere!"

Dr. Jean-Baptiste continues:

These Mellons are remarkable. They're not just rich people. This is their home. We had a lot of trouble convincing Dr. Mellon when he was sick to go to the States for treatment. When he had to go for radiation therapy because he had a tumor in his neck, he didn't want to. The minute he got the last treatment, boom—"Okay, we're going back now." They tried to get him to stay a few days to see if complications developed. No. He wanted to come right home to Haiti, and he did.

It's a real challenge for us to keep his spirit alive. This is not just "a great hospital." There are many great hospitals in the world, in Boston, New York, Pittsburgh. But there's only one like this. It's unique because of the people who founded it and the people who work in it, especially the Haitians, who don't get much credit. The foreigners get the credit. Somebody comes for a year or so, and people say, "What a wonderful job!" They forget the guys who've worked in the lab, doing the smears, for fifteen years.

.   .   .

EACH OF THE THOUSAND Deschapelles stories is unique, but one of the most compelling belongs to Dr. Marcella Scalcini. An Italian citizen, she trained entirely in the United States, including a postgraduate degree in tropical medicine at Tulane. There, undecided about where to practice, she consulted Dr. Margaret Smith, a distinguished pediatrician who had been one of Dr. Mellon's teachers.

"I was thinking about Africa," she said, "but Dr. Smith told me about Dr. Mellon and said Deschapelles was one of the most beautiful places in the world—'You live well, nice house, swimming pool, good food.' When I got there, it was a little disappointing. Why did she tell me all that? Well, I guess it was important to assure me in that way."

Dr. Scalcini came to HAS in 1982 and remained through the 1990s, becoming chief of medicine.

"I was only planning to stay one or two years. Then you decide you like it and stay on, year by year. When you feel your time is over, you leave. But you can really stay as long as you want. You stay if you're happy about being here. For me, the lifestyle is right. It's a quiet life without many distractions. You have a lot of time for yourself. I come from the big city—Milano—I'm a city woman. In the States, I lived in New York. But I don't miss many things.

"I tell the new residents, 'This is essential work.' There are very few situations in life where you know you are doing essential work. In the United States, you know there are plenty of other doctors a patient can go to. Here, when they come in the middle of the night, you know this is the only hospital for miles and miles. Here, you give essential care to people who have nowhere else to go."

Like everyone else at HAS, Dr. Scalcini had to adjust to certain deprivations in Deschapelles, most notably the lack of telephones, which Dr. Mellon regarded as an intrusive nuisance. "If I'd had a phone here," he once told Michel Jean-Baptiste, "I would not have been able to do half the work." In Scalcini's view, satisfaction or discontent in Deschapelles is a matter of priorities and personality:

"Some people have to be on top of things. When I first went to the United States, my father said, 'Marcella, buy the Italian newspaper every day. You must know what's going on in Italy!' It was easy in New York, but in Haiti the paper comes four or five days old, at best. To some that is unacceptable, but for me it fits. We live in a close community here. Many people now have a VCR, but I don't. I read. It's like nineteenth-century life: reading and walking, and little else.

"The first two years, you go to the beach, you want to see Haiti, you do a lot of things. Then you do less and less. I go to Port-au-Prince rarely now, only when I have to get a visa from the Italian embassy. Mrs. Mellon says when couples come here, they become very close because it is a trial of their marriage—they have no distractions."

It is also a trial of personal convictions and emotional responses, as Dr. Scalcini's experience attests:

"I adopted a little Haitian, who crossed the path of my life. His name is Carlo. He will be five soon. He was six months old when he was abandoned by his family in pediatrics. I took him home for a weekend and said, 'I'll return him Monday,' but Monday never came. You do things here that you would never do in the States. My friends said, 'Why didn't you adopt an Italian child?' First of all, I couldn't. Single people usually can't adopt there. Exceptional things happen in your life, and in Haiti—everything is exceptional. A person comes to your door in rags, no food. That doesn't happen in the U.S. Here, if you find a child in the street, who is going to take care of him?"

Blame it on Larry Mellon's contagious principles.

"Dr. Mellon was very much impressed by the gospels," says Dr. Scalcini, "especially the passage in Mark where the rich man asks, 'What should I do to get to heaven?' and Jesus says, 'Honor your parents, don't steal—' all the commandments. The man says, 'I've been doing all this,' so Jesus says, 'Give all your money to the poor and follow me.' The man became sad and left. He could not separate himself from his riches.

"Once Dr. Mellon told me, 'If I gave all my money away to the

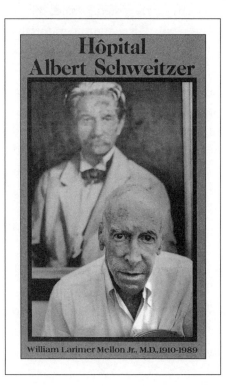

Hôpital
Albert Schweitzer

William Larimer Mellon Jr., M.D., 1910-1989

LARRY TOOK NOTE OF THE PASSAGE IN MARK WHERE THE RICH MAN ASKS: "WHAT SHOULD I DO TO GET TO HEAVEN?"

Haitians, each one would get maybe five dollars, ten dollars—it would be useless. Better to use it to build a hospital. But I can't bring health to the whole of Haiti. I don't have enough money to bring health to six million people. I have to restrict myself to one district.' He was extremely realistic."

Scalcini frowns and falls silent for a minute. But soon enough, her smile returns:

"Dr. Mellon liked life, like Mrs. Mellon. They were not like some benefactors who become sour or bitter. They saw the misery and pain and injustice here, but they were happy in their own souls. They were full of humor. Many times I would see the patients and Dr. Mellon laughing together.

"Once when I was doing the tuberculosis clinic, there were certain patients who were delinquent—never showed up for their appointments. I became outraged that day and I said to one of them, 'I don't want you here anymore! You are wasting my time and medication. I am disgusted with you!' The patient said, 'No, no, don't be disgusted.' I said, 'Go to some other hospital!' The patient said, 'No, I feel more comfortable here.' When I told Dr. Mellon this, he laughed and laughed. He was so full of the joy of life."

Marcella was fascinated by the way Larry and Gwen worked together and complemented one another, despite—or because of—their very different personalities: "Dr. Mellon was more community-oriented, Mrs. Mellon more interested in the hospital. Initially, I think they both wanted to become doctors, but it was too hard for her with three children. Dr. Mellon told me that if he had to re-do his life, Mrs. Mellon would become the doctor."

.   .   .

ALBERT SCHWEITZER ONCE SAID in an address to the students of Silcoates School in Yorkshire:

"You ask me to give you a motto. Here it is: *service*. Let this word accompany each of you throughout your life. May it be recalled to your minds if ever you are tempted to forget it or set it aside. It will not always be a comfortable companion, but it will always be a faithful one. . . . Never have this word on your lips, but keep it in your hearts, and may it teach you not only to do good, but to do it simply and humbly. So many drift into the misery of indifference because they did not start out with the vital power that comes from helping others. . . .

"The interior joy we feel when we have done a good deed, when we feel we have been needed somewhere and have lent a helping hand, is the nourishment the soul requires. Without those times when man feels himself to be part of the spiritual world by his actions, his soul decays.

"I don't know what your destiny will be. Some of you will perhaps occupy remarkable positions. Perhaps some of you will become famous by your pens or as artists. But I know one thing. The only ones among you who will be really happy are those who have sought and found how to serve. Happy only are those who let themselves be guided by their hearts, because the heart is the great reason, the reason that always is right in life."

His most receptive student was thousands of miles away across the Atlantic Ocean. "People tell me what I am doing is noble," Larimer

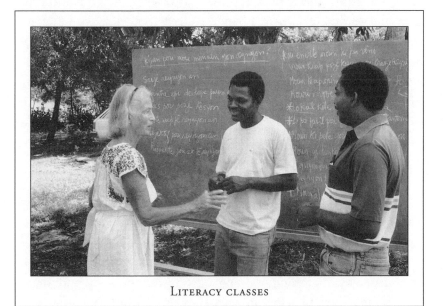

LITERACY CLASSES

Mellon told a journalist, "but I really know it is selfish. I have found happiness in helping people no one else was helping. It was worth everything I had to get to do this. I have sacrificed nothing."[7]

What does it mean to give and care?

"The first time you send a man home to die of pulmonary tuberculosis—and probably infect his family—you feel sorry," said René St. Léger, HAS physician. "Then you have to do it a second time, and you're just a little less sorry because you've done it before . . . So you go on doing it again and again. By the hundredth time you feel nothing. You've become a monster."[8]

He had despaired. Temporarily. But many others, like Dr. Harold Lear, a visiting surgeon for three tours of duty in the 1960s, considered HAS the most satisfying experience of their lives. In Deschapelles, he said, "One felt at least within shouting distance of the Hippocratic Oath."

Dr. Lucien Rousseau assesses his years at l'Hôpital Albert Schweitzer thus:

"Before, I was practicing a specialty. In Deschapelles, I was not a specialist. I was a doctor. I worked in the out-patient clinic, the operating room, the wards, everywhere. I had to go back to my books and refresh my memory—and I never regretted it. I had the opportunity to practice medicine with peasant patients, who are much different from urban ones: Simple people, ready to accept, who believe in you as a doctor. People here in Port-au-Prince are more 'sophisticated': They expect this and that from the doctor and are annoyed if they don't get it. But in the country, a peasant will accept and understand what you say, because he sees what you are trying to do for him."[9]

Nurse Paul Vissers said after his HAS experience:

"I have to find out for *myself* what it means to have compassion for every living thing, to take care of this world and its creatures. Did I really feel compassion for the poor lady with the sick child from the mountains? For the suffering babies? For the dirty hungry beggars? Or did I just enjoy the feeling of doing a good work, of being important? What is the motive to help someone? How much selfishness is there involved? These are the issues I'm struggling with.

"I think it is very good Dr. Mellon didn't leave a legacy, nor did he write any statement about how we should cope with these problems. We'll have to find out ourselves. Deschapelles is better than five years in a university or 100 books on morality. It urged me to look at my own motives, my own way of life, to observe the complexity of helping people."[10]

Dr. Jaime Ollé, who first visited HAS as a tourist in 1975, worked with the World Health Organization in the sub-Saharan region of Africa before signing on for two years at HAS in 1989. He went from a monthly salary of $5,000 to a fifth of that amount:

"The madness in Haiti that really touches some people got to me too. Many people, it doesn't touch at all, or touches them negatively. I have a friend who was here for two days and left. He couldn't stand it. But I loved it.

"When something functions in this country twenty-four hours a day, 365 days a year, it's quite unique. It's unique anywhere in poor countries. You see lots of things that work for a while and then disappear. What counts is if it *always* functions, and that's what was most valuable about HAS: no grand discourse, just hands-on. I've been through all these big international bureaucracies and they always have a plan to save the world—blah, blah, blah, then nothing. Here, it was the opposite: No big talk. Just do fifty patients, and *then* we'll talk about the philosophy. Practice, not theory. You can spend your life asking questions. In a place like this, if you ask too many questions, you'll go crazy.

"The questions are obvious, but the answers are not so obvious. Recently, I had a heart patient here—a girl who was thirteen but looked like ten—in my clinic. It was obvious she was going to die, so I did everything to organize surgery for her. For me, it was a symbol of HAS: The fact that she was here meant I was going to try and do something. She happened to *be* here. A guy in Spain said, 'What you're doing is stupid. With the money you're spending to save one girl, you could vaccinate 1,000 people.' I said, 'The airline's giving me a free ticket, the surgeon's doing the surgery free. No one's going to give me vaccine for 1,000 Haitians.' The end of the story is that she died a year and a half later. You can say it was useless; on the other hand, you can say that she lived pretty happily and gained another year and a half of life."

Was there something particularly important about her case that motivated such extraordinary intervention?

"No," Dr. Ollé replies. "All the cases are important. That's why you
can go crazy. You have to be able to get involved, but not too involved.
It's a very difficult balance to keep. That's why I had to leave HAS,
though I'd like to come back. To keep balance, I have to take a step back
now and then. People come here short term, for a month or so, and
they leave and say, 'We've done something.' And they have. But what's
more difficult is the everyday business. The short-termers are very important to us, but I think what they take away is more important than
what they leave behind.

"It's the same story everywhere: The people are here today and they'll
be here tomorrow and the day after tomorrow. You're here today, but tomorrow you're gone. When I was with WHO, I had arguments with my
boss, who was from Burundi. We were going around preaching the
gospel of primary health care, and this guy who'd had six months of
training said, 'Don't try to treat specific problems—it costs too much.'
Well, all of a sudden, this guy gets hypertension. I said, 'I can treat you
right here. I have the drugs, I know how to treat hypertension.' But he
took the first flight out to Geneva for a three-month treatment at the
best hospital in Switzerland!

"The point is, people in Africa or Haiti don't know if I or some other
doctor, as soon as he gets hypertension, is going to stick around or get
the hell out. It's hard to maintain an island, and this is an island, but it's
functioning pretty well. It's a big show and a difficult show to maintain.
That's its strength and also its weakness. I'm a perfect example myself:
I'm going to Bolivia for two years now. I plan to come back here, but
the pay is so lousy, I have to go and make a little money somewhere else
to be able to afford it."[11]

.   .   .

HAS MIRACLES OVER THE YEARS include the virtual eradication of
tetanus and an overall improvement in the health of the entire district.
Life expectancy was about thirty when the hospital was established;

now it is fifty-three. Typhoid has been greatly reduced. The Artibonite Valley is now almost free of vitamin A deficiency and measles—and it's a little freer from ignorance, too.

"When we first came to Haiti," says Gwen, "hardly anyone could read. One of our first projects was to teach people to read and write their names. We held night classes with kerosene lamps and a blackboard and chalk. After one or two lessons, most of the local farmers could do it. I never had such a thrill—seeing how pleased they were to be able to write their names, and not to have to use their thumb prints to sign papers."

The education picture has changed radically for the better. In the Deschapelles area, there are now fourteen schools. There are myriad other social-development problems, but also myriad potential solutions—integrally related to public health.

Some 65 percent of illnesses in the Artibonite stem from the lack of food and clean water. If those two problems, both intertwined with irrigation, were solved, half of HAS's caseload would be eliminated. The first challenge is to repair and preserve existing dams and canals, such as the great Tapion, which have become so clogged that the water in them hardly moves.

"We were on a jeep trip once and had two flat tires," Gwen recalls, "and Larry said, 'Oh, well, let's go down to the canal and take a swim.' When we jumped in, it was silt and mud up to our waists! We had trouble getting out. There are beautiful irrigation projects like this all over Haiti—reservoirs and dams filled with silt and rocks washed down by the rain. It's feasible to do something about it and a lot of people are ready to help, but it can't be up to us anymore."

Instead it's up to the government and private philanthropy. In the Tapion Dam's case, thirty years of spring floods seriously damaged the masonry pillars holding up its dalles. Finally, a sizable grant from the International Rotary Club subsidized the purchase of sand, cement, and gasoline (at inflated prices) needed to repair and restore the project to full effectiveness.

The medical challenges are increasing, too, due to the daunting tuberculosis and AIDS epidemics, and there are still only 1.4 doctors for every 10,000 Haitians.[12] HAS treats some 50,000 patients a year, and HAS doctors see more people in twenty-four hours than most American doctors see in a year. The strain and pain gets to some of them, but not to Gwen Mellon.

"The staff is more stable today than it's ever been," she says. "The main reason for that is Michel Jean-Baptiste—and the fact that most of our doctors and nurses are now Haitian, which makes for less coming and going." Dr. Jean-Baptiste had the unusual advantage of his Haitian birth and excellent Harvard education, a combination of the best American credentials and deep understanding of Haiti that served the hospital well.

All in all, HAS history is remarkable for its dearth of internal strife. "We've had our bad days and our staff problems, and we've had to let certain people go," says Gwen, "but institutions close if they don't do that. People come from all over the world to find out what makes HAS work. They just *arrive*. Henri Ménager will call me up at 7 P.M. and say, 'Five people have just come and want to spend the night.' I say, 'Henri, we have no rooms.' He says, 'We have to find some. It's the price you pay for being successful.'"

If and when the awful road to Deschapelles is ever paved, that trouble will be compounded, says Marie-Thérèse Menos:

"Dr. Mellon said he didn't want to fix the road because there would be even more accidents and because even more visitors would get off the plane in Port-au-Prince and come straight to Deschapelles. If the road stays bad, a lot of them will just say, 'Oh, it takes four hours, forget it.'"

Dr. Jean-Baptiste has a sly last word on the subject: "That bad road never kept the good folks out."[13]

.   .   .

WHAT ENABLED AN extraordinary man named William Larimer Mellon Jr. to create such an extraordinary institution?

"Larry did not have the fear of failure or ridicule that govern most of us," says Michael Rawson. "What separated him from many others is that his goals were attainable. To found, build, and operate a hospital in the tropics is not a goal most of us would consider feasible. But once the physical plant was completed, he stayed within the boundaries of the services HAS could manage without stressing the resources.

"It was having the self-discipline to stay within attainable goals that made Larry Mellon the most spiritually at ease person I have known. His goals were on higher planes than most men's. And what made the experience of knowing Larry so valuable is that he was willing to bring all of us along with him."[14]

Among those brought along was LeGrand Mellon Sargent, Billy's widow. All trips to Deschapelles are "working visits" and, on one of LeGrand's many, she and Gwen spent a particularly grueling day dealing with planned and unplanned urgencies. For their reward at the end of it, LeGrand recalls, they staggered to the tiny swimming pool behind the house:

Gwen wore her biggest sunglasses and wide-brimmed hat and perched under the wide green ginger leaves. I was doing my "laps"— which consisted of lying cross-wise in the pool, pushing off from one side with my toes and floating six inches to the other side. From there I would push off with my fingers to float six inches back to my starting point . . .

Relating the horrors of the day, Gwen enumerated the number of patients who had chosen to throw up on her. I was whimpering about lugging heavy cameras while trying to keep up with the work teams as they scampered up mountains and across ditches and fields. Over and over we groaned, "You think that's bad—listen to this!" After going back and forth many times, almost in unison we blurted out, "What the hell are we doing here?" That outburst was followed by whoops of laughter. Somewhere between howls we came out with, "Those damn Mellon boys. They lured us to this godforsaken place, dumped all of this work on us—then left!"

When we could again speak without cracking up, Gwen asked, "Would you want to be anywhere else?" I answered, "Nope. Would you?" She answered, "Nope."

So much for that.[15]

Gwen Mellon, as always, remains an optimist.

"I've never lost faith in Haiti. But what we need more than visitors are ways to raise the economy. The land is potentially rich to produce, and the people are ready to work. They can accept all the adversities if they see a change possible."

But there is a cold, ugly question to be asked: In a country with such terrible overpopulation and disease, isn't the high mortality rate, especially infant mortality, nature's way of seeking a balance? Did it ever disturb the Mellons that, by saving children's lives (or adults', for that matter), the great economic food-chain struggle was made even harder?

"No," says Gwen, without a beat. "It may bother other people, and I've heard many say it about Haiti and about the famines in Africa. We teach planned parenthood—we urge it and speak of the ideal family as two or three children, and we explain *why* it's ideal. We offer most kinds of contraception. But I know too many people who've survived tetanus and other things to become very valuable people."

Were the Mellons never discouraged?

"Neither of us ever were," says Gwen. "We had many disappointments, but we always could think of something else to be done and we did it and it made a difference. We were more fortunate than a poor person sitting in his house with no food. There's not much he can do. For us, it was different. We could try another program, ask someone else for help—do *something*."

In the face of overwhelming obstacles, they refused to be overwhelmed. "It's never too late and it's always too late to start helping others," Larry once said. "The trick is not to do too much at once. If you get discouraged, you become impotent."[16] Dr. Robert Wells, a forty-year veteran of unpaid orthopedic-surgical visits to HAS, took that advice to heart long ago:

"Haiti has had such a turbulent history and doesn't seem able to make a smooth transition into a government that can support the people in a way they deserve. I don't know the answer to that. I try not to get too involved with things I can't do much about. I just try to go down and help the people who show up. I don't spend a lot of time concerning myself with whether the whole place is going to get straightened out."[17]

HAS pediatrician Jack Wiese summed it up simply: "Look after the little picture, and the big picture will take care of itself."[18]

Dr. Mellon's granddaughter, Kate Grant Kellogg, recalls that Larry "always seemed so comfortable and at home with his life in Haiti," and it was true.[19] Once, in a lighthearted thank-you note to a contributor, Larry admitted that Haiti's "atmosphere of 'laissez-faire' or 'The will of God' or 'mañana'" often frustrated his efforts to plan ahead. Even so, he assured the donor, determination kept them going, and "of course the other thing which keeps us here is your dough! Wish you would stop off some day and see the fun we're having spending it . . .

"This work which Gwen and I do here never fails to amaze us! Today is so much like yesterday that I'd have to think a long time before being able to distinguish the difference. We get up before sunrise, eat the same breakfast from the same table while watching the Artibonite Valley come to life. The morning scene at all seasons year in and year out is practically identical. The slanting rays of sunlight on the rice paddies,

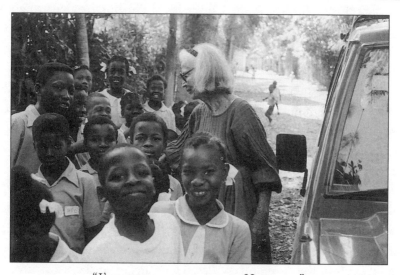

"I'VE NEVER LOST FAITH IN HAITI . . ."

which are thickly dotted with large green trees—mango, mapoo, royal palm—remind me daily of an illustration in the front of my grandmother's Bible, entitled 'The Garden of Eden.'"[20]

But surely he needed a vacation now and then.

"Why would I want a vacation from Paradise?" was his reply.

.   .   .

EDGAR STOESZ—longtime Mennonite central committeeman, HAS board member, and close friend of the Mellons—wrote Gwen: "I am always amazed at how first you and Larry, and now you alone, move over and let the rest of us participate in what was originally your dream, and what has become the dream of many. . . . This is what will permit the work to go on. It is this dimension that Albert Schweitzer, for all his wisdom, neglected and which now limits his well-intended successors at Lambaréné."[21]

The work of Albert Schweitzer Hospital indeed continues unabated, with the help of an international medical network that provides concrete assistance instead of long-distance sympathy. One of its most important elements is Eye Care Inc., founded by Dr. Gérard Frédérique, the first black admitted to the University of Pittsburgh's Department of Ophthalmology. He had attended medical school in Port-au-Prince, where his family was so poor that he borrowed and copied out all his medical books by hand because he couldn't afford to buy them.

"Dr. Frédérique mopped up most of the eye pathology in this valley of a couple hundred thousand people," says Dr. Maimon. "Once I asked what his follow-up was for patients he'd operated on, and he said about 5 percent. He virtually never saw people after he operated on them—which means he did superb work."

Dr. Frédérique's patients were beneficiaries of HAS' *raison d'être*. "It is not there for the purpose of changing the overall rural way of life," said Dr. Wells. "It hasn't made the overall living standards a lot different. But it has made an enormous difference in the lives of thousands of individuals in the Artibonite Valley. There are 250 orthopedic surgeons in Atlanta, and for me not to be there won't make any difference. In Haiti, it does make a difference, and that is a very good feeling.

"This hospital is one of very few places where people who otherwise would have no health care at all have a combination of both preventive public health and curative medical services. It is a unique institution in the world—a place of hope for the people it serves."[22]

Despite, or because of, the crushing weight of its needs and demands, HAS manifests another phenomenon that doesn't exist in many other medical communities in the world. "Everybody seems to be very kind to everyone else," says Dr. Maimon, "with a heightened sense of awareness." Bill Dunn has observed that something about Haiti in general and Deschapelles in particular tends to simplify people once they get there:

"The people that make up L'Hôpital Albert Schweitzer are unique. Dull people don't come here. We all have different reasons for being here, but you become pretty honest with one another, because you can't be phony when you live and work together in this close of an environment. You can be phony for two days, but by noon of the third day, somebody finds you out. So much needs to be done, and phoniness just gets in the way. Pretty soon, you find it's simpler and more productive to be yourself. The Mellons set the example for that here.

"There were no fancy words with Dr. Mellon; it was straight, accurate and simple, and his style permeated the organization. He had an uncanny ability to cut through the fluff, and he didn't deal with 'situational ethics.' Things were right or they were wrong. His goal was to simplify.

"There is virtually no lag time here. You can make a decision at noon and implement it by four in the afternoon, as opposed to the United States with its planning agencies and state health departments, where it takes months and months for approval to get things going. It was a professional rebirth for me here because of the freedom, the ability to create change. It's an extremely refreshing thing."

Gwen Mellon called her husband's spirit "a real and living thing." Former HAS medical director Bob Hollister provided the most moving vignette:

"We saw about fifty patients each Saturday from eight A.M. to noon. I was working at a table under a tree, mostly talking to the patients and dispensing paper sacks with a three-month's supply of tuberculosis medication. Dr. Mellon pulled his jeep up in the driveway. He had been out in the countryside helping villagers build a new well. Just as he climbed out of his vehicle, a tearful Haitian woman rushed up to him, wailing with grief. She had just lost a child. Without a word, but with the most concerned look of compassion and understanding, Larry took her hand, looked into her tear-stained face and said, 'Awww, awww.'

"I cannot put into words on paper the feeling in his voice. He didn't cry, he didn't talk, he just stood there with her hand in his and listened as she poured out her sorrow. Whenever she paused for breath, he said, 'Awww, awww,' with deep feeling, his facial expression mirroring hers without the tears. She gradually subsided and they walked away together, with his arm around her shoulders. He never said a word, no Bible verse, no verbal message, just the deepest feeling of compassion, of concern. I learned that day what fifteen years of 'higher education' had never taught me—how to care, and how to express that care."[23]

He was capable of infinite concern for people in all walks of life, Bob Wells reflects: "I don't know a better word than *gentle*. Dr. Mellon was a gentle man, gentle in his relationships with other people. He comes about as close to fulfilling the qualifications of a saint as anybody I have ever known."[24]

Larry heard that term more than once, and it galled him. "Whatever you wind up writin' about me," he told Burton Hersh in the '70s, "don't make me sound as insipid as the others have. We're not sacrificing anything. We'll run the place as long as we can. We intend to die here, because we really can't see anything better to do."[25] Edgar Stoesz calls him neither saint nor secularist but "an ordinary man who loved God and served others."[26] When Art Maimon once complimented him on what he and Gwen had done, Larry's reply was, "Anybody could do it."

Anybody could, perhaps, but nobody else did. Ninety-two-year-old Acelom Congo who, as a foreman, helped build the Tapion Dam with the Mellons thirty years ago, says:

"They are *blancs* who participate in the life of Haitians. They are a gift. I never knew whites would come and work with Haitians. When Mrs. Mellon comes to visit, her presence makes me want to dance. [He does a little dance around his courtyard to demonstrate.] We are all her children. On the Tapion, Dr. Mellon worked physically. Others would be lazy, but he showed by his example. He carried water pipes on his own shoulders. He was like a little piece of God. He is an example of what a king should be for his people. Some people don't deserve to die."[27]

Albert Schweitzer wrote that anyone contemplating a course of action similar to his own should have no thought of heroism, only of a spiritual adventure: "There are no heroes of action, only heroes of renunciation and suffering. There is no reward for the work except the privilege of doing it."

Contributions to the Albert Schweitzer Hospital of Deschapelles, Haiti, are tax-deductible and may be made in care of the Grant Foundation, Three Mellon Bank Center, 525 William Penn Place, Suite 3901, Pittsburgh, Pennsylvania 15219-1709.

ACKNOWLEDGMENTS

THE MELLON EXTENDED FAMILY

Gwen Grant Mellon

Ian and Lucy Rawson and children: Nicole, Rachel, Andrew, and Ed Rawson

Jenifer Rawson Grant and Ron Noe and children: Dr. Gwendolyn Grant (Wendy) Bowers, Dr. John P. (Jeff) Grant III, Susannah Grant Henrickson, and Katherine Grant Kellogg

Michael Rawson and Rosemary Azar and family: Carine, Tate, Grant, and Glen Rawson

LeGrand Mellon and Herb Sargent

Rachel Mellon Walton

Paul Mellon

Lisa Cox

Farley and Josh Whetzel

Will Whetzel

Louise Stephaich

Dr. John P. Grant, Jr.

Margaret C. Hill

Carolyn Payne Langfitt

William and Kathleen Simpson

Bill and Irene Dunn

Tahirah Duncan

Jenny Miller

Rachel Laff

Manité Boussicaut

THE PARIS EXTENDED FAMILY

Myrna Paris

Merica Claire Paris

Wyoming B. (Ben) Paris III

Wyoming B. Paris I

Wyoming B. and Nancy Paris II

Pamela and David Loyle

Todd, Heather, and Paris Loyle

Genevieve and Reid Fletcher

Karen and Larry Guggisberg

Bill Bollendorf and Dr. Madeline Simasek

John and Margie Barba

Mary Pat Brennan

Kate and Evan Brennan

Cathy Henkel

Judson Klinger

Cynthia and José de Almeida

THE RESEARCHERS AND ARCHIVISTS

Maria Ciaccia

The *Pittsburgh Post-Gazette*: Stephen Karlinchak, Lizabeth Gray, Mark Murphy, Marylynn "ZaSu" Pitz, James and "Queen" Christina O'Toole

The Grant Foundation: LeGrand Mellon Sargent, Stephen Midouhas, Ted Chastain, and Hertha Isaac
Carnegie-Mellon University: Dr. Herbert Simon and Teresa Thomas
Peter Michelmore
Leland Scruby
Antje Lemke (Albert Schweitzer Fellowship)
The Albert Schweitzer Center, Great Barrington, Massachusetts
The Albert Schweitzer Collection, Syracuse University
Fondation Haïtienne de Reconnaissance du Merité

PUBLICAFFAIRS BOOKS

Peter Osnos

Lisa Kaufman

Robert Kimzey

Mary-Claire Flynn

Erica Brown

Kate Darnton

Evan Gaffney

Jenny Dossin

INTERVIEWEES

Pierre Allen

Gesner Armand

Luquèce Bélizaire

Drs. Gretchen and Warren Berggren

Drs. Renée and Art Bergner

Saint-Louis Blaise

André Cassius

Newt Chapin, Jr.

Garry and Lise Charlier

Acelom Congo

Maître Delenois

Alix Dorleus

Katherine Dunham

Tim and Carol Dutton

Dr. Keith Flanagan

Anny Frédérique and John Chew

Dr. Gèrard Frédérique

Dr. Jacqueline Gautier

Aristeman "Ti Blanc" Jacques

Dr. Michel Jean-Baptiste

Aubelin Joliecoeur

Dr. John Judson

Gottfried Kräuchi (College Suisse, Jacmel)

Fritzner Lamour

Dr. Frank Lepreau

George Lockhardt

Carroll Long

Stivenson and Ramfis Magloire

Dr. Arthur Maimon

Dr. Florence "Skeets" Marshall

Dr. Harold and Agnes May

Gustave Ménager

Henri Ménager

Marie-Therèse Menos

Dr. Sonny Miller

Michel and Tony Monnin

Dr. Jaime Ollé

Gerald Orr

Dr. Richard Pantelone

André Pierre

Frédérique Pierre-Jules

Louise Rémy
Selden Rodman
Nicole Roumer
Dr. Lucien Rousseau
Renée Rousseau
Issah El-Saieh
Dr. Marcella Scalcini
Jean-Louis Sénatus
Dr. Margaret Smith
Pastor André Sonnal

Edgar Stoesz
Dr. Julian Strauss
Ray and Randy Strothman
Dieutel Toussaint
Antoine Véus
Dr. Robert Wells
Dr. Steve and Karen Williams
Dr. Peter Wright
Frantz Zéphirin

. . . plus countless l'Hôpital Albert Schweitzer patients, staff members, people of the Artibonite Valley, and the Mysterious Guillaume. . .

Support Troops

Daniel A. Strone,
    William Morris Agency
James and Carole Donahue,
    Mellon Bank
Janet Yobp, Heidi Oman, and
    Theresa Morrissey, Mellon Bank
Victoria Wilson, Knopf
Judith Regan, HarperCollins
Michael Drohan, Haiti Solidarity
    Committee
Jeffrey Schaire

Lorraine Glennon
Annie Schmidt and Shelley Rohe
Kathleen Imhoff
Mary Jo and Chris Capizzi
Elaine Levitt
Frances Debroff
Natalie Taaffe
Arthur Albrecht
Frederick W. Burr
Eric Utné
Mark Erickson

Special thanks to legendary University of Pittsburgh Press editor Frederick A. Hetzel for the encouragement—and Cynthia Miller for the discouragement—that led me to PublicAffairs.

CHAPTER 1: ANDANTE: PRINCES AND PAUPERS

1. Cheryl McCall, "A Mellon from Pittsburgh Gives His Life and Fortune to Help the Poor of Haiti," *People*, April 28, 1980, pp. 24, 28.
2. David E. Koskoff, *The Mellons: The Chronicle of America's Richest Family* (New York: Thomas Y. Crowell Company, 1978), p. 90.
3. Ibid., pp. 91–93.
4. Ibid., pp. 94–97.
5. Ibid., pp. 89, 106.
6. Ibid., p. 59.
7. Burton Hersh, *The Mellon Family: A Fortune in History* (New York: William Morrow and Company, 1978), pp. 164, 182–184.
8. Henry La Cossitt, "Miracle of the Spirit," *Reader's Digest*, March 1956, p. 183.
9. McCall, *People*, p. 28.
10. Gwen Grant Mellon, *My Road to Deschapelles* (New York: Continuum, 1997), pp. 35–36.
11. Hersh, *The Mellon Family*, p. 182.
12. Ibid., p. 30.
13. Bill Dunn to BP, Deschapelles, October 1, 1992.
14. Rachel Mellon Walton to BP, Pittsburgh, February 6, 1993.
15. Ibid.
16. Hersh, *The Mellon Family*, p. 182.
17. George Lockhardt to Bill Bollendorf, Pittsburgh, April 14, 1994.
18. Newton Chapin Jr. to Bill Bollendorf, Edgeworth, PA, April 6, 1993.
19. Ibid.
20. Koskoff, *The Mellons*, p. 244.
21. Mellon, *My Road to Deschapelles*, p. 181.
22. Paul Farmer, *The Uses of Haiti* (Monroe, Maine: Common Courage Press, 1994), p. 16.
23. Ibid., p. 20.
24. Erica Anderson, ed., *Albert Schweitzer: Thoughts for Our Time* (New York: Pilgrim Press, 1975).
25. Newton Chapin Jr. to Bill Bollendorf, Pittsburgh, April 14, 1994.
26. Hersh, *The Mellon Family*, p. 460.
27. Rachel Mellon Walton to BP, Pittsburgh, February 6, 1993.
28. Hersh, *The Mellon Family*, p. 461.
29. McCall, *People*, p. 28.

30. Hersh, *The Mellon Family,* p. 461.
31. McCall, *People*, p. 28.
32. Hersh, *The Mellon Family,* p. 459.
33. Ibid., p. 462.
34. Ibid.
35. Ibid.
36. Ibid., p. 463.
37. McCall, *People,* p. 30.
38. Aline Griffith Romanelli, *The Spy Wore Red* (New York: Random House, 1987), pp. 60–67.
39. Ibid.
40. Ibid.

CHAPTER 2: ALLEGRO VIVACE: HOMES ON THE RANGE

1. Cheryl McCall, "A Mellon from Pittsburgh Gives His Life and Fortune to Help the Poor of Haiti," *People*, April 28, 1980, p. 29.
2. Gwen Grant Mellon to BP, Deschapelles, October 1, 1992. All unattributed Gwen Mellon quotations hereafter are taken from interviews with the author in Haiti on October 1–5, 1992, January 10–16, 1993, October 5–7, 1993, and April 4–8, 1995.
3. Burton Hersh, *The Mellon Family: A Fortune in History* (New York: William Morrow and Company, 1978), p. 463.
4. Jenifer Rawson Grant to Lucy Rawson, Essex, CT, February 3, 1999.
5. Gwen Grant Mellon, *My Road to Deschapelles* (New York: Continuum, 1997), p. 40.
6. Ibid., pp. 35–36.
7. Hersh, *The Mellon Family,* p. 463.

CHAPTER 3: LARGO: ROAD TO DAMASCUS

1. Henry La Cossitt, "Miracle of the Spirit," *Reader's Digest*, March 1956, p. 184.
2. Albert Schweitzer, translated by Antje B. Lemke, *Out of My Life and Thought* (New York: Henry Holt, 1990), p. 155.
3. Albert Schweitzer letters to Larimer Mellon, February 27 and March 3, 1948.
4. Albert Schweitzer letter to Larimer Mellon, March 3, 1948.
5. Burton Hersh, *The Mellon Family: A Fortune in History* (New York: William Morrow and Company, 1978), p. 464.

6. Dr. Arthur Maimon to BP, January 11, 1993, Deschapelles, Haiti.

7. Albert Schweitzer letter to Larimer Mellon, March 3, 1948.

8. Larimer Mellon letter to Albert Schweitzer, May 16, 1948.

9. Larimer Mellon letter to Albert Schweitzer, December 18, 1947.

10. Gwen Grant Mellon, *My Road to Deschapelles* (New York: Continuum, 1997), p. 47.

11. Larimer Mellon letter to Albert Schweitzer, May 16, 1948.

12. Hersh, *The Mellon Family*, p. 447.

13. Henry La Cossitt, *Reader's Digest*, p. 186.

14. David E. Koskoff, *The Mellons: The Chronicle of America's Richest Family* (New York: Thomas Y. Crowell Company, 1978), p. 353.

15. Burton Hersh, *The Mellon Family*, p. 465.

16. Albert Schweitzer letter to Larimer Mellon, April 20, 1950.

17. Larimer Mellon letter to Albert Schweitzer, May 28, 1950.

18. Albert Schweitzer letter to Larimer Mellon, July 26, 1948.

19. Larimer Mellon letter to Albert Schweitzer, May 16, 1952.

20. Mellon, *My Road to Deschapelles*, p. 116.

21. Ibid, pp. 115–116.

22. Jenifer Grant, *The Spirit of Hôpital Albert Schweitzer* (New Haven, CT: Jenifer Grant, 1992), pp. 37–38. Hal Krizan was the storeroom manager at l'Hôpital Albert Schweitzer from 1988 to 1990.

23. Hersh, *The Mellon Family*, p. 447.

24. Albert Schweitzer letter to Larimer Mellon, April 23, 1953.

25. Larimer Mellon letter to Albert Schweitzer, November 30, 1952.

26. Albert Schweitzer letter to Larimer Mellon, April 23, 1953.

27. Larimer Mellon letters to Albert Schweitzer, February 12 and June 15, 1954.

CHAPTER 4: PRESTO: MIRACLE-WORKING

1. Erica Anderson, *The Schweitzer Album* (New York: Harper & Row, 1965), p. 52.

2. Dr. Sonny Miller to Lucy Rawson, January 6, 1999.

3. Albert Schweitzer letter to Larimer Mellon, March 3, 1948.

4. Larimer Mellon letter to Albert Schweitzer, June 15, 1954.

5. Gwen Grant Mellon, *My Road to Deschapelles* (New York: Continuum, 1997), pp. 122–124.

6. Gay Sutphin, "The Good Samaritan of Haiti," *The Saturday Evening Post*, January/February, 1976, p. 36.

7. Burton Hersh, *The Mellon Family: A Fortune in History* (New York: William Morrow and Company, 1978), p. 467.

8. Undated Larimer Mellon letter to Albert Schweitzer, c. January 1954.

9. Jenifer Grant, *The Spirit of Hôpital Albert Schweitzer* (New Haven, CT: Jenifer Grant, 1992), p. 40.

10. Larimer Mellon letter to Albert Schweitzer, June 15, 1954.

11. Mellon, *My Road to Deschapelles*, p. 145.

12. Ibid., p. 131.

13. Grant, *The Spirit of Hôpital Albert Schweitzer*, p. 13.

14. Norman Cousins, "The Business of Larimer and Gwen Mellon," *Saturday Review*, December 10, 1960, pp. 26–27, 36.

15. Grant, *The Spirit of Hôpital Albert Schweitzer*, pp. 33–34.

16. Hersh, *The Mellon Family*, p. 468.

17. Larimer Mellon letter to Jessie May Hill, January 30, 1970.

18. Peter Michelmore, *Dr. Mellon of Haiti* (New York: Dodd, Mead & Co., 1964), p. 48.

19. Dr. Florence "Skeets" Marshall to Lucy Rawson, January 10, 1999.

20. Julian Strauss, quoted in Jenifer Grant, *The Spirit of Hôpital Albert Schweitzer*, p. 25.

21. David E. Koskoff, *The Mellons: The Chronicle of America's Richest Family* (New York: Thomas Y. Crowell Co., 1978), pp. 404–405.

22. Joe Alex Morris, "Doctors vs. Witchcraft," *Saturday Evening Post*, September 16, 1961, p. 59.

CHAPTER 5: MODERATO: "GO TO THE PEOPLE"

1. Renée Bergner to Lucy Rawson, November 12, 1998.

2. Dr. Harold May to BP, Boston, June 21, 1998.

3. Jenifer Grant, *The Spirit of Hôpital Albert Schweitzer* (New Haven, CT: Jenifer Grant, 1992), p. 42.

4. Ibid., pp. 31–32.

5. Ibid.

6. Gwen Grant Mellon, *My Road to Deschapelles* (New York: Continuum, 1997), p. 134.

7. Burton Hersh, *The Mellon Family: A Fortune in History* (New York: William Morrow and Company, 1978), p. 469.

8. Julian Strauss to Lucy Rawson, January 10, 1999.

9. Grant, *The Spirit of Hôpital Albert Schweitzer*, p. 26.

10. Farley Walton Whetzel to Bill Bollendorf, Pittsburgh, May 28, 1993.

11. Grant, *The Spirit of Hôpital Albert Schweitzer*, p. 10.

12. Ibid., p. 17.

13. Mellon, *My Road to Deschapelles*, p. 159.

14. Grant, *The Spirit of Hôpital Albert Schweitzer*, p. 15.

15. Dr. Harold May to BP, June 21, 1998, Boston.

16. Joe Alex Morris, "Doctors vs. Witchcraft," *Saturday Evening Post*, September 16, 1961, pp. 48–64.
17. This account and quotations concerning Billy Mellon's death are compiled from Mellon, *My Road to Deschapelles*, pp. 315–316, and David E. Koskoff, *The Mellons: The Chronicle of America's Richest Family* (New York: Thomas Y. Crowell Company, 1978), p. 555.
18. Grant, *The Spirit of Hôpital Albert Schweitzer*, p. 53.
19. Ibid., p. 50.
20. Ibid., p. 27.
21. Ibid., pp. 34–35.

Chapter 6: Scherzo: "Mon Pays Est L'Haïti"

1. Jenifer Grant, *The Spirit of Hôpital Albert Schweitzer* (New Haven, CT: Jenifer Grant, 1992), p. 39.
2. Albert Schweitzer, *Memoirs of Childhood and Youth* (New York: Macmillan Co, 1949).
3. Grant, *The Spirit of Hôpital Albert Schweitzer*, p. 20.
4. Erica Anderson, ed., *Albert Schweitzer: Thoughts for Our Time* (New York: Pilgrim Press, 1975), p. 38.
5. Grant, *The Spirit of Hôpital Albert Schweitzer*, p. 41.
6. Herb Sargent to BP, March 14, 1999.
7. Renée Bergner to Lucy Rawson, November 12, 1998.
8. Jenifer Grant to Lucy Rawson, February 3, 1999.
9. LeGrand Mellon to BP, March 12, 1999.
10. Grant to Lucy Rawson, February 3, 1999.
11. Peter Michelmore, *Dr. Mellon of Haiti* (New York: Dodd, Mead & Co., 1964), p. 31.
12. "Financier Turns Physician, Builds Hospital in Haitian Village," *Medical News*, July 8, 1959, p. 12.
13. Grant, *The Spirit of Hôpital Albert Schweitzer*, p. 36.

Chapter 7: Adagio: "When the Roll Is Called Up Yonder"

1. Jenifer Grant, *The Spirit of Hôpital Albert Schweitzer* (New Haven, CT: Jenifer Grant, 1992), pp. 27–28.
2. Renée Bergner interview with Lucy Rawson, November 13, 1998.
3. Grant, *The Spirit of Hôpital Albert Schweitzer*, p. 30.
4. Larimer Mellon letter to Albert Schweitzer, May 16, 1948.
5. Edgar Stoesz letter to Gwen Mellon, August 13, 1995.

6. Dr. Marcella Caldi-Scalcini to BP, January 10, 1993, Deschapelles, Haiti.
7. Erica Anderson, *Gift of Friendship* (New York: Harper and Row, 1964), p. 83.
8. Grant, *The Spirit of Hôpital Albert Schweitzer*, p. 18.
9. Ibid., p. 16.
10. Ibid., p. 19.
11. Erica Anderson, ed., *Albert Schweitzer: Thoughts for Our Time* (New York: Pilgrim Press, 1975), pp. 52–61 (excerpted).
12. Gwen Grant Mellon, *My Road to Deschapelles* (New York: Continuum, 1997), p. 205.
13. LeGrand Mellon to BP, March 22, 1999.
14. Grant, *The Spirit of Hôpital Albert Schweitzer*, p. 71.
15. Paul Farmer, *The Uses of Haiti* (Monroe, Maine: Common Courage Press, 1994), p. 20.
16. Ibid., p. 20.
17. Max Blanchet interview with Jonathan Pitts, Assistant Executive Secretary, The Haitian Advocacy Platform for an Alternative Development, Washington, D.C., September 6, 1998.
18. Dr. Florence "Skeets" Marshall to Lucy Rawson, January 10, 1999.
19. Dr. Richard Pantalone to BP, Pittsburgh, May 25, 1999.
20. Blair Calvert Fitzsimons, "An Heir's Mission," *Washington Post Magazine*, June 15, 1986, p. 11.
21. Grant, *The Spirit of Hôpital Albert Schweitzer*, p. 21.
22. Herb Sargent to BP, March 14, 1999.
23. LeGrand Mellon to BP, January 13, 1999.
24. Joe Alex Morris, "Doctors vs. Witchcraft," *Saturday Evening Post*, September 16, 1961, p. 61.

CHAPTER 8: FINALE: REVERENCE FOR LIFE

1. Jenifer Grant, *The Spirit of Hôpital Albert Schweitzer* (New Haven, CT: Jenifer Grant, 1992), p. 76.
2. Dr. Michel Jean-Baptiste to BP, Deschapelles, October 5, 1992.
3. Ian Rawson to BP, Pittsburgh, November 12, 1998.
4. Farley Walton Whetzel to Bill Bollendorf, Pittsburgh, May 28, 1993.
5. Jean-Baptiste to BP, Deschapelles, October 5, 1992.
6. Dr. Julian Strauss to Lucy Rawson, January 10, 1999.
7. Cheryl McCall, "A Mellon from Pittsburgh Gives His Life and Fortune to Help the Poor of Haiti," *People*, April 28, 1980, p. 24.
8. Peter Michelmore, *Dr. Mellon of Haiti* (New York: Dodd, Mead & Co., 1964) p. 68.
9. Dr. Lucien Rousseau to BP, Port-au-Prince, January 18, 1993.

10. Grant, *The Spirit of Hôpital Albert Schweitzer*, p. 58.

11. Dr. Jaime Ollé to BP, Deschapelles, January 13, 1993.

12. Blair Calvert Fitzsimons, "An Heir's Mission," *Washington Post Magazine*, June 15, 1986, p. 8.

13. Grant, *The Spirit of Hôpital Albert Schweitzer*, p. 69.

14. Michael Rawson to Lucy Rawson, November 10, 1998.

15. LeGrand Mellon to BP, March 22, 1999.

16. Grant, *The Spirit of Hôpital Albert Schweitzer*, p. 3.

17. Dr. Robert Wells to Lucy Rawson, November 13, 1998.

18. Grant, *The Spirit of Hôpital Albert Schweitzer*, p. 57.

19. Kate Grant Kellogg to Lucy Rawson, November 11, 1998.

20. Grant, *The Spirit of Hôpital Albert Schweitzer*, pp. 44–45.

21. Edgar Stoesz letter to Gwen Grant Mellon, May 24, 1996.

22. Dr. Robert Wells to Lucy Rawson, November 13, 1998.

23. Grant, *The Spirit of Hôpital Albert Schweitzer*, p. 9.

24. Dr. Robert Wells to Lucy Rawson, November 13, 1998.

25. Burton Hersh, *The Mellon Family: A Fortune in History* (New York: William Morrow and Company, 1978), p. 459.

26. Edgar Stoesz letter to Gwen Mellon, August 13, 1995.

27. Grant, *The Spirit of Hôpital Albert Schweitzer*, p. 17.

BOOKS

Abbott, Elizabeth. *Haiti: The Duvaliers and their Legacy.* New York: McGraw-Hill Book Company, 1988.

Anderson, Erica, ed. *Albert Schweitzer: Thoughts for Our Time.* New York: Pilgrim Press, 1975.

Anderson, Erica. *Gift of Friendship.* New York: Harper and Row, 1964.

Anderson, Erica. *The Schweitzer Album.* New York: Harper & Row, 1965.

Baldeck, Andrea. *The Heart of Haiti.* Blue Bell, Pennsylvania: Hawkhurst, 1996.

Bentley, James. *Albert Schweitzer: The Enigma.* New York: HarperCollins, 1992.

Davis, Wade. *The Serpent and the Rainbow.* New York: Warner Books, 1985.

Farmer, Paul. *AIDS and Accusation: Haiti and the Geography of Blame.* California: University of California Press, 1992.

Farmer, Paul. *The Uses of Haiti.* Monroe, Maine: Common Courage Press, 1994.

Grant, Jenifer. *The Spirit of Hôpital Albert Schweitzer.* New Haven, Connecticut: Jenifer Grant, 1992.

Hersh, Burton. *The Mellon Family: A Fortune in History.* New York: William Morrow and Company, 1978.

Jeanty, Edner A., and Brown, O. Carl. *Parol Granmoun: 999 Haitian Proverbs in Creole and English.* Port-au-Prince: Editions Learning Center, 1976.

Koskoff, David E. *The Mellons: The Chronicle of America's Richest Family.* New York: Thomas Y. Crowell Company, 1978.

Mellon, Gwen Grant. *Letters from St. Marc.* Sarasota, Florida: Gwen Grant Mellon, 1995.

Mellon, Gwen Grant. *My Road to Deschapelles.* New York: Continuum, 1997.

Michelmore, Peter. *Dr. Mellon of Haiti.* New York: Dodd, Mead & Co., 1964.

Picht, Werner. *The Life and Thought of Albert Schweitzer.* New York: Harper & Row, 1964.

Rodman, Selden. *The Miracle of Haitian Art.* Garden City, New York: Doubleday & Company, 1974.

Romanelli, Aline Griffith. *The Spy Wore Red.* New York: Random House, 1987.

Schweitzer, Albert. *Memoirs of Childhood and Youth.* New York: Macmillan Co., 1949.

Schweitzer, Albert. *Out of My Life and Thought.* New York: Henry Holt, 1990. (Translated by Antje B. Lemke.)

Schweitzer, Albert. *The Quest for the Historical Jesus.* New York: Macmillan Co., 1948

Shacochis, Bob. *The Immaculate Invasion.* New York: Viking, 1999.

Simon, Charlie May. *All Men Are Brothers: A Portrait of Albert Schweitzer.* New York: E.P. Dutton & Company, 1956.

Thomson, Ian. *Bo'jou' Blanc: A Journey Through Haiti.* New York: Penguin Books, 1993.

Watts, Harold, and Lilly Lessing. *I Am His Wife,* a dramatized portrait of Helene Schweitzer. Typescript, 1981.

Wolkstein, Diane. *The Magic Orange Tree and Other Haitian Folktales.* New York: Schocken Books, 1978.

ARTICLES

Bergner, Renée and Arthur. "Hôpital Albert Schweitzer." *Resident Physician,* February 1963, pp. 86–114.

Cousins, Norman. "The Business of Larimer and Gwen Mellon." *Saturday Review,* December 10, 1960, pp. 26–27, 36.

"Financier Turns Physician, Builds Hospital in Haitian Village," *Medical News,* July 8, 1959, p. 12.

Fitzsimons, Blair Calvert. "An Heir's Mission." *Washington Post Magazine,* June 15, 1986, pp. 7–17.

La Cossitt, Henry. "Miracle of the Spirit." *Reader's Digest,* March 1956, pp. 182–187.

McCall, Cheryl. "A Mellon from Pittsburgh Gives His Life and Fortune to Help the Poor of Haiti." *People,* April 28, 1980, pp. 24–31.

Morris, Joe Alex. "Doctors vs. Witchcraft." *Saturday Evening Post,* September 16, 1961, pp. 48–64.

Sutphin, Gay. "The Good Samaritan of Haiti." *The Saturday Evening Post,* January/February, 1976, pp. 34–109.

Photo Credits

PUBLICAFFAIRS is a new nonfiction publishing house and a tribute to the standards, values, and flair of three persons who have served as mentors to countless reporters, writers, editors, and book people of all kinds, including me.

I.F. STONE, proprietor of *I. F. Stone's Weekly*, combined a commitment to the First Amendment with entrepreneurial zeal and reporting skill and became one of the great independent journalists in American history. At the age of eighty, Izzy published *The Trial of Socrates*, which was a national bestseller. He wrote the book after he taught himself ancient Greek.

BENJAMIN C. BRADLEE was for nearly thirty years the charismatic editorial leader of *The Washington Post*. It was Ben who gave the *Post* the range and courage to pursue such historic issues as Watergate. He supported his reporters with a tenacity that made them fearless, and it is no accident that so many became authors of influential, best-selling books.

ROBERT L. BERNSTEIN, the chief executive of Random House for more than a quarter century, guided one of the nation's premier publishing houses. Bob was personally responsible for many books of political dissent and argument that challenged tyranny around the globe. He is also the founder and was the longtime chair of Human Rights Watch, one of the most respected human rights organizations in the world.

.   .   .

For fifty years, the banner of Public Affairs Press was carried by its owner Morris B. Schnapper, who published Gandhi, Nasser, Toynbee, Truman, and about 1,500 other authors. In 1983 Schnapper was described by *The Washington Post* as "a redoubtable gadfly." His legacy will endure in the books to come.

Peter Osnos, *Publisher*

About the Author

Barry Paris is an award-winning biographer, film historian, music and art critic, translator, and contributor to *The New Yorker* and *Vanity Fair.* His biographies include *Louise Brooks* (named Film Book of the Year), *Tony Curtis* (a number one paperback bestseller), *Garbo* (hailed as the definitive text), and *Audrey Hepburn* (translated into six languages worldwide).

Paris's involvement with Haiti began in the early 1990s when, as a contributing editor for *Art & Antiques* magazine, he traveled there to write about Haitian art. In subsequent trips, his interest shifted from Haiti's art to its public health—in particular, the phenomenal work of L'Hôpital Albert Schweitzer, founded by members of the Mellon family, his fellow Pittsburghers.

Paris's original article, "Song of Haiti," written for the *Pittsburgh Post-Gazette* in 1993, was awarded First Prize by Eric Utné on behalf of the Sunday Magazine Editors Association that year, and was widely reprinted. On the basis of its success, Paris and Gwen Grant Mellon entered into a collaboration that resulted in this book.

Paris has been a performing arts critic and investigative reporter for the *Pittsburgh Post-Gazette* since 1980, feature editor of *The Miami Herald,* editor-publisher of *The Prairie Journal* of Wichita, and since 1981, the co-creator of the Peabody-winning Sunday Arts Magazine at NPR's classical station, WQED-FM. He is a 1969 graduate of Columbia University and of the Institute for the Study of the USSR in Munich. Fluent in Slavic as well as several Romance languages, he is a translator of the plays of Chekhov. His biographical projects include profiles of silent-film star Lina Basquette and novelist Marcia Davenport for *The New Yorker,* and the forthcoming *Pierce in Oblivion,* a biography of the tragic fourteenth president of the United States, Franklin Pierce.

Paris lives in Pittsburgh with his wife, singer-actress Myrna Paris, and their two faultless children, Merica and Wyoming Benjamin Paris III.